To/
Pauline. E. Smith.

I hope this book will be
encouraging to you. These words
are designed to bless you one
day at a time, Because, you
are a blessing to me!

All my Love
Selina
xx

fitforever

Other books by Kay Kuzma:
60 Ways to Energize Your Life
Easy Obedience
Energized!
In Praise of Children
Mending Broken People: 3ABN Miracle Stories

To order, call 1-800-765-6955.

Visit us at www.reviewandherald.com for information on other Review and Herald® products.

fitforever

One-a-day devotionals for Body, Mind, and Spirit

kaykuzma

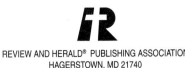

REVIEW AND HERALD® PUBLISHING ASSOCIATION
HAGERSTOWN, MD 21740

The author assumes full responsibility for the accuracy of all facts and quotations as cited in this book.

This book was
Edited by Ray Woolsey
Cover designed by Genesis Design
Cover photos by Getty Images
Interior design by Candy Harvey
Electronic makeup by Shirley M. Bolivar
Typeset: Bembo 11/12.5

PRINTED IN U.S.A.

09 08 07 06 05   5 4 3 2 1

R&H Cataloging Service
Fit forever. Contributions from
        184 health professionals and inspirational writers.
        Compiled by Kay Kuzma.

        1. Devotional calendars.   2. Health.
I. Kuzma, Kay Judeen Humpal, 1941-   , comp.

                        242.2

ISBN 0-8280-1838-3

Dedication

FORTY-TWO YEARS AGO the incredibly gifted man I married encouraged me to write an article for the *Adventist Review*. I did, he edited it, and it was published. When I saw the article in print, something happened to me. It was as if God said, "Write! I have given you an education; share what you have learned with others." I continued writing—and my husband continued editing—until the last few years when medical challenges dominated his life.

While my field was family, his was health. With a Ph.D. in biostatistics, he and his college buddy and School of Public Health colleague, Dr. Roland Phillips, received funding for the first Adventist Health study. My husband has dedicated his life to providing information that can help people live a healthful lifestyle. For 27 years he taught and did research at Loma Linda University. He wrote a health science biostatistics textbook and a book for the general public, *Live 10 Healthy Years Longer,* published by Thomas Nelson. For five years he developed and sponsored *Got a Minute for Your Health,* a syndicated radio broadcast. In 1997 he coedited the health devotional, *Energized!* with DeWitt Williams and me.

And now it's time to honor this man who has done so much for me and for the promotion of a healthy lifestyle. So,

JAN W. KUZMA,

I dedicate this book to you—

the love of my life,

my inspiration,

and the wind beneath my wings!

Why a Devotional Book
That Focuses on Health?

THERE IS MUCH WE can learn about God's creation and what our bodies and minds need in order to experience the abundant life Jesus came to give us. The first Seventh-day Adventist health devotional, *Energized,* was published in 1997. In the foreword of that book DeWitt S. Williams, director of health ministries for the North American Division, wrote, "We need to be reminded that there is an inexplicable tie between our physical, mental, and spiritual health. Our bodies are the temples of the Holy Spirit (1 Cor. 6:19), but some of our bodies need a little cleaning up and refurbishing before they are fit dwellings for the Deity" (*Energized!* p. 9).

The same is true today. Once more it is time to focus on the abundant life that God has promised.

—*Kay Kuzma, Ed.D.*
Founder and Speaker
Family Matters Ministry

How Human Beings Live Well

*How good and pleasant it is when brothers
[human beings] live together in unity! Ps. 133:1, NIV.*

HERE'S MY TAKE on being human and, beyond that, living well. It is the nature of being human that we make mistakes, that we occasionally offend one another, and that we sometimes fail in our efforts to live well. Genetics, temperament, environment, and habit may each play a role in our clumsy behaviors. Nothing, however, exceeds the fact that we are, first of all, human beings. Fundamentally, being human is what we're designed for. It's our generic self, much like the automobile we drive away when we pay only the base price.

For a human being to live well, however, requires something more. It implies physical, emotional, and spiritual health, none of which carries a particularly high price tag. It has to do with our desire to rise above generic living and above our ability to simply exist. It implies at least a measure of physical fitness. It involves emotionally healthy relationships, intimacy, and genuine forgiveness. It involves connecting with a God who says: "Here I am. Trust Me. We need each other. I hope you'll accept Me and let Me be a part of your life."

A wise and loving God created within us the gifts to succeed and the ability to fail. As human beings, we do plenty of both. Out of the balance of success and failure, however, we derive character, humility, integrity of mind and spirit, and we experience both joy and grief. Living well is not so much about success or achievement, nor is it about the absence of humiliation or sadness; we need all of those experiences. Living well spiritually, emotionally, and even physically is all about process. Golfers have a saying: "It's not how you drive, it's how you arrive." The process between the tee and the green is what matters.

Living well is about correcting mistakes while trying to avoid their repetition. Living well is about apologizing to those we offend while trying to avoid repeated offenses. Living well is about making choices that reduce the magnitude, frequency, and consequences of our failures.

Living well is to view, to behave, and to respect all others as we would have them view us, behave toward us, and respect us. This is the plain and simple golden rule of a human being's life well lived. It is Christ's life reflected in our lives.

Thank You, Lord, for creating us human, with all the potential of living well.

LEONARD L. BAILEY

The Incredible Creation Process

You watched me as I was being formed in utter seclusion, as I was woven together in the dark of the womb. You saw me before I was born. Ps. 139:15, 16, NLT.

GOD'S PROCESS BY which a human being is created is probably the greatest wonder of the universe. It starts with a few million sperm swimming, pollywog-like, toward a released ovum in the fallopian tubes. One lone swimmer arrives shortly before the rest. It penetrates the mucosa layer covering the cell and delivers its half of the DNA required to give the ovum the potential to create a child. As a result of this penetration, in an instant a cascade of chemical changes occurs that block the entry of other sperm cells, ensuring the proper development of the embryo.

Within hours the fertilized ovum is implanted in the uterine wall and begins to replicate, forming stem cells. All are clones of each other—exact copies of the original ovum. Yet within a few more hours each of them will "decide" to make something different from the others.

Ponder for a moment that one of these stem cells "decides" to be a certain organ—perhaps it will make the heart. For a few hours it appears to be dividing simply at random, but as one watches, as it were, under the microscope, the early shape of a heart materializes before your eyes. The cells continue to divide, making muscle, vessels—arteries and veins—valves, tendons connected to the valves and muscles, neural network structure—all in the most perfect and marvelous order. In about two weeks there is a kind of twitching of muscle tissue that in about three more weeks will be detectable by the gynecologist as the infant's heartbeat. It's not pumping blood yet, but it's beating.

Another stem cell "decides" it will become an eye. It forms the only completely transparent tissue in the body—cornea and lens. It makes an iris to respond to changes in light intensity or brightness by automatically operating miniature muscles. It creates the beautiful eye color, muscles, tendons, rods, cones, vessels—all in the right places and in the right sizes. Perhaps most remarkable of all is the nerve bundle that grows from the back of the eye and penetrates the growing brain near the rear of the head. It turns, dives, and twists back, and then connects to a few billion precisely chosen brain nerve cells so there will be vision!

And this same precise, intricately engineered process happens as each of the different organs is formed. Incredible, isn't it?

Once more, Lord, I have to exclaim, as did the psalmist, "I am indeed wonderfully made!"
                                                                JIM BRACKETT

A Mind-boggling Communication System

Let this mind be in you, which was also in Christ Jesus. Phil. 2:5.

THE KEY TO clear thinking has to do with the healthy communication of billions of neurons (nerve cells) that conduct impulses from one part of the body to another.

Let me give you a small idea of how mind-boggling the process is: Each neuron in your brain can carry on several million different conversations at the same time. No, you're not going crazy. This is normal. A single neuron can receive signals from more than 1,000 other neurons. And these electrical impulses take differing routes and speeds. Some take express routes. Light is bright—you squint your eyes. The dish is hot—you remove your hand quickly. Reflex actions like these travel first to the spinal cord, where the nerve impulse to pull your hand away is initiated; then it travels to the brain. Interestingly, messages sent through pain receptors can travel as slowly as 2 mph, whereas the signal from a kiss travels at an amazing 140 mph! We were created for love!

To picture the working brain, we might think of viewing New York City from the sky, with cars going in all directions and yet all is orderly and each part is in tune with the others. However, the perfection with which our minds function can become damaged, blunted, or shattered. In addition to injuries or illnesses, the type of stimuli we feed into our systems can distort the perception or interpretation of the information. The communication within can go awry. Neurons (including the chemicals, neurotransmitters and hormones that regulate them, their circuitry, and the electrical impulses that flow through them) make you, *you* and me, *me*. We're not all wired the same. Each nerve pathway and connection has been constructed experience by experience, choice by choice.

We were created for an incredible amount of communication or stimuli reception. Not only are our brains capable of immense amounts of storage, but their programming and reprogramming occur largely as a result of information, chemicals, and stimuli that enter through the avenue of the five senses. What we do with this information or stimuli plays a part in shaping our lives.

The Lord desires to infuse our senses with information that will cause our hearts to beat with His, our minds to long for His will, and our love to be set upon Him.

Lord, help me to guard my senses so I can have what You created me to experience: Your mind in me—as it was in Your Son, Jesus. RISË RAFFERTY

God's Home Run for You

For all the promises of God in Him are Yes, and in Him Amen,
to the glory of God through us. 2 Cor. 1:20, NKJV.

SHAWN BUTLER WAS dying of cancer at age 7. His frail, weak body was sinking into a coma. Cancer had infiltrated 90 percent of his brain. On August 9, 1982, Shawn's father agreed with the physicians that if he stopped breathing they would not try to revive him.

But four days later something remarkable occurred. Red Sox first baseman Dace Stapleton, Shawn's hero, paid him a visit. Upon hearing the voice of the sports champion, Shawn actually awoke from his comatose state and talked for a few minutes about baseball. Then Stapleton leaned over the bed and made a promise. "Tomorrow," he stated, "I'm going to hit one over the fence just for you." Shawn's eyes lit up. During the Red Sox game the following day, when Dace Stapleton first came up to bat he had a determination in his gait. With a steely gleam in his eye he knocked the ball over the left field wall for a home run.

Five months later, Shawn's doctors were mystified. They could find no trace of the malignancy. The boy seemed almost completely recovered. His family was even planning a trip to Disney World.

What made the difference? Some believe it was hope. Shawn's hero made a promise and fulfilled that promise. Possibly, by doing so, he opened a door of hope for Shawn.

As we begin a new year, it stands before us full of hope. New beginnings and new opportunities. But sometimes optimism fades into disappointment. We discover our lack of ability to make lasting change. We fail to seize the moment. At those times we need to remember that "the Lord is not slack concerning his promise" (2 Peter 3:9). And His promise is "I will not fail thee, nor forsake thee" (Joshua 1:5). In addition, Psalm 37:4, 5 offers the assurance that God will give us the desires of our hearts.

In 2 Corinthians 1:20 the apostle Paul says that all God's promises find their "yes" in Jesus. He is the key. Jesus imparts power to live a new life and makes hope a reality. Rivet your eyes on Him. He will never disappoint you.

What changes do you want to make in your life? Put your hope in Christ and rejoice as He hits a home run for you this year! MICHAEL CAULEY

Getting in Gear

*Beloved, I pray that you may prosper in all things and
be in health, just as your soul prospers. 3 John 2, NKJV.*

STARTING A FITNESS PROGRAM—and sticking with it—may be one
of the most challenging tasks you'll ever face. To be successful, you must
commit to get fit. Humans are creatures of habit. Adopting a new lifestyle
requires breaking old, ingrained habits and forging new and perhaps unfamiliar ones. Many meet their Waterloo on this first step because their decision is based on emotional enthusiasm rather than a disciplined
commitment. When the going gets tough (it will) and the emotional highs
fade (they will), the strength of your commitment must carry you through.

Decide that you will be a person of your word—with your reputation
on the line. Put your resolution in writing and place it where it will continually remind you.

Ask for divine strength to support you. Remember that your body is
a temple of the Holy Spirit. As you strengthen your physical body He is
better able to communicate with you spiritually. The Lord has promised
His power to those who ask for it. Develop an awareness that He is beside
you when the going gets difficult. Claim God's promise in Jeremiah 30:17:
"I will restore you to health and heal your wounds" (NIV).

Ask others to help keep you accountable. Make your decisions public. Public pledges are difficult to break because you don't want to let
others down.

What else do you need in order to keep your commitment? Here's a
list of essentials: (1) Have a definite plan, but avoid inflexibility. (2) Make
modest beginning goals. Drastic changes may be necessary if serious health
hazards need to be dealt with but, generally speaking, excessive goals set
you up for failure. (3) Make your plan a part of your daily life. (4) Go for
moderation and balance. (5) Expect progress to be gradual. If it took years
to get out of shape it will takes months to get it back. (6) Enjoy the process, not just the end product. (7) Don't be too hard on yourself. Old
habits die hard. (8) Monitor your progress on a regular basis, but don't be
obsessive. (9) Follow the 90/10 rule rather than the 100/0 rule. Go for 90
percent compliance. Cut yourself a little slack, rather than wallow in guilt.
(10) Give credit where credit is due; thank the Lord for your success.

*What lifestyle changes would you like to make this year to help you become the
person you really want to be? Today's a great day to start getting in gear!*

ELMAR P. SAKALA

15

Sleeping the Sleep of the Righteous

Now when He got into a boat, His disciples followed Him.
And suddenly a great tempest arose on the sea, so that the boat
was covered with the waves. But He was asleep. Matt. 8:23, 24, NKJV.

DOES IT SEEM to you that more and more is required of you every day? That the demands of work, family, your children's school—not to mention the burgeoning red-tape that business bureaucracies as well as government are piling up—are just too much?

Sometimes it reminds me of that story about Jesus asleep in the boat in the midst of a storm. Usually when we preachers tell this story, we go to the part where Jesus commands the winds and the waves to "be still." But it seems to me there is an even larger lesson in the simple fact that He was sound asleep in a sinking boat that was taking on water, with the wind howling and the stinging rain all around Him! "He slept the sleep of the righteous," an older deacon once told me after I preached on this topic. Christ had placed Himself in the hands of His Father, and He could sleep completely, deeply, and untroubled no matter the commotion and fear all around him.

The transforming grace of Jesus is just like that. With all of the muddled demands of supervisors (or your staff), requirements of clients and vendors, corporate switchboards with excessive telephone trees and disembodied voice mail, and unexpected emergencies of your children (or your parents)—with all of that, the transforming grace of the Lord Jesus Christ can help you sleep "the sleep of the righteous." There can be peace on the inside if we allow that transforming grace to permeate our heart and mind completely.

Frankly, I think Jesus would probably tell us that multitasking is a tool of the devil. The Creator did not make human beings to be pushed to the limit, sucked dry of every bit of energy in order for employers to increase productivity. We have a pandemic of degenerative diseases in America that are the direct result of trying to get too much out of life without putting the same investment back in. Everyone wants to win the lottery; everyone wants to get more than they pay for. Very soon Jesus is coming back to tell us, "Enough is enough!"

We can live in the promise of that coming Kingdom of Peace every day, no matter the storms around us, no matter the excessive demands of bosses, corporations, and institutions.

May the peace and the grace of the Lord Jesus Christ be with you today and every day!   MONTE SAHLIN

Common Sense in Diet Reform

And every man that striveth for the mastery is temperate in all things.
Now they do it to obtain a corruptible crown; but we an incorruptible. 1 Cor. 9:25.

THOSE WHO UNDERSTAND the laws of health and who are governed by principle will shun the extremes, both of indulgence and of restriction. Their diet is chosen, not for the mere gratification of appetite, but for the upbuilding of the body. They seek to preserve every power in the best condition for highest service to God and man. The appetite is under the control of reason and conscience, and they are rewarded with health of body and mind. While they do not urge their views offensively upon others, their example is a testimony in favor of right principles. These persons have a wide influence for good.

There is real common sense in dietetic reform. The subject should be studied broadly and deeply, and no one should criticize others because their practice is not, in all things, in harmony with his own. It is impossible to make an unvarying rule to regulate everyone's habits, and no one should think himself a criterion for all. Not all can eat the same things. Foods that are palatable and wholesome to one person may be distasteful, and even harmful, to another. Some cannot use milk, while others thrive on it. Some persons cannot digest peas and beans; others find them wholesome. For some the coarser grain preparations are good food, while others cannot use them. . . .

The diet reform should be progressive. As disease in animals increases, the use of milk and eggs will become more and more unsafe. An effort should be made to supply their place with other things that are healthful and inexpensive. The people everywhere should be taught how to cook without milk and eggs, so far as possible, and yet have their food wholesome and palatable. . . .

Carefully consider your diet. Study from cause to effect. Cultivate self-control. Keep appetite under the control of reason. Never abuse the stomach by overeating, but do not deprive yourself of the wholesome, palatable food that health demands. . . .

Eat according to your best judgment; and when you have asked the Lord to bless the food for the strengthening of your body, believe that He hears your prayer, and be at rest.

Wise Creator, give me common sense when it comes to choosing what I should eat.

ELLEN G. WHITE—*The Ministry of Healing*, pp. 319-323

The Green Machine

To everything there is a season, a time for every purpose under heaven. Eccl. 3:1, NKJV.

I HIT THE CAR'S brakes, but nothing happened. I pumped them three or four times, but each time the pedal went straight to the floorboard. My passenger, the conference publishing secretary, let out an involuntary "Oh, no!" as he and I careened toward Main Street.

My aging car, dubbed "The Green Machine," had been in serious need of repair for some time. I relied on several somewhat dubious reasons for delay. As a college student I could hardly afford toothpaste, much less a trip to the garage. Also, my frenetic schedule didn't allow for such sensible pauses. Lastly, I took a perverse, macho delight in seeing how much could go wrong and still have the car get me to where I wanted to go. No wimpy trips to the mechanic for this rugged auto. My only concessions were to carry a few cans of oil and brake fluid in the trunk, plus several jugs of water.

As Main Street loomed before us, I steered hard right onto a side road that had a gentle incline; that slowed us until I could yank on the emergency brake. I took in a deep breath, filled the master brake cylinder with fluid, and headed off to our next appointment.

For years I treated myself the very same way. I drove myself until a visit to the repair shop was long overdue. The warning signs were all there—increased anxiety, inability to sleep well, upset stomach, a short emotional fuse, frequent headaches, and overdoses of junk food.

Then I discovered the simple truth that we need to balance input and output. Our ability to produce depends to a large extent on the time we take to renew. Hours spent replenishing ourselves, physically, emotionally, and spiritually, are just as important, just as valuable, as the time we actually spend working. Not an easy message for a long-time workaholic.

The Scriptures taught this truth centuries ago with the observation "To every thing there is a season, and a time to every purpose . . . : a time to plant, and a time to pluck up that which is planted; . . . a time to keep and a time to cast away" (Eccl. 3:1-6). We ignore at our peril life's God-given cycles of receiving and giving. I am now much more sensitive to trying to maintain that balance in my own life and keeping my inner brakes from letting go.

How are your inner brakes? Are they in need of some repair?

KIM ALLAN JOHNSON

Meaning in Suffering

These trials are only to test your faith, to show that it is strong and pure.
It is being tested as fire tests and purifies gold—and your faith is far
more precious to God than mere gold. So if your faith remains strong
after being tried by fiery trials, it will bring you much praise and glory and
honor on the day when Jesus Christ is revealed to the whole world. 1 Peter 1:7, NLT.

WHEN YOU'RE SUFFERING, it's easy to lose hope. Dr. Victor E. Frankl, who lived through the horrors of the concentration camps in World War II, was asked to make a presentation to his fellow sufferers in the last dreadful days before liberation. He began with the hypothesis that "our situation was not the most terrible we could think of." Here are the points he made to instill hope within the hopeless (from his book *Man's Search for Meaning*).

1. Very few of their losses were irreplaceable. Most could be restored or achieved again, such as health, family, happiness, professional abilities, fortune, or position in society.

2. Although their chance of survival seemed small (perhaps 1 in 20), there was always the possibility that a great opportunity would come their way quite suddenly.

3. What they had experienced, no power on earth could take from them.

4. Human life always has a meaning, and this includes suffering, privation, and death. Regardless of circumstances, life must be lived with dignity and meaning. Even the sacrifice they were forced to make could have meaning if they chose to see that by their suffering someone else might suffer less. Or perhaps by their courage, others would be blessed.

5. Life is still expecting something out of them. To give up would mean that someone in the future would suffer because they weren't there; the word of kindness would not be said, a friend would not be helped, the book would not be written. They could never be too sick, too disabled, or too old that God does not need them and what they have to offer.

Many are angry at God because they think He allowed bad things to happen in order to work out His master plan for the universe, perfect our characters, teach us important lessons, or punish us for our mistakes. But God doesn't make planes crash or boats sink; He doesn't cause children to be born with AIDS, or sentence thousands to die from starvation. The basic truth is, bad things happen to us because we are living in Satan's territory. And the consequence of sin is death.

If you are suffering, ask God to help you find meaning in it. KAY KUZMA

19

Laughter Is Good for Your Health

A cheerful heart is good medicine. Prov. 17:22, NIV.

PERHAPS YOU HAVE heard some of these misstatements that have appeared in church bulletins:

- "Don't let worry kill you. Let the church help."
- "Thursday night: potluck supper. Prayer and medication to follow."
- "For those of you who have children and don't know it, we have a nursery downstairs."
- "The ladies of the church have cast off clothing of every kind, and they may be seen in the church basement Friday."

If you fail to see the humor in these announcements you may have a serious problem (pun intended), because there is hardly a system in your body that a good laugh doesn't stimulate. Laughter benefits the entire cardiovascular system through dilation and increase of blood flow. As you gulp in large amounts of air it creates a rich, highly oxygenated flow of blood. Sometimes this extra flow will make your face flush and you feel refreshed all over.

While you are laughing your blood pressure and heart rate increase (much like when you exercise), but after the laughter subsides both your blood pressure and heart rate return to levels lower than when you started. According to one expert in the field of humor, your daily laugh total should equal at least 15 chuckles a day or you are under-laughed.

Have you ever laughed until your sides hurt? Such an experience gives new meaning to the old adage, "No pain, no gain." As your diaphragm convulses it sets up a chain reaction in your body that shakes up your stomach and other vital organs, providing an internal massage. Some call it internal jogging.

Smile a lot! The Bible reminds us that "a happy heart makes the face cheerful" (Prov. 15:13, NIV). Comedian Fred Allen once quipped, "It is bad to suppress laughter. It goes back down and spreads to your hips." Perhaps, with enough practice, you may identify with little Freddie, who was scolded by his third-grade teacher for laughing out loud in the classroom. "Teacher," replied Freddie apologetically, "I really didn't mean to. I was just grinning and my smile broke."

Have you gotten in your 15 chuckles today? If not, let your smile break, and reap the reward of better health! LEN MCMILLAN

The Significance of a Marshmallow

So I say, live by the Spirit, and you will not gratify
the desires of the sinful nature. Gal. 5:16, NIV.

IMAGINE YOU ARE 4 years old. Picture yourself in a strange room; a strange person gives you a marshmallow and promises you a second one if you don't eat the first one until he returns from a short errand. What do you do? Do you gobble down the marshmallow, not thinking about the possibility of another? Or, with nothing to do but stare at the marshmallow, do you muster all the self-control available to you as a 4-year-old and wait until the giver returns?

That question has proved to be a classic in a research study conducted on a group of 4-year-olds. When the researchers tracked down the children 14 years later they found that this test was an amazing predictor of how the children would do in school. The ones who had waited in the test scored significantly higher—210 points higher—on their Scholastic Achievement Test. In addition, the kids who had patiently waited were, later, more stable emotionally than the other group, better liked by their teachers and their peers, and were still able to delay gratification in pursuit of their goals.

The children who had eaten the marshmallow immediately were, 14 years later, less emotionally stable, more irritable, more likely to pick fights, not as well liked, and fell apart under stress.

The Bible talks about the importance of self-control. Galatians 5:22, 23 says, "But the fruit of the Spirit is love, joy, peace, patience, kindness, goodness, faithfulness, gentleness, and self-control. Against such things there is no law" (NIV). While our society places great emphasis on scholastic success—defined as how much knowledge you can pack into your brain in a given amount of time—God, as usual, has an entirely different way of measuring success.

Now science has caught up with what the Bible has always presented to us. God promises us success, not based on worldly standards, academic achievement, or measures of wealth, but upon His Spirit working in us. When He develops the fruits of the Spirit in our characters we will be healthier and happier, our relationships will be more satisfying, our academic pursuits more successful, and our jobs more fulfilling. Better yet, we will be successful not only in the physical world but in the spiritual world as well. That's where it really counts.

Isn't it interesting that one character trait—self-control—can have such a widespread effect on a person's success in life? How healthy is your self-control?

CAROLE BROUSSON ANDERSON

JANUARY 12

The Father Factor

My prayer for all of them is that they will be one, just as you and I
are one, Father—that just as you are in me and I am in you,
so they will be in us, and the world will believe you sent me. John 17:21, NLT.

IT'S HEALTHY WHEN dads are involved in parenting. Here are the facts: kids with dads have healthier social relationships and higher achievement motivation and therefore do better in school. They are more able to defer immediate gratification for later rewards. They have higher self-esteem and are less susceptible to group influence and to juvenile delinquency. In fact, "All the elements of mental health are better," states Dr. Robert Moradi, a psychiatrist at the University of California at Los Angeles's School of Medicine. After analyzing census figures, Dr. Loren Moshen, of the National Institute of Mental Health, concluded that absence of the father was a stronger factor than poverty in contributing to juvenile delinquency.

But of all the findings the most incredible was Dr. Kyle Pruett's that men who have been involved in the physical care of children under the age of 3 are significantly less likely to become involved in the sexual abuse of children. Apparently, the very intimacy of feeding, changing diapers, and bathing seems to inoculate men against subsequent sexual arousal, not just in relation to their own children but to others as well. The concluding statement in a special issue of *Newsweek* Magazine (spring/summer, 1997, p. 73) put it this way: "Few forces are as powerful, and as underused in our culture, as this sacred bond between father and child, the magnetic attraction of strength for weakness, the 'attachment' that begins with dependence and grows into love."

But there's more: In a study of 1,337 medical doctors who graduated from Johns Hopkins University between 1948 and 1964, lack of closeness with parents was a common factor in hypertension, coronary heart disease, malignant tumors, mental illness, and suicide. In a study of 39 teenage girls suffering from the anorexia nervosa eating disorder, 36 had one common factor: lack of closeness with Dad. In a study done at John Hopkins University, white teenage girls living in fatherless families were 60 percent more likely to have premarital intercourse than those living in two-parent homes.

Fathers, if you want healthy kids, get involved with them—and with God!

My heavenly Father, may my family see You in me through my actions and my words.   KAY KUZMA

Drinking Living Water

*Jesus answered and said to her, "Whoever drinks of this water
will thirst again, but whoever drinks of the water that I shall give him
will never thirst. But the water that I shall give him will become in him
a fountain of water springing up into everlasting life." John 4:13, 14, NKJV.*

WATER IS ESSENTIAL to life and makes up 60 to 75 percent of our body's weight. It is a solvent. Nutrients, such as glucose, are dissolved in the blood plasma and transported to body cells, thanks to water. Without water, waste products wouldn't be dissolved and excreted in the urine. Plus, the sense of taste depends on water.

Water is a lubricant. It prevents friction where surfaces meet and move; it's part of the synovial fluid in the joint cavity that prevents friction as the bone moves. And because the digestive tract mucus (mostly water) is slippery, our food has a smooth passage through the intestinal tract.

Water changes temperature slowly—it absorbs a great deal of heat before the temperature rises significantly; conversely, it releases a great deal of heat before the temperature drops significantly. This is one of the factors that help our bodies maintain a constant temperature. Plus, without water we wouldn't be able to sweat, which is the evaporation process that helps keep the body cells from overheating.

These are just a few vital body functions that water makes possible. Yet it's surprising how many people have no idea that their body's health is dependent on getting adequate water.

In 1991, I was a member of an evangelistic team sent to Lvov, Ukraine, formerly part of the U.S.S.R. I was shocked to learn that as part of the treatment for various diseases, the people had been told to restrict the drinking of water! In one of my first lectures, I talked about the importance of water, stressing that at least eight glasses of water was essential for proper kidney function, which removed wastes from their bodies. Then I asked the audience to try to drink eight glasses of water daily for the next three weeks. At the end of this period, when I asked if they had followed this practice, they gave me a standing ovation. Apparently, water had made a significant difference in their lives!

Similarly, you can experience a significant difference in the quality of your life by drinking the "living water" of Christ's salvation.

Are you drinking enough water to keep healthy—both physically and spiritually?

ALEX P. BOKOVOY

Managing the Monkeys in Your Life

Sow for yourselves righteousness; reap in mercy; break up your fallow ground, for it is time to seek the Lord, till He comes and rains righteousness on you. Hosea 10:12, NKJV.

THINGS THAT NEED to be done are like monkeys. Feed them and they'll never go home. They cling to you. They chatter incessantly. They vie for your attention. They multiply until they've taken control of your life. They cause stress!

If your life has become a zoo, follow these monkey-managing rules:

Rule 1: You're not the only zoo keeper in the world—or in your family. You don't have to do everything. To show your family that you love them, you don't have to cook from scratch or always be the one who does the laundry.

If you think you are indispensable to your family, you'll always have too many monkeys. You must believe that your family *can* get along without your "working" for them. Encourage others to do what they are capable of doing, even if it's not done exactly the way you'd do it.

Rule 2: Don't feed other people's monkeys. Make sure each person keeps his own monkeys. Don't allow others to dump their monkeys on you. Learn to put responsibility back on others. Learn to feel OK about disappointing others by saying, "That's not my monkey!"

Rule 3: Keep your monkey population under control. It may sound cruel, but you need to kill the excess ones. Let them starve to death. I've found that things to do tend to expand to fit the amount of time you'll give them. That's why you must prioritize (determine what's really important) and schedule. Allow only a certain amount of time for a project and let the rest "starve"; for example, washing windows every time it rains! Learn to just say *no*.

Rule 4: Monkeys come in the mail, over the telephone, and via the Internet. Control your mail by reading and processing it immediately. Control the telephone by using an answering machine. Don't be quick to answer yes when someone asks, "Do you have a minute?" Set a time when you are available for calls. Budget your time on the Internet.

Rule 5: Don't start the weekend with a cage full of monkeys. Instead, plan fun and family into your weekend. Take the Fourth Commandment seriously. Instead of spending your week putting things off until the weekend, plan your week so that you'll have time to enjoy the weekend.

How can you reduce the monkeys in your life so you have time for the Lord—and your family?   KAY KUZMA

The Other Side of Violence

So perish all thine enemies, O Lord; but let all who love
thee be like the sun rising in strength. Judges 5:31, NEB.

IN ONE OF THOSE determined-to-read-the-Bible-through projects, we're likely to get as far as Judges. By this time we can note the genius of the Bible writers to condense more than 2,000 years of history into some 200 pages. We reach Judges 4 and encounter a graphic account of an attack spearheaded by Deborah, prophetess and judge in Israel. Once the enemy troops are routed, the story ends like the 6:00 news: Sisera, the fleeing general, accepted the hospitality of Jael, who gave him milk to drink; then as he slept, she hammered a peg thorough his head. "His brains oozed out on the ground, his limbs twitched, and he died" (Judges 4:21, NEB).

Then we move on to Judges 5. What has happened to the pace of the book? Deborah has composed a song about the battle, and it's inserted into the biblical record—the same story all over again. Why?

Judges 5 reads like a pitch for a documentary movie. Imagine a director creating the opening scene—people traveling fearfully because of enemy ambush on the road: "In the days of Jael, caravans plied no longer; men who had followed the high roads went round by devious paths" (Judges 5:6, NEB). For Israel, the recapitulation came in a song that climaxes with the enemy routed. But at the end we detect a new feature: Deborah is creating a scene she has not witnessed but, with the heart of a mother, can imagine.

At the home of Sisera, the enemy general, his mother must be waiting for her son's return. Deborah sings: "The mother of Sisera peered through the lattice, through the window she peered and shrilly cried, 'Why are his chariots so long in coming?'" (verse 28, NEB).

The princesses answer: "They must be finding spoil; . . . booty of dyed stuffs for Sisera, . . . two lengths of striped stuff—to grace the victor's neck" (verse 30, NEB).

This is no amateur production. Deborah knows her characters. We have been transported through her eyes. The retelling is worthy of a pause in the biblical record, as Deborah reminds us of the other side of violence.

As you hear the news today, pause and rerun in your mind the heartache of those who have lost loved ones because of violence—even though they might have been the "enemy"! EDNA MAYE LOVELESS

Energized by Space

*When I consider Your heavens, the work of Your fingers, the moon
and the stars, which You have ordained, What is man that You are
mindful of him, and the son of man that You visit him?
For You have made him a little lower than the angels, and You
have crowned him with glory and honor. Ps. 8:3-5, NKJV.*

I'M ENERGIZED BY thoughts of outer space. Our earth is one of nine planets in our solar system. Billions of solar systems, perhaps similar to ours, make up our galaxy, the Milky Way. And there are billions of galaxies! I wonder, *Surely there are other planets, with other life forms.*

Our closest star, Proxima Centauri, is about four light years away—right next door, relatively speaking. But four light years is the distance light travels in four years, at 186,000 miles per second! Even that near neighbor is a long, long distance from us.

Telescopes are being built that will be able to see objects that are 12 billion light-years away. Each group of pictures from the Hubble Space Telescope reveals marvelous new and unexpected treasures in space. The heavenly skies, which only a few years ago seemed so static and defined, are now indicating new mysteries and revisions of old ideas about the great universe. The stars and star clusters—their colors, their shapes—are so beautiful and so varied; the more we see the more breath-taking the heavens become!

God, why is there so much space? When You created the universe, what existed before? Are there other kinds of universes? Are there other planets such as Earth? If so, what would life be like there? Is Earth the only planet that needs a Savior? I ponder things such as:

• The universe is unimaginably gigantic; our solar system and our earth are but tiny specs in Your eyes. What is man that You are mindful of him? Considering space, how insignificant we are. Yet, You walk and talk with us! You even number the hairs on our heads. This I cannot comprehend.

• You have given us life, the ability to reason, and the ability to consciously consider context beyond our daily lives. You have crowned us with undeserved glory and honor. You have made us rulers of all other animals—just a little lower than the angels who live somewhere in the heavens with You.

• In this massive universe, You sent Jesus to remind us that we are of far more value than sparrows, yet You care for them. You care what happens in our lives. You died for us. How valuable we are!

When you feel insignificant, look up into space and remember that the God of it all loves you!
FORREST BAILEY

A Whale of a Lesson

Then Jonah prayed to the Lord his God from inside the fish: . . . "When I had lost all hope, I turned my thoughts once more to the Lord. . . . I will never worship anyone but you! For how can I thank you enough for all you have done?" Jonah 2:1-9, TLB.

IT WAS ALMOST 8:30 when Marilyn invited me to walk down the beach with her. I was planning to power walk with another friend—as I did religiously each morning—so I was about to decline when the phone rang and my walking partner said she couldn't make it. "Marilyn," I called, "I'll join you."

That's why I was on the beach when it happened. It was the first time in three years of living next to the ocean that I had seen anything like it. Just past the breakers, about 100 feet away, a pod of whales were spouting, cavorting, breaching, and crashing into the water.

"Look over there. Wow! It's incredible!" we shouted to each other as again and again the whales rose into the air, flapped their tails, and disappeared beneath the surface. We were wild with excitement!

Later, I thought about Jonah. I imagined myself entombed in a fish's belly enduring the internal roller-coaster ride as it dove to the bottom of the ocean and then rose to breach and dove again. I would have screamed to God, "Get me out of here!" But that's not what Jonah prayed. Instead, he recognized that this was God's way of saving him from death. And right there, in the midst of half-digested food, Jonah thanked God. Then he promised that He'd do what God wanted him to do.

All of us have days when we feel we're in the belly of a whale. Instead of feeling sorry for ourselves, blaming God, or screaming "Get me out of here," maybe we should accept the experience as God's wake-up call—His way of saving us—and then choose to do what we know we should.

You're in the hospital after by-pass surgery: "Wake up and change your lifestyle." Your pants are too tight: "Wake up, watch what you eat, and exercise!" Persistent cough: "Wake up and stop smoking!" Chest pains: "Wake up and make that doctor's appointment!" Headache: "Wake up, increase your water intake and reduce the stress!"

I hope it doesn't take something as drastic as a ride in the belly of a whale to teach me it's always better to do it God's way.

God, please soften my stubborn will so I don't have to ride in the belly of a whale to learn the lessons You want me to learn.　　　　LAURA LE SALISBURY

Rebuilt by the Lord and LLUMC

"And God will wipe away every tear from their eyes; there shall be no more death, nor sorrow, nor crying. There shall be no more pain, for the former things have passed away." Then He who sat on the throne said, "Behold, I make all things new." Rev. 21:4, 5, NKJV.

IT WAS OCTOBER 15, 1994. She was crying tears of joy as she was swept off her feet by Brian Robertson, No. 55 on Riverside (California) Christian School's football team. You see, Mary Van Dyke had just been crowned homecoming queen.

Born July 12, 1977, with 23 physical and neurological anomalies, Mary was not supposed to survive infancy. It was thought she would never be able to do more than lift her head. Mary was born with the Mary Van Dyke syndrome, a condition so rare that her doctors at Loma Linda University Medical Center in Southern California later named it after her. But Mary was born a fighter. With encouragement from her big sister, Alice, and her parents, Pete and Pat Van Dyke, Mary learned to crawl, climb stairs, and eventually to walk with the help of a tiny aluminum walker.

When Mary was just 3, her mother made a T-shirt with a message emblazoned over the chest, "REBUILT BY THE LORD AND LLUMC." When she was 8, her medical records weighed more than she did. Mary has had heart surgery to repair a hole in her heart. She has undergone hip construction, hand surgeries, ear surgeries, and all kinds of facial reconstruction.

Just before her thirty-first operation, before a cheering crowd, 17-year-old Mary Van Dyke walked onto the field to be named homecoming queen of Riverside Christian School. The determined teenager has earned an "A" average and the admiration of an entire school. Many fought to maintain their composure as an astonished Mary was crowned and handed a bouquet of red roses. That's when her escort, Brian, swooped her into his arms and carried her off the field.

"After everything she's gone through," said school administrator Vance Nichols, "I just can't stop crying." In a feature published the next day in the Riverside *Press Enterprise,* Nichols said, "Our school is a better place because of her. My faith is a stronger one because of her."

According to her mother, Mary faces a lifetime of periodic surgery for various problems. For strength, Mary will continue to rely on her faith in God. Mary Van Dyke is a royal inspiration.

Thank You, Lord, for the day when we can all wear the message on our heavenly robes, "Rebuilt by the Lord!"   RICHARD A. SCHAEFER

Keeping Your Reservoirs Full

You anoint my head with oil; my cup runs over. Ps. 23:5, NKJV.

I'M A STATISTICIAN. I'm the one who looks at the results of research and determines the probability of a person getting certain diseases. Working in the School of Public Health at Loma Linda University, I knew what the risk factors were for stroke, and I was sure I would never have one. I was lean, exercised daily, ate a mostly vegan diet, had low blood pressure, was living a fairly stress-free life, and had never smoked or drank.

But on February 8, 1996, the improbable happened. I was not taking enough blood thinning coumidin for my heart's irregular beat (caused by a heart defect at birth), and my heart threw a clot straight to the core of my brain. It knocked out the control panels for my left-side movement, analytical thinking, directionality, time concepts, and my initiation and inhibitory responses. In short, it was very bad. I was not expected to walk again—or think straight!

Three years later, if you were to meet me on the street, I doubt if you'd know I'd had a stroke unless you caught my slight limp or noticed my crooked smile. What happened?

I call it the Reservoir Effect. If your life is empty and a crisis hits, you don't have any reserves to battle the illness. But my life was full to overflowing with three things to which I credit my incredible recovery: faith in God's grace, a loving and supportive family, and a healthy lifestyle.

Reservoir 1: *A healthy faith in God's grace.* When crisis hit, I put my fate in God's hands and relaxed. I was anointed and never doubted His love and miraculous healing power. If you don't have faith, hopelessness can settle in. It's easy to give up. Stroke patients can't give up! They've got to work to rebuild the destroyed connections that make movement, thinking, and talking possible.

Reservoir 2: *Healthy relationships.* I was never alone. My wife and daughter were there, loving me, supporting me, encouraging me, and nudging me on to exercise my reluctant muscles. I had something to live for. I got well for them.

Reservoir 3: *Healthy lifestyle.* Yes, I had a stroke that affected my brain, but my body was healthy; my veins were clean; my immune system was strong. My physical health gave me the stamina to will myself to walk, to climb stairs, to swim, and to play tennis once again.

What could you do today to make sure your reservoirs are full?

JAN W. KUZMA

Miracle on Monarch Pass

For he shall give his angels charge over thee, to keep thee in all thy ways. Ps. 91:11.

NANCY AND I WERE heading home through the Colorado Rockies after vacationing with Nancy's family. Her folks, brother, and his wife had taken the jeep up over the pass, so Nancy and I were driving the two motor homes with all the kids. Everything was fine until we started up Monarch Pass. The altitude affected the carburetors in our motor homes— they kept flooding out. Two miles from the 11,000-foot summit we pulled over again. After I got Nancy's motor home running, I couldn't get mine started. We had a quarter tank of gas but we were parked on a slant and gas couldn't get to the engine. So I got the bright idea that if I could just get some gas in the carburetor it would start.

I siphoned some gas into a pressure cooker and placed it between the two front seats. I asked Isadora, my oldest niece, to help me while her sister Alisha watched the dogs in the back. She began to pour gas slowly into the carburetor. The motor started for a moment and quit. Slowly I went from neutral to drive, back and forth, as she poured the gas slowly into the carburetor. Everything was going as planned! We were actually moving when all of a sudden the engine backfired and flames shot up through the carburetor. Isadora dropped the tin cup with gas in it beside the pressure cooker full of gas.

Instantly I knew we were in trouble. We both jumped up and headed for the door. I grabbed her and threw her out but as I kicked the pressure cooker out, gas went all over me. Just as I was ready to jump out, I noticed the motor home was rolling backward—and Alisha was still in the back. I climbed back over the fire to the driver's seat, hit the brakes, and jammed the gear into park. But when I got back to the door, the heat of the fire had swollen it shut. I yanked but it wouldn't budge.

By now I was fully ablaze and as I looked out the little window and saw Nancy and our kids I thought, *I'm not going to make it!* Just then the door opened on it's own! I jumped out and started rolling to put out the fire. All of a sudden I felt two hands grab my shoulders, stopping me just as a part of my right leg went over a 200-foot cliff. I ran back to check on the motor home. By then the kids had put the fire out and everyone was safe. It was a miracle I was alive. It had to be my guardian angel who opened that door and then grabbed me when I was about to roll off the cliff.

Aren't you glad God sends His angels to protect us, even when we do foolish things that get us into trouble? Can you think of a time when your angel saved you? Why not thank the Lord!   TERRY NELSON

A Life-saving Exchange

If anyone desires to come after Me, let him deny himself, and take up his cross, and follow Me. For whoever desires to save his life will lose it, but whoever loses his life for My sake will find it. For what profit is it to a man if he gains the whole world, and loses his own soul? Or what will a man give in exchange for his soul? Matt. 16:24-26, NKJV.

DID YOU KNOW that the average meat-eating American will consume 21 cows, 14 sheep, 12 hogs, 900 chickens and 1,000 pounds of swimming and flying animals in a lifetime?

It was once believed that the more meat a man ate the healthier he would be. But that all changed when the American Cancer Society made the following recommendations that would significantly lower the risk of cancer: A diet high in fruits, vegetables, and whole grains but low in high-fat foods, especially those containing animal fats; the maintenance of a healthy weight and exercise program; and limited or no alcohol intake.

The scientific support for this recommendation is strong: Here are a few examples concerning meat eating: A study of 35,000 women found that those with diets high in meat and animal fat, especially hamburgers, had double the risk for lymph node cancer. Norwegian men who ate the most processed meat had the highest rates of colon cancer. In a 14-year follow-up study of Swedish men, meat (beef and lamb) was the only food linked to higher rates of colon cancer. A six-year Harvard study of 90,000 women showed that no amount of red meat was safe when it came to colon cancer. Women who ate a main dish of meat daily (beef, pork, or lamb) were 250 percent more apt to develop colon cancer than those eating meat less than once a month. And the more they ate, the greater the risk. Even women who ate red meat infrequently, once a week or once a month, were still 40 percent more apt to get colon cancer than those who ate red meat less than once a month.

Isn't it time to trade in some of those 21 cows for a truckload of soy-derived protein, swap some of the 14 sheep for a few bushels of beans, totally eliminate the 12 hogs and substitute a couple wheelbarrows of fresh carrots and apples?

But even more important, I hope you will try the spiritual exchange that Jesus suggested in Matthew 16:24-26. What a strange exchange this sounds like—losing your life only to find it? It seems so opposite to the way we are used to thinking, but the exchange is worth it.

To follow Christ, is there something in your life that you should be exchanging for something better? RISË RAFFERTY

The Sin of Hurry

For there is a time there for every purpose and for every work. Eccl. 3:17, NKJV.

ONE MORNING I GOT caught hurrying again. I was on my way to coach our college football team. As usual, I'd tried to cram too much into the early morning hours. The blinking lights of a car made me pull over, and a somber man in blue gave me a copy of a yellow form marked "Municipal Traffic Court." The charge: I had broken the law. I had been hurrying too fast.

As I drove on, the Lord spoke to me, "You broke the law." I agreed.

"No," He continued., "You don't understand. You broke *The Law."* Breaking a man-made law was serious enough, but I was guilty of breaking a far greater eternal rhythm. I had submitted to the sin of hurry.

Nikos Kazantzakis, in his book *Zorba the Greek,* relates a life-changing event. "I remembered one morning when I discovered a cocoon in the bark of a tree, just as the butterfly was making a hole in its case and preparing to come out. I waited a while, but it was too long appearing and I was impatient. I bent over it and breathed on it to warm it. I warmed it as quickly as I could, and the miracle began to happen before my eyes, faster than life. The case opened. The butterfly started slowly crawling out, and I shall never forget my horror when I saw how its wings were folded back and crumpled before its time. It struggled desperately and a few seconds later died in the palm of my hand.

"That little body is, I do believe, the greatest weight I have on my conscience. For I realize today that it is a mortal sin to violate the great laws of nature. We should not hurry. We should not be impatient. But we should confidently obey the eternal rhythm. If only that little butterfly could always flutter before me to show me the way."

Time is a holy mystery. It doesn't matter what kind of time it is— Greenwich, Daylight Savings, Standard, Mountain, or Pacific. We just never seem to have enough of it.

How can we avoid the sin of hurry? By being absolutely surrendered to Him, releasing our self-imposed deadlines, and living in the rhythm of "All to Jesus I surrender, all to Him I freely give," with no apologies, no excuses, no regrets, living in moment-by-moment obedience to His timing.

Lord God, Creator of time and eternity, forgive me for submitting to the sin of hurry. TIM HANSEL

Sugar in the Morning?

It is not good to eat too much honey. Prov. 25:27, NIV.

SUGAR IN THE MORNING? You bet. Millions of us start the day with dessert, whether it's frosted Pop-Tarts, marshmallow-laden cereal, chocolate yogurt, or a muffin the size of a small TV. Then we spend the next 14 hours chugging more sweets, from a mid-morning Danish to a vanilla shake at lunch to cookies after dinner. Meanwhile, soft drinks rise around us like flood waters: we're swigging nearly 54 gallons a year per person.

Americans are consuming more than three-fourths of a cup of sugar a day for each man, woman, and child. We can't seem to get enough of the white stuff, even as science warns of obesity and other health risks. Are we off to a sweet hereafter?

People don't realize how much sugar they are consuming because most of it is hidden sugar. For example, soft drinks are the biggest source of refined sugar in the U.S. diet, carrying eight to 12 teaspoons per 12-ounce can. A frozen yogurt contains 12 teaspoonfuls of sugar.

Sugar is also hidden in most prepared foods such as canned soups and fruits, pot pies, ketchup, TV dinners, and many brands of peanut butter. Most ready-to-eat cereals contain sugar, and some, such as Fruit Loops and Sugar Smacks, carry 50 percent or more of their calories as sugar.

Refined, concentrated sugars enter the bloodstream quickly. Up goes the blood sugar, resulting in a quick energy boost—a sugar high. But the high is only temporary because it triggers a surge of insulin. Insulin brings down blood sugar levels and, in the absence of the modulating effects of fiber, sometimes pulls it down too fast and too far.

A falling blood sugar level often mimics symptoms of hypoglycemia, producing feelings of weakness, hunger, fatigue, and let-down—the sugar blues. The usual reaction is to reach for another sugary snack, and then another, leading to a sort of *grazing* all day long. Try eating an apple, a banana, or a bowl of brown rice. The fiber in these foods slows down the absorption of sugar into the bloodstream. The sugar levels won't jump around so much, your energy will stabilize, and you'll feel satisfied longer.

The wise man warned us that even a natural food such as honey can be abused. The lesson? Too much of a good thing is a bad thing.

Lord, I know my body is a temple. Help me to treat it that way.

AILEEN LUDINGTON

Changing Your Heart Changes Your Head

*Then Peter came to Him and said, "Lord, how often shall my brother sin against me,
and I forgive him? Up to seven times?" Jesus said to him, "I do not say to you,
up to seven times, but up to seventy times seven." Matt. 18:21, 22, NKJV.*

THERE IS A REASON Jesus told Peter to forgive 490 times. The human brain is a complex organism, with many conscious and unconscious connections. Forgiveness, however, is the catalyst that gets rid of the negative connections. Here's an example:

Rebecca had been married to a man who had a dark side—he dabbled in pornography and on his trips to other cities he solicited prostitutes. In time, he left Rebecca for another woman. Rebecca felt humiliated and angry. Just the sight of her ex-husband coming to see their children made the adrenalin rush through her system, causing her heart and breathing rates to increase. Anything that reminded her of him, such as his car or even his parents, caused the same reaction.

Why was this happening? Neurons that memorized her ex-husband were constantly associating with the noradrenalin neurons, so anything that reminded her of her ex-husband caused her to subconsciously release noradrenalin. As long as there is this association, forgiveness is impossible. That's why Rebecca's first prayers were vengeful: "God, give my ex-husband what he deserves."

Then she realized this unforgiving spirit was making her feel worse. She could not break the connection between the neurons that memorized her ex-husband and the noradrenaline neurons. As Paul wrote to the Romans, "Righteousness by works does not work at all!" (Gal. 2:21). And in Isaiah 64:6 we are reminded that "all our righteousnesses are as filthy rags."

So Rebecca changed her prayer and asked God to give her a forgiving heart. Immediately she experienced a "heart transplant." The connection of her neurons that memorized her ex-husband was switched to the endorphin neurons that gave her peace of mind. Changing her heart changed her head! She did not forget what her husband had done to her, but the bitter feelings were gone. And with that, the process of forgiveness was completed.

C. S. Lewis put it this way: "To be a Christian means to forgive the inexcusable, because God has forgiven the inexcusable in you."

If our loving God is willing to forgive our iniquities in order to bring healing, shouldn't we as His children do likewise to the ones who have wronged us?

KATHLEEN H. LIWIDJAJA-KUNTARAF

Crack Crazy

When the hour had come, He sat down, and the twelve apostles with Him. Then He said to them, "With fervent desire I have desired to eat this Passover with you before I suffer." Luke 22:14, 15, NKJV.

CRACK COCAINE IS made by heating a concoction of cocaine hydrochloride, baking soda, and water. Vaporization leaves behind a small rock. When this rock is smoked by an individual, within eight seconds 80 percent of the cocaine goes to the brain, causing the brain to release dopamine, a pleasure hormone. This results in a massive high that lasts for one or two minutes.

Upon having that first high, 60 to 80 percent of users are addicted immediately. Within hours they go back for another dose. When they try for a second high, they can't reach the level of the first because their brains have less dopamine to release. So they try more drugs and get less stimulation, finally falling into depression. Because the crack crash is very painful, addicts use other drugs to break the fall, such as marijuana, alcohol, or heroin. Addicts get high from anything that reminds them—money, jewelry—and they must have their high, even if it means killing someone.

What can be done? Dr. David F. Allen, a psychiatrist who has made the behavior of users of illegal drugs his lifelong study, sees that a spiritual approach holds the most hope for helping addicts. He uses as a model the Lord's last supper with His disciples.

The first component must be love. Jesus said, "I love you to the uttermost." If we are to help, we must open ourselves to become a vehicle of God's love. Second, Jesus had a time of communion with His disciples. It takes time, but we must meet the addicts' need for food; eat with them, listen.

Third, we must expect resistance. Judas resisted Jesus' love, but that didn't stop Jesus from His mission. We must not get discouraged. Fourth, Jesus took off His outer garments and did the work of a slave. We must not act "better than you." Fifth, simplicity. Our Lord took a basin of water, something very simple. Programs don't have to be expensive and complicated to be effective.

Sixth, service. Jesus washed His disciples' feet—even Judas'. Could it be that the real test of the healing power of God is when we can wash the feet of those who would destroy us?

Seventh, transcendence. This means simply that in spite of terrible problems, God is still on His throne—and if God is for us, who can be against us?

Lord, help me to model my life after Jesus and reach out to help others as He did. Amen. KAY KUZMA

Finishing the Race

*I have fought the good fight, I have finished
the race, I have kept the faith. 2 Tim. 4:7, NKJV.*

FOR MY FORTIETH birthday I wanted to prove that I wasn't getting older but getting better! So I decided to do a marathon.

Preparation began a year before the big day. The first step was to find a book that told me how to safely train for a marathon. The second step was to start the training program, and the third step was to actually implement the training.

My brother, a veteran marathoner, sent me the book *4 Months to a 4-hour Marathon,* by Dave Kuehls. I realized that my experience would be more like "10 Months to a six-hour Marathon," but my goal was to finish not to break records.

I started walking five miles a day, four days a week. Then I increased a mile or two each week. Soon I was up to five to 10 miles a day, for five or six days a week. During this time I added running a mile for every two miles walked. Two months before the marathon I increased my long day to 15 to 18 miles. I was logging in 35 or more miles a week.

The day of the marathon I felt ready. I felt I had "fought the good fight" with a regular training schedule. I would soon find out if I could "finish the race"—all 26.2 miles of it!

At 7:30 a.m. I was off, running/walking in the cold, drizzly Seattle morning. I stopped and refueled at every aid station to keep up my energy. At mile 8, I joined another runner/walker novice marathoner and stayed with her the rest of the race. We encouraged each other and had a great time socializing. At mile 20, my knees started hurting, but I pressed on. After five hours and 45 minutes I limped over the finish line!

I didn't make headline news or even have a crowd cheering for me, but I have a medal to prove I finished!

The Christian life is like running a marathon. You need to read the Bible for instruction, make a plan on how to live a Christian life, implement that plan, then finish the race and keep your faith—and your reward will be much greater than a medal!

What would you like to do to live a healthier lifestyle? Make a plan, work it, and celebrate when you've "finished your race." SANDRA CLAY

Sweeten the Health Message

And you must commit yourselves wholeheartedly to these commands I am giving you today. Repeat them again and again to your children. Talk about them when you are at home and when you are away on a journey, when you are lying down and when you are getting up again. Deut. 6:6, 7, NLT.

AFTER CHERYL ATTENDED a lifestyle seminar she went home and turned her kitchen upside-down. Out went the hamburger, ice cream, refined sugar, white flour, margarine, processed foods, candy bars, and caffeinated drinks. She put the family on an exercise program and lectured them about health reform.

Most health buffs would applaud Cheryl for her zeal, but the way she went about it was anything but healthy. Why? Her family became so angry at her for taking away all the "good" stuff and imposing on them a "restrictive" lifestyle that they didn't understand, that they turned away in disgust. Just as you can't come home from church a saved person and require all your family to read the Bible and pray, so you can't force health reform on people who haven't yet caught the vision.

Make health reform attractive. Sweeten it a little. Motivate and make it fun. Persuade; don't push. Here's what I've learned from families who have made the transition successfully:

1. *Live what you believe.* You can't expect others to live healthily if you don't! Your actions will speak louder than words. Do your children see you putting on your jogging shoes and heading out into the brisk morning air? Do they see you choosing an apple instead of a piece of pie, or water instead of a soda? Pray that God will give you the will power to act on your beliefs.

2. *Know why you're doing what you're doing.* Living healthily should make sense. Keep it simple. If something depresses your immune system, clouds your thinking, or puts you at risk for heart disease, stroke, or diabetes—it's bad.

3. *Be flexible and balanced.* Don't be so health-conscious that you make your family miserable. Don't be so concerned about what you put into your mouth that you forget to watch what comes out in terms of criticism and faultfinding. (And if you feel a sermon coming on, bite your tongue!)

4. *Make changes slowly.*

5. *Be happy and praise God.* A healthy grouch appeals to no one.

Consider one healthy lifestyle change you'd like your family to make. What could you do to make it appealing rather than appalling? KAY KUZMA

It Takes a Lot of Faith to Not Be Healed

*For to you it has been granted on behalf of Christ, not only
to believe in Him, but also to suffer for His sake. Phil. 1:29, NKJV.*

AS MY WIFE was driving me to a speaking appointment, she asked, "What are you preaching about today?"

"I thought I'd talk about how it takes more faith not to be healed than to be healed."

"What?" she exclaimed, driving a little erraticly.

I tried to explain, "Some people don't have enough faith to not be healed, so all God can do is heal them!"

I continued, "We have always thought that if we have enough faith, we will be healed. But, in fact, the opposite may be true. If we have lots of faith perhaps we will not be healed."

If you question this thesis, as my wife did, here's Bible evidence: All Jesus' disciples but one died a martyr's death, and that one was banished to Patmos. John the Baptist perished alone in the dungeon. Elisha received a double portion of God's Spirit, but died after a lingering illness. Why? It is not God's will that people suffer. But it is His will to have an honor guard of those who continue to trust Him during a devastating illness or terrible trial, and say like Job, "Though He slay me, yet will I trust Him" (Job 13:15, NKJV).

We tend to ignore the stories where God's dedicated people didn't get the miracles they prayed for. Instead we tell the ones about the grasshoppers that stopped at the fence of the tithe payer but ate all the crops of the neighbors. Or if the grasshoppers ate the tithe payer's crops, we tell about him saying, "If the Lord wants to graze His creatures on His property, that's OK."

Reality is, the vast majority of people who ask for a miracle don't get what they ask for! Instead, these people prove that they do not serve God for what they get out of Him. They serve Him regardless of what happens. This is what real faith is all about.

One of my favorite writers, "Anonymous," put it this way, "There is a peace that cometh after sorrow, of hope surrendered, not hope fulfilled, peace that looks not on tomorrow but on the tempest. A peace that does not find peace of successes, but of conflicts endured. A life subdued, from will and passion free. That peace triumphed in Gethsemane. Thy will be done."

May you find the peace that God offers, regardless of whatever may come your way today.   MORRIS VENDEN

God's Broomstick Scripture

"Sanctify them by Your truth. Your word is truth." John 17:17, NKJV.

AN OAT BRAN muffin or a glazed doughnut?

Brown rice or French fries?

It was not very difficult to make those decisions, right?

How about the Oprah Winfrey talk show versus reading the Bible? Getting a little more difficult?

These choices illustrate something important to our spiritual health as well as to our physical health. You've probably heard that oat bran and brown rice are the better choices because of their high fiber content. Fiber is there not just to make the food brown. It plays a vital role in the intestines of our digestive system. It's like the brooms in our houses. It goes in and sweeps out the innermost parts and removes the remains of the food that our bodies could not use. It also purifies our systems of harmful carcinogens (agents that cause cancer) and other microorganisms that, if left, would make us sick from such diseases as colon cancer, diverticulitis, and ulcerative colitis.

The Word of God is also vital, and plays a role similar to fiber. Reading it must be our number one choice. It is not there to look pretty on our shelves or to carry to church in attractive binders, but to be eaten, to be digested, and to become a part of us.

Jesus, when praying to His Father for His disciples and us, prayed that we would be sanctified by His truth. He said that His Word, the Word of God or the Bible, is truth.

The Greek word for sanctify is *haziago* (haz-ee-ahd-go), which means to purify. The Word of God is our spiritual broom. As we read it, it goes to the innermost parts of our beings, our hearts, and shows us our need of Christ.

Through the Holy Spirit, the Word sweeps our soul temples clean of habits, desires, appetites, and character traits that if allowed to remain would leave us sick with the disease of sin. We must be purged of these things to make it through the final moments of earth's history. Our Saviour will return soon. The Word of God, spiritual fiber, was given to us so that we do not die both a physical and a spiritual death.

Have you used your spiritual broom today? It's the only way to keep spiritually healthy!   TABASURI CHAPMAN

Anger and the Adrenaline Connection

*If you are angry, don't sin by nursing your grudge. Don't let the sun
go down with you still angry—get over it quickly; for when you
are angry you give a mighty foothold to the devil. Eph. 4:26, 27, TLB.*

ON RARE OCCASIONS as a child I heard my folks speak angry words—
usually when Dad was driving one way, and Mom thought we should be
going another! It wasn't hostile; they weren't trying to hurt each other.
They were just trying to get their points across. But the loud voices and
negative words made an impact on me. After the passion blew over, which
usually happened quickly, I felt the hurt in my sensitive heart. And I figured there had to be a better way to settle differences.

Psychologists have observed the destructive effects of long-term anger
and have erroneously come to the conclusion that you've got to get it out,
regardless of whom you hurt. But it's never appropriate to hurt another in
order to heal yourself! Instead, the Bible admonishes us to be kind, tenderhearted, and forgiving (Eph. 4:32)!

Now studies are proving the psychologists were wrong—and the Bible
right. The answer is in prevention, early recognition, and educated control.
It's not wrong to feel angry as a temporary emotion that produces needed
energy to correct injustice, but how you express that emotion—the behavior that follows—is what matters. If it hurts yourself or others, it's wrong!

If you stuff it, you're going to mess up the way God intended your
body to work. Anger produces an adrenaline rush that God designed for
your survival—to fight or flee. Stuffed anger keeps the adrenaline motor
running—flooding body tissue and organs with unnecessary chemicals that
damage the arteries, elevate blood pressure, and cause headaches, ulcers,
and premature heart disease.

But the same thing happens if you express anger with angry words and
behavior! Dr. Carol Tavris reviewed anger research, then wrote the book
Anger, the Misunderstood Emotion. Her conclusion was that freely venting
doesn't relieve anger but increases it and establishes a hostile habit. She says
it is better to "keep quiet about your momentary irritations and distract
yourself with pleasant activity until your fury simmers down."

This method is good for your health because it avoids the unnecessary
adrenaline rush that poisons your system. You'll feel better faster and be able
to think more clearly about how to solve the problem so no one gets hurt.

Lord, help me to handle my anger in healthy ways so it won't hurt me—or others.

KAY KUZMA

There Is a God!

O Lord, You have searched me and known me. . . . Your hand shall lead me, and Your right hand shall hold me. . . . For You formed my inward parts. Ps. 139:1-13, NKJV.

THIRTEEN YEARS AGO my life was a mess. I did drugs, smoked, drank alcohol, was fat, skipped high school classes, had a horrible attitude, and was mean to my family. When I was a junior I dropped out and wasted a year of my life watching TV and partying.

I believed in the power of self. If I wanted something, I got it. So when I decided to go back to high school, I crammed and graduated with my class, even though my grades were terrible! Who cared; none of my family had ever gone to college.

When I met and married Rick I began cleaning up my lifestyle, but it was not until my grandpa died of colon cancer at 63 that I became a vegetarian. His daily diet of bacon and eggs had probably killed him. Grandpa was the only father I really knew and his death was devastating.

Shortly after, when Grandma had a serious stroke, I came unglued. Why was this happening to me? Then as I took her to all her therapy sessions, I became impressed with the importance of physical therapy (PT) and decided to apply to the PT Assistant program at Michiana College. I was turned down! I couldn't handle not getting what I wanted, so I moved to our summer cottage in Tennessee to take the PTA program at Roane State in LaFollette.

That's where I met Kari, who had taken her physical therapy training at Andrews University, a Seventh-day Adventist school just a few miles from our home in South Bend. When I was running 10 to 12 miles a day training for a marathon, Kari would bike or run beside me and tell me Bible stories—something I'd never heard before. As our friendship grew, she encouraged me to apply to the physical therapy program at Andrews University. No way! My grades were lousy! But as it turned out, Kari's confidence in me gave me the confidence to apply—and they accepted me!

One day in anatomy class as I was studying the skull, it hit me: *God was real!* Evolution just couldn't explain the tiny holes in the chin that were exactly the right size for the trigeminal nerves to go through the skull so that we could chew. There had to be a God! And this personal God was directing my life even though I didn't know anything about Him. Amazing!

Think back on how God has led you in the past, and let the reality of God energize your life!   GRETCHEN TURNER

My Journey to Spiritual Health

To the angel of the church in Laodicea write: . . . I am about to
spit you out of my mouth. You say, "I am rich; I have acquired wealth
and do not need a thing." But you do not realize that you
are wretched, pitiful, poor, blind and naked. Rev. 3:14-17, NIV.

IT WAS A COLD night in Michigan. A social visit with good friends. I was sharing what was on my mind—our new house, latest purchases, dreams of cruises—when Peter gently asked, "Donna, what are you going to do with your pride?"

Peter's friendship refrained me from instant anger and rebuttal. Instead, I saw not just the crackling fire in the hearth, but the lake of fire—the final resting place of Laodicea.

Internally I wept for the next 10 months. It brought "eyesalve" that helped me see my miserable condition. Yes, I carried a Bible to church and regularly lead out in beginners' Sabbath school and the social committee. Vegetarianism and tithing were ingrained in my DNA structure. But I did not have a heart for lost people—only for myself!

My journey from lukewarm, ho-hum Christianity to being on fire for the Lord began when I begged God to give me whatever it would take to have a personal 15-minute morning devotional time. Since my mind was lethargic spiritually, I knew I couldn't do it on my own.

Beginning in Genesis, I discovered that a God big enough to create the universe could re-create me. I marveled at Abraham's journey, the foolish things he did, only to realize that God has called each of us to a similar journey toward complete trust. I shook my head to realize there were Israelites who didn't want to leave Egypt's bondage—only to recognize I felt the same about leaving my comfortable lifestyle.

As I became aware of my condition; the spiritual battle intensified. The more God opened my eyes, the clearer I saw Satan and his strategies and plans for my life, but also the stronger pull back to Egypt—tennis at the club, shopping, instant gratification.

In Gethsemane I faintly heard His voice, "Stay awake and pray," and began praying through my day and walking through the wilderness sanctuary. My priorities began to change.

Today I realize Laodicia is not a place one visits. It is a place in the heart—a heart chained to self. I praise God for my journey to spiritual health, and a new heart that beats for lost people!

Precious Father, close my eyes to self and open my heart to lost people.

DONNA WILLEY

Dying for a Cigarette?

But thanks be to God, which giveth us the victory
through our Lord Jesus Christ. 1 Cor. 15:57.

DURING THE 28 YEARS that David smoked he had thought about quitting many times, but never did. His best friend, 45-year-old Larry, who had smoked for more than 25 years, was recently diagnosed with lung cancer. This was a "wake-up" call for David; he enrolled in a smoking cessation program.

David learned that the medical consequences of smoking are the number one health problem in the United States, with more than 450,000 deaths annually. That is more than 37,000 deaths a month, 1,230 deaths a day, 51 deaths per hour, and almost 1 death per minute. It's the equivalent of eighteen 747 jumbo-jet airliners crashing every week, with no survivors.

The prospects of suffering from a long, painful, terminal illness, such as emphysema or cancer, were frightening to David. Although the most common smoking-related cancer is lung cancer, there is also cancer of the lip, mouth, throat, voice box, esophagus, stomach, liver, pancreas, colon, and bladder. Then there is the possibility of heart disease or stroke. It is estimated that smoking is a causal agent in 30 to 40 percent of all coronary heart disease deaths in the U.S., as well as 15 percent of the nearly 150,000 stroke deaths. He learned that the risk of having atherosclerotic peripheral arterial disease is 10 times or more common in smokers, and death from rupture of an abdominal aneurysm is two to five times more common.

Obviously, the cost of smoking-related misery is incalculable. And yet, the tobacco companies gross more than $50 billion dollars a year from the agonies they inflict!

The question is, will David be successful in kicking the habit? Yes, he will be, because he has realized that he cannot gain victory by himself. Instead, he has chosen 1 Corinthians 15:57 as his victory text and has claimed the promise that with Christ he can do anything (Phil 4:13). David has determined that smoking is a sin—because it slowly kills, and God's law is clear, "Thou shalt not kill." So David is cutting cigarettes out of his life, "cold turkey." He's flushed away his cigarettes and has determined to stay away from smokers to lessen the temptation. Plus, he's got a group of friends praying for him, and his classmates in the smoking cessation program are holding him accountable. It's only been a few days since he quit, but he is already thanking God for the victory.

If God can give David victory over his addiction after 28 years, He can do the same for you.   ELMAR P. SAKALA AND KAY KUZMA

When Childhood Problems Grow Up

If anyone desires to come after Me, let him deny himself,
and take up his cross, and follow Me. Matt. 16:24, NKJV.

EMOTIONAL PROBLEMS OF adults usually stem from unresolved problems in childhood. That's why it's best to help children resolve their emotional problems when they are young and impressionable, and when people are sympathetic and helpful.

Lynn is always late for work, meetings, and appointments. When she was a child, no one required her to be on time. Lynn finds it hard to break her bad habit and develop good work ethics.

Bob is overweight, suffers from ill health, and has difficulty in developing proper eating habits. It started when his mother fed him snacks, comforted him with food, and permitted him to raid the refrigerator. He was indulged and pampered under the sobriquet, "I love you." Today, Bob acknowledges that his obesity does not stem from big bones, inheritance, or glandular problems, but is the result of unresolved childhood emotional problems.

Jane drops her clothes on the floor and leaves them there until she trips over them. Her untidy habits spill over to her work place. She is bright and hardworking, and could advance at her child-care agency, but management knows that a disorganized supervisor is a negative role model. Jane's unresolved emotional problem is holding her back.

When childhood problems grow into adult ones, is there any hope?

Here's the good news: You can overcome all inherited and cultivated emotional problems when you are truly converted, accepting Christ as your Savior, for you can do all things through Christ who will strengthen your self-control and determination to change. (See Phil. 4:13.)

Satan, however, wants you to believe you are hopeless and are too far gone to get help. When you're tempted to believe Satan's lie, consider this declaration from one of God's messengers: "In the whole Satanic force there is not power to overcome one soul who in simple trust casts himself on Christ" (Ellen G. White, *Christ's Object Lessons*, p. 157).

Jesus cast out devils, raised the dead, and healed the sick. He told the crippled man at the pool to take up his bed and walk. The man obeyed and walked without any follow-up therapy.

What are you waiting for? Follow the instructions: drop your burdens, deny yourself, take up His cross, and follow His example—for with Christ all things are possible. BLONDEL E. SENIOR

A Day of Delight

*If you call the Sabbath a delight and the Lord's holy day honorable,
and if you honor it by not going your own way and not doing as you please
or speaking idle words, then you will find your joy in the Lord. Isa. 58:13, 14, NIV.*

I GREW UP IN a Sabbathkeeping home in Catholic Poland. My father, even as a child, had a heart for truth and an intense love for Christ. His greatest desire was to have a Bible so that he could read God's Word for himself. One night he had a dream about a book salesman who had a Bible in his briefcase. Father never forgot the dream. One day while he was visiting a friend, a salesman came to the door. The man was sent away when they learned he was selling Protestant books. Father immediately followed the man and asked, "Do you have a Bible?" He not only bought the Bible but all his other books as well. And that's how Father learned about the Sabbath.

Once you read the Bible it's not hard to find out about the seventh-day Sabbath. The second chapter of Genesis (verses 1-3) tells how God rested, blessed, and sanctified the seventh day. Then in Exodus 20:8 the recently released Israelite slaves were commanded to "remember the sabbath day." Obviously, worshiping on the seventh day was important to God—and therefore precious to my father. It was a memorial in time, to remember and praise the Creator he loved.

For as long as I can remember, the Sabbath was a delight to me. I recall as a young boy putting on my Sabbath shirt and pants and standing in the sunshine, waiting for the rest of the family to get ready, and then walking with them to another church member's home for worship services.

We never missed church—not even during the war, when it was illegal to hold religious meetings in Nazi-occupied Poland. We took gifts and flowers to the house, pretending to be attending a party. Then we'd speak the words of hymns, fearing if the neighbors heard us singing they would report us. After a special Sabbath lunch Father would take us to the park overlooking the Wistula River, or we'd play on the sandy shore of Lake Lansk. I think that's why my childhood memories of Sabbath are always associated with Father. That was the day he spent with us.

Much later in life—when English became my language—I discovered that the word *abba,* the Bible term for daddy, was in the middle of the word *Sabbath.* No wonder the Sabbath is a delight!

Keep the Sabbath day holy and see if it doesn't bring you closer to your heavenly Abba.   JAN W. KUZMA

The Song of the Bird

Rejoice in the Lord. . . . Sing to Him a new song; play skillfully with a shout of joy. For the word of the Lord is right, and all His work is done in truth. Ps. 33:1-4, NKJV.

ELLEN WAS A GIFTED child. She had a buoyant, hopeful disposition; she was social, courageous, resolute, and persevering. And with her love of studying, quick perception, and retentive memory, her parents held high hopes for her future. Then when she was 9, an angry classmate threw a stone, breaking her nose and disfiguring her face. She lay in a coma for three weeks and nearly died.

In 1836 there was little that could be done to repair such an injury. Ellen herself wrote: "Every feature of my face seemed changed. The sight was more than I could bear. . . . The idea of carrying my misfortune through life was insupportable. I could see no pleasure in my life. I did not wish to live, and I dared not die, for I was not prepared" (*Spiritual Gifts,* vol. 2, p. 9).

Instead of a strong, self-reliant child, she became feeble, timid, and despondent. Her friends turned away. Her health was so frail that she couldn't attend school for long, and then she couldn't remember what she had learned. Her hand trembled so much she couldn't write, and when trying to read, the letters of her book would run together, and she became dizzy and faint.

Some 50 years later she visited the site of the accident and wrote, "This misfortune, which for a time seemed so bitter and was so hard to bear, has proved to be a blessing in disguise. The cruel blow which blighted the joys of earth was the means of turning my eyes to heaven. I might never have known Jesus had not the sorrow that clouded my early years led me to seek comfort in Him." She then tells the story of a bird who wouldn't sing the song of his master when his cage was full of light, but when the master covered his cage, the bird listened to the song until he could sing it perfectly. Ever after, he could sing it in the light. "Thus God deals with His creatures. He has a song to teach us, and when we have learned it amid the deep shadows of affliction we can sing it ever afterward" (in *Review and Herald,* Nov. 25, 1884).

Ellen became a spiritual leader and prolific author. Look up her name, Ellen G. White, and you'll find she has the distinction of having more books published than any other American author in history. Incredible, isn't it?

God can take whatever disability you have and turn it into an opportunity. Trust Him!   KAY KUZMA

New Teeth, New Life

For there are many . . . [who are] the enemies of the cross of Christ.
These men are heading for utter destruction—their god is their own
appetite. . . . But we are citizens of Heaven. . . . He [Christ] will change
these wretched bodies of ours so that they resemble his own glorious body, by that
power of his which makes him in command of everything. Phil. 3:18-21, Phillips.

LOSING ONE'S TEETH is always a traumatic experience, whatever the cause. There are several reasons for such loss, the most common of which is gum disease. In this case, persons are often totally unaware they are in trouble until they notice their teeth are starting to loosen, or they visit their dentist for a check-up and discover it is too late to save their teeth.

Another cause of tooth loss is extreme decay. People with this problem are aware that a problem exists, but they are afraid to visit their dentist so they put off treatment until they are in pain. In the case of trauma, persons may see the damage coming, but can't do anything to stop it—can't get out of the way in time to avoid being hit, or they may not see it coming at all.

People with gum disease may be likened to those who are in denial about sin disease. They look good on the outside but their roots are being insidiously weakened from within. Their pride is in that which they should be ashamed of.

The person with tooth decay may be likened to one who is outwardly rebellious and refuses to ask God for help—their god is their own appetite.

The person who meets with trauma is in the wrong place at the wrong time and can't escape the disastrous consequences of another's actions.

When people combine an unhealthy diet with lots of sugar, lack of dental hygiene, and neglect of regular exams, they can get into serious trouble. If the problems persist they may come to the point where the only solution is to start all over!

Whether implants, partials, bridges, or dentures, new functioning teeth can give one a whole new lease on life! A person can finally chew again, digest better, and look better! Sometimes we have to experience utter destruction before we are ready to look beyond the narrow horizons of our own pain and ask Jesus to remake these wretched bodies of ours to resemble His own glorious body! When we are willing to do this, He promises to give us a whole new life.

Lord, please give me a new life today. JERRY MUNCY

If Your Life Depends on It—Change!

Jesus said to him, "Rise, take up your bed and walk." . . . Afterward
Jesus found him in the temple, and said to him, "See, you have been
made well. Sin no more, lest a worse thing come upon you." John 5:8-14, NKJV.

THOSE WHO TRY to make too many major lifestyle changes at once, often burn out from discouragement. But if you're sick, your life may depend on rapid change.

Take diabetes, for example. Average type 2 diabetics think that if they are following their doctor's orders they will be all right. But even with the best medical care and medication, their blood sugar is not under optimal control. Virtually every organ and tissue in their body is slowly being damaged. If this were not the case, diabetics wouldn't have the horrible side effects they suffer. Diabetes is the number one cause of blindness. One hundred fifty legs are amputated every day in the United States because of diabetes. Heart disease risk is increased 10 times.

What is needed is rapid change. By exercising (walking about four miles a day or the equivalent) and eating only plant foods and no refined products, within three to six weeks more than 50 percent of type 2 diabetics can get well enough to not need medication. Eighty to 90 percent of diabetic neuropathy will be completely "healed."

Heart disease also requires rapid change. The most common sign of a heart problem is sudden death! So don't wait for angina (pain) before making some changes. It has been shown that if the fat in the diet is reduced to 10 percent of caloric intake, along with exercise and other changes, a 5.5 percent average decrease in atherosclerotic plaque occurs in 12 months. Most heart attacks do not occur from a buildup of plaque that finally closes off the artery. Rather, because plaque buildup is inherently unstable, the "cap" over the plaque can rupture, allowing the cholesterol gruel inside to ooze into the bloodstream. This causes a clot to form and occlude the artery, even when the plaque is not large. Dramatically changing one's diet can cause the cap to become stable in a few weeks.

So, if you're healthy and want to stay that way, decide what goals you'd like to achieve and put yourself on a progressive life-improvement plan. But if you're not healthy, don't wait! Whether or not you have tomorrow depends on how you live today!

To keep spiritually healthy, put yourself on a spiritual progressive life-improvement plan. But if you've got a sin "disease," ask God for will-power to make a rapid change today. JIM BRACKETT

Lessons I Learned on Surviving Crises

Yet there is one ray of hope: his compassion never ends. It is only the Lord's mercies that have kept us from complete destruction. Lam. 3:21, 22, TLB.

ON FEBRUARY 8, 1996, my husband had a massive brainstem stroke. He lost all left side movement, his speech slowed, and he had difficulty with spatial perceptions and analytic thinking. The neurologist told me he would never work again.

Before the stroke Jan and I were professional people, each with our own careers, organizations, daily radio programs, seminars, and writing projects; his area was health, mine the family. Then on that fateful night, the page abruptly turned and a new chapter of our lives began.

"Lord," I prayed, "couldn't I have learned what you wanted me to learn in a less stressful, less devastating way? Wasn't there a good book I could have read or a sermon I could have heard?" And God's answer came back: "My grace is sufficient for you."

I hope the lessons about life, love, and relationship I learned will give you perspective and courage. Here are the top seven:

Lesson 1: Nothing is forever. Praise God, He has promised to make everything new (Rev. 21:5).

Lesson 2: Relationships are more important than productivity. It would be nice if Jan could fix household appliances, bicycle, and swim like he used to, but it's not necessary. What is important is our love—and that has only gotten stronger.

Lesson 3: You can survive crises; you can adjust to major change. I once thought I wouldn't be able to cope if something happened to Jan. Now I know I will survive. I can adjust to change.

Lesson 4: Don't put off living, saving it for the future. Today is all any one of us has been given. Continue to live each day to the fullest, with no regrets.

Lesson 5: Live one day at a time. Don't worry about the future, but keep dreaming. Dreams keep hope alive. And hope is a welcome companion in tough times.

Lesson 6: There's incredible power in prayer. Within minutes after Jan's stroke, prayer chains were formed across the world on his behalf. Jan's recovery has been miraculous.

Lesson 7: God is good. Although crises and pain may dim our view, God is with us, and His Word offers comfort and encouragement. His compassion never ends!

Thank God that His compassion never ends.   KAY KUZMA

Are You as Lucky as Kyle?

Be always joyful; pray continually; give thanks whatever happens;
for this is what God in Christ wills for you. 1 Thess. 5:16-18, NEB.

"KYLE'S A VERY lucky kid," his mom said with a smile.

"Why do you say Kyle's lucky? I thought being disabled was always bad."

"Oh, no," she replied. "Just think, if Kyle had been born a generation ago he wouldn't have had a voice-activated computer!"

I was amazed that neither Kyle nor his mom were bitter toward the "system" that demanded Kyle be immunized as a baby, which had caused the allergic reaction that resulted in his suffering severe physical disabilities. Despite being confined to a wheelchair and having to endure countless surgeries, Kyle was a bright, straight-A sixth grader in regular school, and class president.

When I first met Kyle, he was in the hospital for more surgery and not doing well. He had become critically ill but hung on to life. His mom and dad stayed by his side 24 hours a day, assisting the staff whenever possible. It was at this time, when things were so bad, that his mom had made the comment about Kyle being a lucky kid.

As it turned out, Kyle was lucky. He recovered. It took him more than three weeks in Pediatric ICU, but he eventually made it home and back to school.

Was Kyle grumpy and complaining about having to spend time in the hospital? No. Did he bemoan his lot when he compared himself with his buddies at school? No, at least not often. Did he try his best to work with the seemingly impossible requests of his physicians? Yes, he did all he could to cooperate.

That made me think. *What if Kyle had given up? What if his mom had not had an attitude of gratitude? What if his dad had blamed others for his son's problems?*

Kyle reminded me that my reactions are a choice. First of all, my frustrations are only momentary—not for a lifetime. For that alone, I should be thankful!

How is it for you? When you get angry, grumpy, or mean, consider what you could do next time to respond more positively. Remind yourself how very lucky you are. Say with the apostle Peter, "For I have learned to find resources in myself whatever my circumstances" (Phil. 4:11, NEB).

List 10 reasons that you are a lucky person—and praise the Lord!

TABITHA ABEL-COOPER

The Captain's Question

*So the captain came to him, and said to him, "What do
you mean, sleeper? Arise, call on your God; perhaps your God
will consider us, so that we may not perish." Jonah 1:6, NKJV.*

THE SETTING: A VICIOUS storm on the Mediterranean. Terrified seamen jettison the cargo, to no avail; then turn from salty curses to crying to their gods to still the raging water and save their lives.

Sensing the absence of one of the passengers, the captain goes searching and discovers him in the hold—asleep, dead to the storm and the shrieks of terror.

The captain's question reveals his astonishment and anxiety. "What are you doing, sleeper? Get up, pray to your God. Maybe He'll save us."

You know the rest of the story. The superstitious sailors cast lots and Jonah confesses that he, a Hebrew who worships the true Creator God, is running away from a God-given mission to warn the inhabitants of Nineveh about their imminent destruction.

"What should we do with you?" they ask. Obviously the cause of this storm must be removed, or they would all perish.

"Throw me into the sea," Jonah insists. They are reluctant, but there seems no other option. So they throw Jonah overboard. The storm calms instantly, and the sailors learn to fear the true God.

What does all this have to do with health? Most people are on a collision course with premature death. Contagious diseases are murdering multitudes, and before cures are found, even more deadly viruses and bacteria erupt. No longer do conventional cures work. The best protection a person can have is a strong healthy immune system. Then there are the lifestyle killers: heart disease, diabetes, cancer. Do people know that what they're eating, drinking, and smoking is killing them? If they don't change their ways, they're at high risk for disease.

God, our heavenly Captain, has a saving message. In the midst of the storm He's asking, "What are you doing, sleeper?" Hopefully we don't have to be thrown overboard before we're willing to share the God-given message of health: the original plant-based diet of Genesis, the clean meats of Leviticus 11, and the Exodus 20 commandments for healthy relationships.

Like Jonah, we're scared to say anything, because we don't think people will change their ways. But Jonah was wrong.

Thank You, Creator God, for the health message. With whom would You like me to share it?　　　　　　　　　　　　　　　MARJORIE V. BALDWIN

Don't Be Fooled by Statistics

The way of a fool is right in his own eyes, but he
who heeds counsel is wise. Prov. 12:15, NKJV.

MY HUSBAND WAS a biostatistician at Loma Linda University for 27 years. As a researcher he applied mathematics to medical data to determine significant factors that influence health. As a teacher he required his students to read *How to Lie With Statistics,* because without carefully looking at all the evidence it's easy to be fooled.

Take, for example, the argument over protein. I had always thought that since protein builds healthy bones, meat and animal products are essential to a good diet. When I met strong, healthy athletes who were vegans (they ate no animal products), I began to wonder. Years later, after an accumulation of research findings, I've learned that a little protein goes a long way, while a high-protein diet stresses the body.

People say, "We need a lot of meat because it builds muscle and gives us energy—and vegetables don't have any protein." The fact is, meat protein doesn't go directly to the muscles. Our bodies process it the same way they do all food. And most vegetables contain some protein, so if you eat a wide variety each day you should have no trouble getting enough protein. And as for energy, carbohydrates are the body's most efficient energy source, not protein.

"OK," people argue, "at least a high-protein diet is the best way to lose weight." There is research that shows people lose weight on a high protein/low carb diet. But is it the *best* way to lose weight? Not exactly. Here are the facts: Proteins can't burn fat, as some have claimed. In addition, proteins have the same number of calories as carbohydrates—four for each gram. And many proteins, such as beef, are high in fat, which has nine calories per gram. Since a high-protein diet isn't balanced, it can strain the kidneys. And it's been found that long-term liquid protein diets may damage heart function. Experts recommend that protein should be only 12 to 15 percent of a healthy diet.

When making lifestyle decisions, you can't take just one study as truth and ignore the volume of evidence to the contrary. The same is true for the Bible. You musn't pick one text, especially out of context, and interpret it in a way contrary to voluminous Bible evidence.

Truth, whether it is spiritual truth or health truth, can mean the difference between life and death. What can you do today to become better informed?

KAY KUZMA

The Miracle of Marcus

I have heard your prayer, I have seen your tears;
surely I will heal you. 2 Kings 20:5, NKJV.

"ARE YOU MOMMY WIGGERS? Your baby is not doing well. He's shutting down on us. We've placed him on a high-frequency ventilator, given him a paralyzing drug, and shaved his head for IV lines. He's blue all over and looks terrible." These were the words I heard as I approached the Neonatal Intensive Care Unit just five hours after Marcus' birth.

The next few hours were agony as Marcel and I watched our precious son struggle to hold on to life. The doctor explained that Marcus' blood gas pH had been too high for too long. Twice she suggested we consider disconnecting him from life-support, as they were not sure how much brain, kidney, and liver damage had occurred.

How could I let them unplug my baby? The doctor suggested that Marcus' last moments be in my arms. I pleaded that they keep trying for just half an hour more. My parents, our pastor, several hospital staff members, and friends gathered around to plead with God for healing. I knew the strict visiting rules in the NICU (two visitors per patient), and knew they were letting us say goodbye. Even the nurses had tears in their eyes. Soon we were ushered out of the room so the surgeon could try for a central IV line. She was successful, and Marcus began to slowly improve.

That night the most incredible thing happened. Marcel started singing a Dutch lullaby to Marcus that he had sung to him during pregnancy. Upon hearing Daddy's voice, Marcus opened his eyes and kicked one foot. This was a great encouragement to us.

The next few days were a roller coaster of emotions. Because of overwhelming infection, Marcus needed the maximum amount of medications to keep his blood pressure high enough to perfuse his brain; he also had seizures, abnormal liver enzymes, and bleeding in his brain. We had him anointed and asked that if it be God's will his little brain be healed completely. He made steady improvements. A week after birth he was taken off the ventilator, his medications were lowered, he became more alert, his swelling decreased, he had a good sucking reflex, and was able to breast feed. Sixteen days after Marcus' birth we were able to take him home.

Before we left the hospital the nurses said to me, "You know, Heidi, babies this sick just don't leave the hospital OK. We've watched an intervention from above." We agreed.

Aren't you glad God hears our prayers and promises to heal? Thank You, God!

HEIDI WIGGERS

Violence and Music

Set your mind on things above, not on things on the earth. Col. 3:2, NKJV.

VIOLENCE, ESPECIALLY AMONG young people, is on the increase and is considered a significant public health problem. The question has been posed that since violence is often glamorized by the musicians and actors in music videos, are these videos contributing to the epidemic?

We know music enters the brain through its emotional regions, which include the temporal lobe and limbic system. From there, some kinds of music tend to produce a frontal lobe response that influences the will, moral worth, and reasoning power (Mozart, for example). Other kinds of music, such as rock and rap, evoke very little, if any, frontal lobe response; instead, they produce a large emotional response with very little logical or moral interpretation.

Researchers at Bowman Gray School of Medicine studied 518 music videos from four cable networks: MTV, Black Entertainment Television, Video Hits One, and Country Music Television. The researchers found a significantly higher percentage of music videos aired on MTV contained one or more episodes portraying overt violence and the brandishing of weapons. Rap videos had the highest portrayal of violence, followed by rock videos. African-Americans were over-represented as engaging in violence or weapon-carrying, compared with the proportion of African-Americans in the general population. Most videos containing violence showed males as the perpetrators. Fifteen percent portrayed a child carrying a weapon.

What effect do these music videos have on behavior? One study exposed 222 patients to seven months of MTV, followed by five months without it. What happened when they took away the music videos? Verbal aggression decreased 32 percent. Aggression against objects decreased 52 percent, and aggression against other people decreased 48 percent.

Does music influence our behavior? Yes, of course! The MTV type of music video programming constantly stimulates the visual senses through its provocative images of rapidly changing scenes. The ear is stimulated as well. This eye-ear combination seems to induce an even more profound shutdown of the analytical processes. Violence results.

Isn't it time we carefully monitor what we hear and see? Isn't it time we quit polluting our brains with audio and video images of violence? Isn't it time to give up the trash?

Lord, help me watch, hear, and see only that which helps me focus on things above.   KAY KUZMA, with ELMAR SAKALA and NIEL NEDLEY

Love Is a Four-letter Word Spelled T-I-M-E

*May your fountain be blessed, and may you rejoice in the wife of
your youth. A loving doe, a graceful deer—may her breasts satisfy
you always, may you ever be captivated by her love. Prov. 5:18, 19, NIV.*

SOME YEARS AGO I accepted a teaching position at an Adventist boarding academy. In addition to my classes I had charge of the counseling and testing program, served as coordinator of religious activities for the campus, and was an advisor for the student association.

The beginning of the school year was intense. Learning and launching all those enterprises and getting to know the many students was time-consuming. For the first six weeks I spent most of my days, evenings, and weekends at the school. Meanwhile, my wife, Peggy, who was recovering from an illness and not employed, was lonely in this new environment far from familiar friends.

One day as I breezed in for a brief supper, Peggy took me by the hand and led me to the sofa. "I need to talk with you a moment," she said softly. Her communication was direct and personal. "I don't feel special anymore." The quiet simplicity of her message pierced my heart. What was really important in life anyway? Could any job be as important as our relationship?

We decided to go away together that weekend. Somebody else would have to take over those duties. (The school survived.) We went to the mountains and spent the most wonderful Sabbath together. We walked woodland trails hand-in-hand, singing every praise chorus we knew, praying together and renewing our commitment to each other.

Deep relationships are built out of time. One of the most fundamental components of a truly rich marriage is time spent together: time to worship together, talk together, work together, play together. We pledged to each other to let nothing prevent us from giving that time top priority in our lives. The years have passed, but we have tried to be faithful to that pledge. Here are some of the things we do:

Every day it is our goal to take a walk together, during which we accomplish several objectives: we share the day's events, we have our evening prayer, and we and our family pet get in two miles of exercise.

Other activities we enjoy sharing are working in the yard, doing household tasks, writing articles, joint speaking appointments, traveling, and going on a date once a week.

Did you know that research reveals that those happily married and those with close support systems live longer and healthier?

Do you have a loved one who needs your T-I-M-E today? ROGER L. DUDLEY

The Creative Potential of Dust

*The Lord God formed the man from the dust of the ground and breathed
into his nostrils the breath of life, and the man became a living being. Gen. 2:7, NIV.*

IN THE MIDDLE of a marathon cleaning event, vacuuming, polishing,
and dusting my house, I wondered, *Will there be dust in heaven?*

Dust. Something so common to each of us, and yet how vital to life itself!

You were made of dust. That's right. Dust, plus God's breath of life.
Right now you are experiencing dust plus life energy: your lungs are in-
haling and exhaling air and mixing life-giving oxygen with your blood;
your heart is pumping this blood through miles of blood vessels, making it
possible for your brain to think. Your brain directs your conscious and unconscious movements and body functions. All this out of dust! Amazing!

The world you live in is also made of dust. There is dust on the
ground, underground, in the water, in the air. Dust can be so fine that you
cannot see it, or it can be large enough to sting your skin should the wind
whip particles at you with enough velocity.

Scientists tell us that there is galactic dust in outer space. Space dust
forms beautiful images that man has captured through photography. Yet a
cloud of such dust rocketing through space at meteoric speeds would instantly vaporize an unprotected human body.

Will there be dust in heaven? Will you have to dust your celestial
house or avoid celestial mud puddles?

The important thing to me is that my beginning wasn't an accident. I
was created out of dust by an Almighty God who gave me life and purpose. The One who created dust and all of its potential properties created
me! My assignment is to journey into the unknown where God Himself
will be my guide. My mission is to reach lost people with the good news
of salvation.

What incredible power God exhibited when He formed man out of
something so common and seemingly useless as dust, and made him with
such unfathomable potential. In God's world even the teeniest speck of
dust is significant. Wow!

*Awesome Creator, thank You for intentionally forming me out of Your amaz-
ing dust.*   SIDNEY L. CRANDALL

I Will Sing a New Song

I will sing to the Lord as long as I live; I will sing
praise to my God while I have my being. Ps. 104:33, NKJV.

I THOUGHT IT WAS my imagination. No, there it was again: Snatches of the old familiar melody, unmistakable though sketchy, floating down the hall of the nursing home. "I will cherish the old rugged cross. . . ." Silence. "Exchange it some day. . . ."

I couldn't believe my ears. Could it be the same little old woman who sat so small, so helpless, so incapacitated in her wheelchair? The little figure had been placed in the hall near the nurses' station so that she could soak up a bit of life as it flowed by—to watch, listen, and be quiet!

I heard her often, usually yelling, crying, and/or babbling incoherently. Could this really be the same voice that poured forth snatches of the old familiar Christian hymn learned in childhood? Yes, my eyes confirmed what my ears had heard! It was she!

Her mind appeared to be gone. Where did this song spring from?

Then I remembered having read that dementia and Alzheimer's patients can be reached with old familiar songs when nothing else seems to penetrate their sadly deteriorated minds.

Praise the Lord! A miracle right before my eyes! An apparently barren mind singing praises to God! Not even dementia could destroy this marvel!

For years, I have been putting scripture to music, a most valuable means of hiding God's Word in my heart. An inspired writer once said, "There are few means more effective for fixing His words in the memory than repeating them in song" (Ellen G. White, *Evangelism*, p. 496). I can say Amen! Because of an attention deficit that has plagued me since childhood, I have reason to praise God for the miracle wrought as He buried scripture in my memory cells through music.

Even though I turned my back on God for years, He knew I would ultimately comprehend His agape love. He knew I would cherish the scriptures waiting, hidden, buried deep in my heart.

Again I recall that little old woman. Her mind was deteriorated but from somewhere in the deep recesses of her memory there emerged praises to her God. I am touched. Deeply touched.

Lord, if my mind becomes impaired, please help me accept as my own David's desire: "I will sing to the Lord as long as I live; I will sing praise to my God while I have my being."

Why not begin memorizing one of your favorite hymns today?

JODI EULENE DODSON

Christ's Healing Presence and Power

Now a certain man was there who had an infirmity thirty-eight years. When Jesus saw him lying there, and knew that he already had been in that condition a long time, He said to him, "Do you want to be made well?" John 5:5, 6, NKJV.

CAN YOU IMAGINE lying by the Pool of Bethesda for 38 years, waiting to be healed? The story ends with: "Jesus said to him, 'Rise, take up your bed and walk.' And immediately the man was made well." It was only when Jesus Christ was present that healing took place.

Philip Yancey, in his book *The Jesus I Never Knew*, tells of a homeless, sick prostitute who rented out her 2-year-old daughter to men for sex in order to support her own drug habit. When this woman told Yancey's friend what she was doing, he was nonplused. Finally he asked, "Have you thought of going to church for help?" With a shocked look on her face the woman said, "Church? Why would I go there? I was already feeling terrible about myself. They'd just make me feel worse!"

If only this woman could have known that Christ's healing presence could have been hers. Christ's healing presence is most often experienced through His Word.

Ellen Dippenar's husband died because of an accident, her sister died from a heart attack, and her only child died of polio. While living alone, Ellen suffered from a heart attack and was admitted to the hospital. While there she had a slight problem with her vision because of corneal dryness, so she asked a nurse to give her some artificial teardrops. Unfortunately, the nurse accidentally gave her carbolic acid, which blinded her. On top of that, she contracted leprosy. One by one, her toes began to ulcerate and became necrotic, causing her feet to be deformed. During 55 years of her life she had to have 57 surgeries.

When Ellen was asked how she could still smile, she answered, "God still loves me. I am still alive. I am looking forward to the day when Jesus comes. Then I will receive a perfect body and will meet again my loving husband, sister, and son."

There are many types of healing. Although Ellen must have longed for Jesus to stop by her house and heal her leprosy, blindness, and crooked feet, it didn't happen. But it will someday. It was the hope Ellen had in Christ that kept her attitude healthy. That, in itself, is a miracle!

Is there some aspect of your life that needs healing? Focus on Christ instead of yourself and see what a difference it makes.

KATHLEEN H. LIWIDJAJA-KUNTARAF

Dying to Live

*In reply Jesus declared, "I tell you the truth, no one can see
the kingdom of God unless he is born again." John 3:3, NIV.*

EACH HUMAN BEING begins with a single cell. That cell divides again
and again, differentiating into different body parts. The adult human body
is composed of more than 60 trillion structural units of living material of
different sizes, shapes, and functions. These are called cells. Do you have
any idea how many that is? About 600 times as many as there are stars in
the Milky Way! That's how wonderfully complex we are.

Every second the cells are full of activity, building, rebuilding, and
boiling with energy. They work around the clock, slowing down and
speeding up, but not suspending operations even while you sleep. And all
except nerve cells reproduce themselves. For example, if a portion of your
liver were removed surgically, the remaining liver cells would multiply
until the organ returns to its original size.

From the time of birth, skin, bone, bone morrow, and connective tissue cells are dying and being reproduced. It is through this constant process of death and rebirth that we enjoy good health.

Good spiritual health requires this same dying and rebirth process.
Two thousand years ago, Jesus gave one of His most profound sermons to
an audience of one—a Pharisee named Nicodemus. His message was,
"You must be born again in order to see the kingdom of God."

Nicodemus was confused. "How can one be born again when he is
old? It is impossible to reenter a mother's womb the second time!"

Jesus explained that the rebirth must be a birth of water (purification)
and Spirit. In other words, we must leave behind our anger, hurt, envy,
jealousy, and pain. Anything that separates us from God must die and be
buried; then the Spirit will re-create us.

This process of dying to sin does not take place during baptism only.
Rather, every day of our lives we must die to sin and recommit ourselves to
God. If cells died and never reproduced we would be in bad shape. So when
we die to sin—or empty ourselves of sin—we've got to replace it with a life-
giving substance. We must be born again with Christlike love. When His re-
deeming grace becomes a part of us, we are, indeed, new creations!

*Lord, is there anything in my life that is holding me back from being born
again today?*						GLADYS HOLLINGSEAD

Following the Recipe

*Delight yourself in the Lord, and He shall give
you the desires of your heart. Ps. 37:4, NKJV.*

IT WAS RARE that my mom ever got sick, but one day she was laid up in
bed, leaving us kids to fend for ourselves in the kitchen. I decided to make
some biscuits just the way Mom did—from scratch. I pulled out the cook-
book and found the recipe. Flour dusted the counter top as I measured out
the required amount. The recipe called for baking powder. *I wonder what
that's for?* I pondered. I scanned the pantry until I found something that
looked close enough—baking soda. *That will do,* I decided. Then salt. *We
can skip that,* I thought. *Whoever heard of salt on biscuits?* And so on.

When the biscuits came out of the oven they looked all right, so I took
a few samples to Mom for the final approval. To my shock she almost spit
out the first bite she took. "What did you put in this?" she gagged.

I had to agree—they tasted terrible. As we retraced my culinary steps,
Mom uncovered the reason—I hadn't followed the recipe, and the result
was disaster.

God has created a universe where happiness, health, and harmony depend on our following the right recipes. In matters of health, God has
pointed out those foods to avoid. In our dealing with others, God gave us
the golden rule. In our search for heaven, God wrote the Ten
Commandments. When we tinker with God's proven plan or scrap it altogether as we experiment with our own ideas for finding joy, we risk a
far greater peril than producing ghastly biscuits. We risk our chances for
true happiness and an abundant life.

Here are two of my favorite Bible recipes. The first one begins with a
statement of why this recipe is important. It says, "He has shown you, O
man, what is good; and what does the Lord require of you"—then comes
the recipe—"but to do justly, to love mercy, and to walk humbly with
your God?" (Micah 6:8, NKJV).

The second recipe is simple. If you delight yourself in the Lord, He
will give you the desires of your heart (Ps. 37:4).

If we just learn to live by God's recipes for health instead of trying to
invent our own, how much better the result!

*Why not search the Scriptures today for one of God's recipes? Write it down,
follow it, and experience the result. "Yum, good!"* LARRY RICHARDSON

Children Coping With Death

*And God will wipe away every tear from their eyes; there shall
be no more death, nor sorrow, nor crying. There shall be no more pain,
for the former things have passed away. Rev. 21:4, NKJV.*

MY LAST DAY of summer vacation ended in a tragedy I would deny for
the next two years. Grandpa came over to tell us that my aunt and uncle
had been in an auto accident and were in the hospital. Ten-year-old Stevie
was dead. *(No!)* Gary, 13, was in critical condition and not expected to
make it. *(It couldn't be true!)*

We didn't know then that "seat belts save lives." Stevie and Gary
hadn't used theirs that day.

Seat belts saved Neil, 15, and my aunt and uncle, who, in turn, saved
his little daughter Lorna by being her seat belt.

The next 36 hours were a blur. My folks got three different families to
look after my three siblings and me, had seatbelts installed in our car, and
drove from Portland to California with my other uncle. I wanted to go,
but they said a 10-year-old was "too little."

Gary died Monday morning before my parents and uncle reached
Fresno. I couldn't accept this. My mind came up with reasons why it
hadn't happened. I never cried—why cry over fiction?

When Mom and Dad returned, they had photos of the car. It had
rolled seven times before splintering a telephone pole. *(I'd seen worse.)*
There were pictures of two flower-draped coffins. *(They could have belonged
to anyone.)* My aunt and uncle's Christmas card came with only four names.
(They had made a mistake.)

Two years later, while visiting their home and taking a careful tour of
every room, I finally acknowledged to myself that Stevie and Gary were
really gone.

Many people don't believe children can cope with death. But children
need to grieve. I needed closure and a chance to say goodbye. My parents,
trying to protect me, meant well. But when I was excluded from experiencing the truth, my fantasies ran wild.

For me now, death is a part of life. I'm glad it's only temporary and
that I'll see Stevie and Gary again one day, along with other loved ones
who left me too soon.

*Father, comfort those who grieve today. And may the day come soon when
there will be no more death. Amen.* THERESE ALLEN

Renovating Routines

On my bed I remember you; I think of you
through the watches of the night. Ps. 63:6, NIV.

EVERY NIGHT MY children know that before they go to sleep they're going to get "good-night lovin'," as we call it. It's a routine. Without it, my kids and I would feel something was wrong—something was missing.

Routines are good for family relationships as well as for health. Take, for instance, the body's need for sleep. Lack of sleep makes a serious impact on our mental health. It impairs our ability to deal with daily stress, to think clearly, to make decisions, and yes, it can even threaten our lives. The sleepy brain makes lots of mistakes, sometimes life-threatening ones.

In the British journal *Occupational and Environmental Medicine,* researchers report that sleep deprivation can produce some of the same hazardous effects as being drunk. Getting less than six hours of sleep a night can affect coordination, reaction time, and judgment. People who drive after being awake for 17 to 19 hours performed worse than those with a blood alcohol level of .05 percent. People who get too little sleep may have high levels of stress, anxiety, and depression, and may take unnecessary risks.

Getting enough sleep is vital. But the benefit of sleep is not just in how much you sleep. What really matters is when and how you sleep. Volunteers who went to bed two hours earlier or two hours later than their usual bedtimes failed to feel refreshed, even when they were allowed adequate sleep time. Another study reported that volunteers who kept to a regular sleep schedule for a couple weeks began to feel more alert, even though they had cut down on their slumber by an average of 30 minutes each night. So take advantage of your natural rhythms and resist the urge to keep different hours on weekends.

Experiment with yourself. At a certain time every night, start shutting down. I've found that having an early morning appointment with God helps me get to bed on time. If I show up late to my appointment I've robbed myself of a "good morning lovin'" time with my heavenly Father.

By the way, if you have insomnia, try what King David did: "On my bed I remember you; I think of you through the watches of the night."

Dear Lord, help me to put some renovating routines into my life, so I will be rested and can enjoy You more! RISË RAFFERTY

Mind Medicine

For as he thinks in his heart, so is he. Prov. 23:7, NKJV.

I DON'T DRINK coffee; don't even know how to make it. But one particular night I had a special need. I was working late trying to finish an important project, and was nearly overwhelmed by sleepiness. Remembering that my secretary kept a jar of instant coffee in her desk, I added several tablespoons of the powder to a cup of cold water, gulped it down, and waited.

Within 10 minutes I felt energized—yes, caffeine mobilizes blood sugar. Then came heightened alertness—yes, it also stimulates the nervous system. I rushed to the bathroom, confirming that caffeine is a diuretic. The boost lasted the three hours I needed to finish the project.

The next morning I confessed to my secretary. She listened and began to smile. "I'm glad my coffee helped," she said. "But didn't you notice? It was decaffeinated!"

I realized I'd been a victim of what is called the placebo effect. Because I fully expected it to work, it did work.

The placebo effect is commonly used to test new medicines. One group of test subjects is given the real thing while another group receives a look-alike without any of the properties of the other. Surprisingly, placebo subjects often report as good, and sometimes even better, results than those who receive the actual medication.

In short, thoughts and emotions directly influence the mind, which, in turn, powerfully affects the body. Reports are on record of people who believed they were going to die on a certain day and they did, even though no direct cause could be found.

This powerful effect that our minds have on our bodies relates directly to our immune system. Every day we encounter hundreds of germs that could make us sick or even kill us. When our immune system is healthy, the bad things that attack us are fought off and our health is preserved.

A healthful diet, physical fitness, and positive emotional states can stimulate and strengthen the body's immune system. On the other hand, illness, negative emotions, drugs, and excessive stress can weaken it. AIDS occurs when the entire immune system has been decimated.

King Solomon advised us a long time ago about some powerful "mind medicine": "A cheerful heart is good medicine, but a crushed spirit dries the bones" (Prov. 17:22, NIV).

Lord, help me to be careful about what I put into my mind today.

HANS DIEHL

What's Your Destination?

*I go to prepare a place for you. And if I go and prepare a place
for you, I will come again and receive you to Myself;
that where I am, there you may be also. John 14:2, 3, NKJV.*

TEENS OFTEN ASK, "What's wrong with alcohol, drugs, tobacco, pornography, or sex outside of marriage?" In response I tell them the story of the little skylark.

Every day Junior Skylark went out into the garden with his mother and father, brothers and sisters, aunts, uncles, cousins, and grandparents to search for worms. They loved worms—big, juicy worms. It wasn't always easy finding enough worms to fill your tummy, unless you worked hard and long.

One day Junior was searching out near the edge of the garden when he heard a little man call, "Two worms for a skylark's feather."

He hopped closer and asked, "Will you really give me two worms if I give you a feather?"

"That's right," said the little man.

Wow, thought Junior. *That's easy.* So he pulled out a feather, gave it to the little man, and received two juicy worms. The next day he went back for more worms, and the next—and the next. His folks told him this wasn't a good idea, that he would need his feathers. But he had so many, what would it hurt if he traded a few away?

As the days went by he began to feel chilly. He asked, "When are we going to fly south?"

"In a couple of weeks or so," his folks replied. "And don't trade any more feathers away." But he didn't listen. Every day he went back to the little man, trading his feathers for worms.

One chilly fall day his mother and father flew into the air, with his brothers and sisters, his aunts, uncles, cousins, and grandparents. "Come on, Junior," they called. "It's time to fly south."

Junior tried. He flapped his wings. He jumped. He flapped some more, but he didn't have enough feathers to get airborne.

What is wrong with alcohol, drugs, tobacco, pornography, and sex outside of marriage? For one thing, you could hurt others with them. Also, they can keep you from going where you want to go. If your destination is heaven, then let me ask you: How do these things help you grow closer to the Lord Jesus Christ, who makes heaven possible?

Are you living the lifestyle that will help get you to where you want to go?

KAY KUZMA

The Dry Socket Story

*But he said to me, "My grace is sufficient for you, for my power
is made perfect in weakness." Therefore I will boast all the more gladly
about my weaknesses, so that Christ's power may rest on me. 2 Cor. 12:9, NIV.*

AS A DENTAL assistant, I learned a spiritual lesson from the patient with
a dry socket—that's a hole where a tooth used to be. A couple days after
an extraction, the patient came into the office complaining of extreme
pain. The dentist found that the patient's blood clot was no longer covering the hole left by the extraction. With the clot gone, the bone underneath was exposed to the air, causing great pain.

When a tooth is extracted, the empty hole must bleed for a while to
cleanse the wound and for a clot to form. The patient is instructed on how
to take care of this tender area. There is usually only a short period of
time—maybe 15 minutes—that the extraction area can bleed. If a clot
doesn't form, or if it forms and comes out later, the area is not going to
bleed again by itself. For normal wounds this is great; but with extraction
wounds the nerve endings in the open bone cry out in pain.

What is the treatment? The dentist must pack the open area with
medicine and dental packing material to form a "substitute" clot. This usually takes care of the problem, except in stubborn cases. If the area continues to hurt, the dentist must scrape the bone to make the wound bleed
again so another blood clot will form.

Many times in our lives we go through traumatic experiences that
cause pain and suffering, as if a "tooth" is being pulled out. What must
happen if you have exposed "bone tissue" and the pain won't go away?

You must let the heavenly dentist, Jesus Christ, take care of the problem. He may have to scrape the area again by allowing you to go through
another painful experience. But just think, while the bleeding is happening, God's grace and mercy will be waiting to cover that hole in your
heart. That empty feeling will disappear if you let the Lord do His medic-
inal work on you. No one will ever know a "tooth" had even been removed, for God's grace will cover it all. His grace is sufficient for every
weakness and pain. That's good news!

*May we be able to say as the apostle Paul did, "I will boast all the more gladly
about my weaknesses, so that Christ's power may rest on me."*

SILVIA JACOBSEN

Breakfast Brain Food

*My voice You shall hear in the morning, O Lord; in the morning
I will direct it to You, and I will look up. Ps. 5:3, NKJV.*

FOR YEARS EDUCATORS have noticed that children who eat a good
breakfast do better in school. That's why breakfast is called "brain food"!
It is considered to be as essential to learning as understanding the three R's
(readin', 'riting, and 'rithmetic)!

A 1998 study on inner-city children who were fed breakfast at school
confirms this fact. Children who ate breakfast had significant gains in academic and emotional functioning.

When children chronically misbehave in school, everyone suffers.
Breakfast was a big factor in helping these children settle down in the classroom. For others, breakfast kept them from falling asleep at their desks.

Both parents and teachers noted the difference. And grades confirmed
the adults' observations. Those children who often ate breakfast had math
grades that averaged almost a whole letter grade higher than the grades of
the students who rarely ate breakfast. There were also significant decreases
in absenteeism and tardiness.

Are children the only ones needing a brain-food breakfast? Studies on
adults have shown that eating breakfast contributes to better health, faster
reaction time, and maximum work output. Regardless of age, breakfast is
the brain food needed to begin the day.

"But I'm not hungry for breakfast," children and adults complain.
That's because they try to eat before their bodies are fully awake! If they
would eat a light supper at least four hours before bedtime (with no midnight snacking), and then get to bed early so they could get up early and
take a brisk walk in the fresh air, and then if they would take a stimulating
shower and enjoy a good towel rub down, I doubt if they would complain
about not being hungry!

But is that the only food your brain needs in the morning? No.
Morning time, before your brain is cluttered with the junk "food" of the
day, is the best time to fill your brain with spiritual food. Your thinking
will be sharper and your memorizing ability more keen. Morning is the
time to renew your mind with the promises and principles that are found
in God's Word. For a healthy brain, pray the words of King David, "My
voice You shall hear in the morning, O Lord!"

Have you enjoyed your spiritual and physical "breakfast brain food" yet today?

GERARD MCLANE

God's Presence in Tough Times

*In all their affliction He was afflicted, and the Angel of His Presence
saved them; in His love and in His pity He redeemed them; and
He bore them and carried them all the days of old. Isa. 63:9, NKJV.*

IT WAS FEBRUARY 1999. My feet barely touched the sidewalk as I briskly walked across the college campus to my car. The afternoon sunshine and the cool breeze that blew on my face elevated my endorphin level to the point where I wanted to twirl, jump, and shout, "I'm alive!" For the first time in years I felt energized enough to register for a continuing education class.

Four years earlier, after five months of unusual headaches, I realized that shear determination of mind over matter would not dissipate the searing pain. A silent, insidious stalker had slowly robbed my health and zest for life. But endless trips to numerous doctors and countless medical tests brought me no relief. With each passing day my strength lessened until I was nearly too weak to walk.

For years, I'd been struggling with an unknown infectious pathogenic disease and it was now so acute that my colon was riddled with tiny abscesses and ulcers. On one of my darkest days I realized that even my will to live had vanished. As tears of despair soaked my pillow, a verse in Isaiah came to my mind, "In all their affliction He was afflicted." Suddenly I pictured my guardian angel sitting on my bed beside me, and I wondered if he was crying with me. Truly, it was a comforting thought.

During those painful months I felt the arms of God through the loving support of many precious family members and friends around the world who encouraged and prayed for me. Gradually, my doctor, with the help of a medical lab, unraveled the complexity of my illness and developed a long-term treatment plan. Now as the amebic and mercury toxins are being eradicated, I am experiencing healing and the ability to concentrate and think clearly.

I have learned that God permits tough times to test the validity of our faith. The way we react in a crisis is a barometer of how much we really believe God is in control and is doing what is necessary to build a strong character in us. The very condition that cripples us can be the inspiration for the "song" we will one day sing to the world!

Thank You, Lord, for being in control and building our characters through the tough times.   CHARLOTTE BOWMAN

A Big Bang?

So God created man in His own image; in the image of God
He created him; male and female He created them. Gen. 1:27, NKJV.

IF YOU'VE EVER questioned whether God created life or if it happened by chance when something went *bang!* I wish you could visit a semiconductor factory where computer "chips" are manufactured.

A chip with its millions of wires, connections, resistors, capacitors, transistors, and diodes, is made by "stacking" layers of wires and other components one on top of another. Each layer of wires is insulated from the one below except in the places where the wires or other parts need to touch to make an electrical connection.

To produce the chip technicians begin with a thin "wafer" of silicone about the size of a large coin. A very thin liquid layer of light-sensitive material is spread over the wafer. It dries quickly and a picture of the first drawing, reduced to a square about 1/16th inch on a side, is photographically "exposed" onto the light-sensitive layer. Then photographic developer is washed over the wafer. All the light sensitive layer washes away except for the lines and shapes from the picture. At that point the technician, using a microscope, can actually see the drawing on the wafer.

These tiny pictures are exposed side by side all over the wafer—about 10,000 of them. Each place where that first picture has been exposed will become a "chip." Several steps (exposing, spreading, liquid, drying, developing, and so forth) are needed, using computer-controlled machines and lightning-fast robots, to put each layer of drawings in place.

After all the layers are "built up" on the chip, someone solders some 20 to 50 very tiny wires to each of the chips (200,000 wires per wafer). Then each chip must be cut out and equipped with bigger wire connectors suitable for plugging into a circuit board. Presto! You have a digital watch with a calculator, stop watch, timer, and phone list. Or put enough of the chips on circuit boards, find a hard disk drive somewhere, and you have a computer!

Could a computer chip come into being by chance? No way! And the human brain is so much more intricate. A big bang? I don't think so. Only God could make a thinking, feeling, creative brain that is smart enough to create a computer chip!

God, the brain You have given me is so incredible. Help me to live a brain-healthy lifestyle! JIM BRACKETT

A Double Standard

There is a way that seems right to a man,
but its end is the way of death. Prov. 14:12, NKJV.

HE SAT IN my office, a seething mixture of teenaged dejection and frustration. "Caffeine is an addictive drug, pure and simple," the teenager said. "But my folks slug it down by the gallon. They can't even open their eyes in the morning until they've had three cups of coffee apiece." He paused and then continued dramatically. "No one gives them grief about their habit. But me? I hate coffee, so I tried nicotine. You'd think it was the end of the world!"

I smiled at his intensity but it was not a laughing matter. There had been a knock-down, drag-out argument with his parents the night before. He had been thrown an ultimatum: "If you want to live under this roof you will never smoke again!"

I marveled at the facts he testily spouted. "Caffeine and nicotine stimulate the brain, increase alertness, decrease a sense of fatigue, and temporarily improve memory. They both trigger the release of dopamine, a neurotransmitter that helps to elevate mood." He shook his head.

My heart ached for him. "Many individuals rarely stop to think about caffeine use," I agreed, "because its use is so common in our culture." (One out of four adults in the United States smokes, while four out of five drink tea or coffee daily, to say nothing of ingesting caffeine in other forms. The average total intake of caffeine is about 400 mg per day.)

Just as there are long-term health risks with smoking, research shows long-term health risks associated with high caffeine intake—it's just not as life-threatening: exacerbation of heart problems, decreased bone density, an increase in PMS and menopausal symptoms, a reduction in iron absorption, bladder irritation, and gastrointestinal symptoms.

The teenager's real problem wasn't the facts about nicotine versus caffeine. It was with role modeling and acceptance. His parents were clearly addicted to caffeine but refused to admit it. Yet they condemned their son for his addiction and threatened him, which made him feel rejected. There is a better way: Let honesty and unconditional love soften the heart.

The double standard is *not* OK! Healthy role models don't put people down for their bad habits while continuing to cherish and justify their own.

What are you modeling? Is the way that seems right to you, really right? Do you unconditionally love others, as God loves you?   ARLENE TAYLOR

Twisters of Death and Destruction

Humble yourselves, therefore, under God's mighty hand, that he may
lift you up in due time. Cast all your anxiety on him because he cares
for you. Be self-controlled and alert. Your enemy the devil prowls around
like a roaring lion looking for someone to devour. 1 Peter 5:6-8, NIV.

ON MARCH 1, 1997, a powerful windstorm hit the state of Arkansas, leaving as its signature a long, winding, 260-mile path of destruction. What was this mighty beast of the sky? A terrifying tornado.

As a cold front lingers in the atmosphere, a massive front of warm air rises up against it. This movement pulls in more warm air, and that, too, begins to rise. As this process continues, the air begins to rotate, gaining momentum and strength. When fully developed, the twister's fierce winds can reach 300 miles per hour or more.

A tornado can cause incredible damage. In a few hours it can easily obliterate an area 2-4 miles wide and 100 miles long. Fragments and debris the size of needles can drill holes the size of bowling balls. The winds in a twister can send a scrawny piece of straw straight through the stump of a tree. Buildings seem to explode like bombs.

Only proper preparation and the kind, loving hand of our heavenly Father can bring us through these agitated "funnels of death." The best protection is a storm cellar or basement. If caught out in the open by an approaching tornado, a person should lie flat on the ground or hide in a crevice or ditch. In the tornado mentioned above, Kathleen Walton, a single mother, held on to her 11-year-old son, Levi, as together they lay under an overpass on Interstate 35. As the tornado sucked her away to her death, she saved her son's life by letting go of him.

Such disasters remind us that there will be even more perilous times ahead. Are you prepared? Occurring irregularly, yet increasing in frequency, these destructive storms exhibit power and capabilities that immensely surpass our control. It is evident that the results of these "acts of Satan" can be associated with the end-time events described in the Bible. Even though there is not much we can do about a tornado, there is someone else in whom we can completely trust for our protection—Jesus. Let us abide in Him that we may "be able to stand" (Rev. 6:17).

Lord, thank You for Your promise of protection. When I'm surrounded by the
storms of life, help me to remember that even the wind and the waves obey Your voice.

ERIC GULLICKSON and KAY KUZMA

Rest Is God's Way of Saying "I Love You"

Come to me, all you who are weary and burdened,
and I will give you rest. Matt. 11:28, NIV.

REST COMES LOADED with smiles and packed with peace. It offers energy for the burned-out and restoration for the broken. Although it is at its peak on Sabbath, it is always ready to perform healing transformations. Rest turns back the powers of weariness, exhaustion, and fatigue, replacing them with peace, energy, and hope.

Maybe that's why the Creator wrapped Rest with Sabbath. Knowing that we would work hard all week, He dedicated an entire day for us to plug into His power, a time when He packs us full of Himself so we can be healthier people next week.

Wayne Muller says, "Sabbath is a time to stop, to refrain from being seduced by our desires. To stop working, stop making money, stop spending money. See what you have. Look around. Listen to your life. Then, at the end of the day, where is the desperate yearning to consume, to shop, to buy what we do not need? It dissolves. Little by little, it falls away."

Why not plan ahead and make your next Sabbath a time of rest, relaxation, and relationship with God. Stay away from sports and other forms of entertainment; instead do something that gives your mind a chance to think deeply while your body is at ease.

Put a little Sabbath into every day by taking 10 minutes for life-stabilizing rest. That doesn't mean, necessarily, that you will go to sleep. It does mean that you'll stop all other activities and concentrate on the Creator for those 10 minutes. Do something special with Him, take a walk and admire His work, test some of His finest beverages, listen to the wind.

Think of all the things that burden you or make you weary. Write those things on individual cards, put them in a basket. And give them to God. Quote the words of Matthew 11:28, where God promises to replace those burdens with rest, and ask Him to perform that personalized miracle for you now!

Remember, "It is not busyness that we should honor in our midst, but love. Busyness and love are not the same. One is speed; the other is God" (Richard A. Swenson, M.D.).

Rest. It's God's personal way of saying, "I love you."

Shut your eyes, breathe deeply, smile, and thank God for loving you with the gift of rest.   DICK DUERKSEN

Beauty for the Mind

*Your word I have hidden in my heart, that
I might not sin against You. Ps. 119:11, NKJV.*

THE NIGHT OF MARCH 3, 1947, was dark and cold. I lay alone in a hospital delivery room. Periodically a nurse would come by to check on me. Labor and delivery was always a battle for me, a long one. To pass the time between contractions I repeated Bible texts to myself until the doctor finally announced, "It's a girl!" The Bible texts that I've hidden in my heart have cushioned the rough times in my life by keeping my thoughts on something other than myself.

Not only during times of pain and stress but also in peaceful times can the Word stored in the mind bring joy and new dimensions of understanding. Learning Bible verses and memorizing poetry was an important part of my early childhood and during my school days. I even learned to defend my beliefs with a "thus saith the Lord."

I have found that the Word "hid in my heart" keeps me from knowingly sinning. There also is a wealth of beauty in the Scriptures. Take for example the line in Psalm 19, "The heavens declare the glory of God." Try to visualize the beauty of the starry sky, glory in the hues of the rainbow, catch a sunbeam through a shiny window, mark the colors in a sunset, trace the path of a snowflake as it falls. There is no limit to the ideas a passage of Scripture can engender.

I like Ellen White's thought: "As we contemplate the great things of God's word, we look into a fountain that broadens and deepens beneath our gaze" (*Education,* p. 171).

The wise man said, "As he [a person] thinks in his heart, so is he" (Prov. 23:7, NKJV), and Paul counsels in Philippians 4:8, "Finally, brethren, whatever things are true, whatever things are noble, whatever things are just, whatever things are pure, whatever things are lovely, whatever things are of good report, if there is any virtue and if there is anything praiseworthy—meditate on these things" (NKJV).

In a world filled with violence, lust, greed, and dishonesty we can escape mental and moral depravity by consciously filling our minds with the Word. His words are life and truth. "The springs of heavenly peace and joy unsealed in the soul by the words of Inspiration will become a mighty river of influence to bless all who come within its reach" (*Education,* p. 192).

Here's a challenge: Memorize one Bible text a day for the next 21 days and see if it doesn't make a difference in your life. VELDA NELSON

God's Way Is Best

Come, all you who are thirsty, come to the waters;
and you who have no money, come, buy and eat! Isa. 55:1, NIV.

WHEN GOD CREATED humans and the rest of the animal world, He created different foods for each kind of animal, each perfectly suited to their bodies' chemistry. Cows eat different food than cats. Birds eat different food than fish. The food God created for each animal is perfect for that animal's optimal functioning. For humans, God created fruits, grains, nuts, and herbs—and for human babies, mother's milk.

Enter man into the food process—and it has generally spelled "nutritional disaster." Human-engineered food generally clogs the arteries, overloads the system with calories, and causes heart disease, high blood pressure, diabetes, elevated blood cholesterol levels, gallbladder disease, osteoarthritis, low back pain, and many cancers. All of these can be food-related diseases!

Humans have even tried to improve on mother's milk by using formulas made from cow's milk. But God designed cow's milk to grow cows, so it has three times more protein, calcium, and sodium, among other things, than mother's milk. Through laboratory processing man has lowered these concentrations to make it similar to human milk, but protein from cow's milk still causes allergies in many babies. And it still doesn't have the factors that help the bowel to mature or to have the white blood cells and antibodies that will protect babies against such diseases as asthma, bacterial infections, constipation, colitis, gastrointestinal infections, eczema, tonsillitis, and urinary tract infections.

Laboratories, trying to make formula nutritionally adequate for babies, add the substances that are missing in cow's milk but present in mother's milk, but mother's milk is a unity of function and nutrition. The interaction that goes on among its elements is amazing. Man can never satisfactorily duplicate that which God created.

Why is it that we have such a hard time accepting God's way as best for us? Not just in diet, but salvation as well. Salvation is free—just as mother's milk—but we try to substitute Jesus' gift for our own works. We try to buy salvation by being good. And in the process we get sick—if not physically ill because of the stress, then emotionally depressed because we're never good enough.

Lord, help me to remember that Your way is always best.   MARTHA A. LEE

Sonlight

For God, who said, "Let light shine out of darkness," made his
light shine in our hearts to give us the light of the knowledge
of the glory of God in the face of Christ. 2 Cor. 4:6, NIV.

THE SUN PROVIDES life and health to the earth. Without the sun we would freeze to death. Without the sun to kill germs, disease couldn't be controlled. And without the light from God's *Son,* there would be no hope for knowing how to live the abundant life He wants for us—and certainly, no hope for eternal life.

I've thought a lot about the sun, and I've come to the conclusion that my relationship with God's Son is something like the earth's relationship with that giant orb in the sky that we call the sun.

For thousands of years, man thought the earth was the center of the universe and that the sun revolved around it. That's what it looked like. When Copernicus said the earth went around the sun, people cried, "Heresy!"

Just as in Copernicus' time, it's hard for us to admit we're not the center of the universe. We're born thinking that life revolves around us. As we grow we learn that's not true, but we're fooled by our selfish natures. We want to do what feels good to us, we want to eat what tastes good to us, we want to listen to what sounds good to us. We deceive ourselves into thinking we can do our own thing and there won't be any consequences. But the more we sin, doing it our way rather than God's Son's way, the more darkness falls over our hearts, until self-deception so clouds our vision that it's almost impossible for the Son's rays of enlightenment to shine through.

Satan (the god of this age) is trying hard to keep the gospel of self-importance alive. He knows it's impossible for us to look in two different directions at the same time. So, if he can keep us distracted with our needs and desires, we're going to keep stumbling around in the dark. We're going to miss the light of the Son who has pointed out the true source of life by telling us to treat people as we would like to be treated, to love others as God loves us, and that the first shall be last.

It's time to put our self-importance in the right perspective and begin revolving around the Son of Righteousness, letting the warmth of His love and the light of His Word heal us from our selfish, cold, dark, sinful ways.

God, help me turn from my own selfish ways and let Your Son shine in my life.

JENNIFER BROMLEY

Freedom From Pain

I will praise you, O Lord my God, with all my heart;
I will glorify your name forever. For great is your love toward me;
you have delivered me from the depths of the grave. Ps. 86:12, 13, NIV.

FOR TWO YEARS I suffered the most excruciating pain from a disease known as fibromyalgia. I had read the Apostle James' counsel: "Is any one of you sick? He should call the elders of the church to pray over him and anoint him with oil in the name of the Lord. And the prayer offered in faith will make the sick person well; the Lord will raise him up. If he has sinned, he will be forgiven" (James 5:14, 15, NIV). But I hadn't considered this for myself. I wasn't at death's door.

Nonetheless, I had often prayed for healing from the chronic pain that racked all four quadrants of my body. Reconciled to the probability of a life of physical agony, I had accepted the situation as a "thorn in the flesh" with which I must continue to live and cope. I even prided myself on my ability to function and have a productive ministry as a leader in the church.

One particularly painful day, I shared my situation with a small group of friends who had met for a committee meeting. I requested their prayers. They immediately took my situation to the Lord. Their prayers included asking God to guide me in considering an anointing service.

As I prayed the matter through, I sensed my need for spiritual as well as physical healing—healing from my own self-reliance to a deeper reliance on my Savior. I also became certain that I would experience healing as an answer to my being anointed. The timing and method would be in God's control, but I knew He would hear and answer our prayers of faith.

As my friends gathered around me for the anointing service, I sensed the peace of God's presence. I was certain that God would do His work. I also trusted His will and the method He would use to accomplish His purpose.

The next day I awakened to my first day without pain in more than two years. Even greater was the awareness of a constant need to rely on my Lord for every aspect of my life, especially spiritually. The need is constant, but so is my awareness of His presence and strength. Each day, as I praise Him for the freedom from pain, I praise Him even more for the freedom of His forgiving grace.

Are you suffering from any type of pain—physical, emotional, or spiritual? Ask the Lord for healing, and praise Him for His love and deliverance.

BEN MAXSON

Is Your Cup Converted?

O Lord, You are the portion of my inheritance and
my cup; you maintain my lot. Ps. 16:5, NKJV.
My cup runs over. Ps. 23:5, NKJV.

IN HIS BOOK *The God Who Would Be Man* H.M.S. Richards tells of the visit of a chaplain-general of the forces, Bishop Taylor Smith, to a military hospital during World War I. He noticed two wounded men sitting by a table on which was a bowl turned upside down. He asked the men, "Do you know the two things that are under that bowl?" They said they did not.

"Darkness and uselessness," the chaplain replied. Quickly he turned the bowl right side up. "Now," he said to the two curious men, "it's full of light, and ready to hold porridge, soup, or anything you might like to use it for. It's a converted bowl."

What a wonderful concept this is. God has assigned us our cup of life (or bowl), but it's our choice to either turn it upside down and be dark and morose and finally useless, or to turn it right side up and fill it to overflowing with His blessings and then to share them with others.

But remember, there may be times when we are asked to drink a cup of sorrow. Rather than inverting or controverting what can be a spiritual lesson for us, we can convert our cup of sorrow into a dessert of comfort.

Psalm 16:5 helps me greatly when I start to feel sorry for myself because of circumstances. If God has placed me in a particular situation, then I am defying Him when I start complaining. The Israelites in the desert complained to Moses when really they were complaining about God. Finally God asked of Moses, "How long shall I bear with this evil congregation who complain against *Me?*" (Num. 14:27, NKJV).

Merlin Carothers, an apostle of praise, wrote something that always gets me back on track: "The turning point cannot come until we begin to praise God *for* our situation instead of crying out for Him to take it all away." Several years ago I was facing surgery to remove squamous cell carcinoma from my face. I was scared witless, so I started saying over and over, "Thank You, Father!" I imaged my cup of life turned over so there would be room to receive what God had for me. And He filled it. Calm came!

Is your cup of life upside down—filled with darkness and uselessness? If so, turn it over and let God fill it with light and usefulness.   PAT NORDMAN

Leave the Grazing to the Cows

You shall keep the Sabbath, therefore, for it is holy to you. Ex. 31:14, NKJV.

GRAZING—EATING throughout the day—is undermining the health of millions. Most snackers, however, never stop to consider that even though they may nibble on healthy foods this practice can harm the body by slowing the digestive process, leaving toxins and fermented food in the stomach and bowel for longer than necessary.

Your body has natural rhythms. One of those rhythms is the digestive system. Every time you snack, you interrupt the digestive process. This was shown in an experiment involving five people, which has been replicated many times. Each of the participants ate a normal breakfast. It took them an average of four and a half hours to empty their stomachs. A few days later, those five people ate the same breakfast. The researchers then introduced some variables.

1. One person ate an ice-cream cone two hours after breakfast. The ice-cream eater needed six hours to fully digest breakfast.

2. Three of the subjects snacked every half hour after breakfast but ate no lunch. Their snacks consisted of a peanut butter sandwich, a piece of pumpkin pie with a glass of milk, and half a slice of buttered bread. After nine hours they still had undigested breakfast foods in their stomachs.

3. The fifth person in this experiment ate two chocolate candy bars between breakfast and lunch and two more between lunch and dinner. In this case, more than half the breakfast remained in the stomach after 13 and a half hours, a well as portions from the other meals eaten.

Whenever you eat anything, you activate the digestive juices that aid in breaking down food. If you put new food into your stomach several hours into the digestion of the first meal, the stomach slows its work as it begins to process the new food. If you snack all day, your exhausted stomach will not get a chance to rest until late into the night.

Your digestive system isn't the only part of your body that needs rest. That's why God created the Sabbath. For 24 hours every seven days we are to rest from our work and our worries. We might think it won't matter if we slip in a load of wash, study for an exam, or mow the lawn on Sabbath. But it does. It slows the restorative process that God designed for your body and soul.

Lord, please give me victory over snacking—and victory over doing work on Your Sabbath—so my body and soul can get the restorative rest needed to operate as You designed. JAN W. KUZMA

Building Your Brain Boutons

You were taught, with regard to your former way of life, to put off your old self, which is being corrupted by its deceitful desires; to be made new in the attitude of your minds; and to put on the new self, created to be like God in true righteousness and holiness. Eph. 4:22-24, NIV.

MESSAGES ARE PROCESSED in the brain and sent to different parts of the body through nerve cells. These cells are made up of a center called the nucleus, the surrounding fluid called the cytoplasm, and a boundary called the membrane. Extending from this membrane are many little fibers called dendrites that receive messages, and one long sending fiber called the axon; it transmits messages to the neighboring cells. Between the sending fiber of one cell and the receiving fiber or body of another, there is a tiny space called a synapse. At this junction are tiny enlargements called boutons (French for buttons) that secrete various chemicals that close the tiny gap and stimulate the next cell to send on the message.

Brain scientists have discovered that any thought or action that is often repeated builds these little boutons on the ends of certain nerve fibers so that it becomes easier to repeat that same thought or action the next time—and thus habits are established. To change a habit one must build new pathways by choosing a different response; this builds more boutons on the new pathway.

Say you are offered a piece of cake when you are on a diet. You think, *That looks good!* Immediately the coded message backed by, say, 30 millivolts of energy, says to your brain action cell, "Fire!" Just then comes the thought, *No, I'd better not!* Immediately the chemical GABA is secreted to your brain action cell. This one is backed by, say, 40 millivolts of energy with the message, "Don't fire!" (The stronger your decisiveness, the more energy will reach the cell.) The hostess hands the cake your way, but you say, "No, thanks." By a margin 10 millivolts of energy your diet wins the day.

What if you yield to temptation? Start working on the new pathway again. You never lose ground on the new pathway—those boutons are not erased by the occasional fall! But every success strengthens the pathway. Eventually you will have developed such a strong response to the right that it's unlikely you'll respond in the old way.

Think about something good, be kind, smile. Isn't it incredible that chemical changes in your nerve pathways are being made that will be a blessing to you when strongly established.

ELDEN M. CHALMERS

Exercise Moved My Mountain

In repentance and rest is your salvation,
in quietness and trust is your strength. Isa. 30:15, NIV.

HAVING MULTIPLE CHEMICAL sensitivity has been a major mountain in my life. Exposure to chemicals and smells so slight others don't notice them makes my life miserable: severe headaches, fatigue, muscle pain, and "brain fog." I prayed for God to help me.

Taking nutritional supplements helped some, but in October God impressed me to do something more, so I began an exercise program: one hour each morning of stretching and breathing exercises. I noticed more flexibility and peace of mind—exactly what I would need for an unexpected challenge: Moving Mom.

In December I flew to Boston to pack my mother's belongings. It would be an enormous job—her apartment was stuffed, and I had less than a week to do it. Would my energy hold out?

I boarded the plane, confident that if God could find a decent priced flight for me during the Christmas season, somehow He would take care of the weather, find reputable movers, keep my used car running, and give me the stamina I would need. So I closed my eyes and napped peacefully during the long trip.

Each morning during that next week I'd talk with God and do my hour of exercising as I focused on God's sustaining power. Then I'd drive to Mom's, feeling renewed and positive about the tasks ahead. Halfway through the week, I was pretty exhausted when my younger sister, who lives 20 miles from Mom, came for two days and packed only six boxes! Anger exploded within me and I left the apartment early to nurse my self-pity. I needed a chat with my Father; I needed to get myself off the throne and put Him on! I needed to remember that the key to my strength was in quietly trusting in the God who moves mountains. (See Mark 11:23.)

Finally, 150 boxes later and countless steps up to Mom's second-story apartment, we were ready for the movers. Both the weather and the car cooperated on our long ride north. The next day, temperatures plummeted and howling winds whirled the snow, but we were safe and cozy.

I've discovered that exercise is one of God's mountain-moving methods: Physical exercise—and the exercise of faith!

Do you have a mountain in your life that you've been trying to get rid of? Maybe it's time to ask God to show you what you should do, then trust Him to do the rest. DONNA PATCH

Beware of Surfeiting

And take heed to yourselves, lest at any time your hearts be
overcharged with surfeiting, and drunkenness, and cares of this life,
and so that day come upon you unawares. Luke 21:34.

DO YOU KNOW what the word surfeiting means? It means intemperance of any kind, such as overeating. Why does Jesus warn us against weighing our hearts down with excesses?

Obviously, excesses such as overeating, drunkenness, and too many worries, dull the senses, making a person more vulnerable to temptation. Jesus warns that intemperate people won't be able to discern that Christ's coming is near, and they won't be ready.

There's a health reason, too. Overeating leads to obesity, and research shows that there's a relationship between obesity and cancer risk. Obesity increases the risk of prostate cancer two and a half times and the risk of colon cancer threefold; a woman who is 50 pounds overweight has 10 times the risk of endometrial cancer, and breast cancer survival time is shortened by both obesity and a high fat diet. In fact, regardless of your weight, reducing fat intake by 25 percent results in 20 percent fewer breast cancers, but reducing calories by 25 percent results in 75 percent fewer cancers!

How can you tell if you have a weight problem? Here's an easy way: Multiply your weight in pounds by 704 and divide by the square of your height in inches. In the metric system your weight in kilograms is divided by the square of your height in meters. It should be between 18.5 and 25. Between 25 and 30 is considered overweight. Above 30 is obese.

A waist circumference equal to or greater than 94 centimeters or 37 inches in men or 80 centimeters or 31.5 inches in women is an indication to lose weight. Fat around your waist is more dangerous than fat around your hips. Determine your waist-to-hip ratio by measuring your waist just under the ribs, and the hips where you have that protrusion of the hip bone. Divide the hip number into the waist figure. The result should be no more than 1.0 for a man or 0.85 for a woman. It's better to be pear-shaped, bigger around the hips than around the stomach. As you get bigger around the waist, the risk of high blood pressure, diabetes, heart attack, cancer of the breast, and endometrium increase.

So for good spiritual and physical health, beware of surfeiting!

Is there an area in your life in which you're struggling with intemperance?
What changes do you feel God would have you make so you'll be ready for
His coming?   JOHN A. SCHARFFENBERG

Gifts From Our Good Shepherd

Because the Lord is my Shepherd, I have everything I need! He lets me rest in the meadow grass and leads me beside the quiet streams. Ps. 23:1, 2, TLB.

I DEARLY LOVE Psalm 23, the shepherd's psalm. As I get older I am more aware of the beauty and pull of this gem. One of the exegetists of this psalm suggests that we may regard everything that brings relief from the ordinary pressures of daily life and revives our drooping spirits as our pastures of meadow grass and refreshing streams.

When I need a quick respite from the moment, I visualize a stream, and I'm standing on the bank. The day is cool and quiet. It's amazing the peace I feel from just a few seconds of holding this picture in my mind.

Another writer points out that the pastures of God are always fresh and green because they are sheltered with the hedge of God's protecting love and law. What a wonderful idea this is when we are tempted to set fire to God's hedge with our own ideas of what is right for us.

We need hedged pastures today more than ever. My private place is a corner of the bedroom. It has a comfortable chair, a good lamp, and lots of wonderful reading material.

Our inner spirit has been assaulted by outer forces that we don't even recognize anymore. I'm talking about the invasion to our senses, something I've noticed in the past 30 years especially. Pascal wrote centuries ago: "Our senses will not admit anything extreme. Too much noise confuses us, too much light dazzles us, too great distance or nearness prevents vision, too great prolixity or brevity weakens an argument, too much pleasure gives pain, too much accordance annoys." Centuries later, this is still true!

This may sound old fashioned in today's climate, but we are not required to be constantly on the run, physically, mentally, or spiritually. To calm down, I recommend this great psalm for daily meditation. Many of us memorized it as children, but now that we have grown far too busy, when we are in a valley and see only dead ends ahead, we need to dust off this psalm and find out what it really means.

In the meantime, let's remember that music, friendship, books, religious privileges, freedom, and love—all these gifts are meadow grass pastures and quiet streams from our Good Shepherd!

Lord, please lead me to a quiet place where my soul can be refreshed today.

PAT NORDMAN

Trials and Trust

But rejoice to the extent that you partake of Christ's sufferings, that when His glory is revealed, you may also be glad with exceeding joy. 1 Peter 4:13, NKJV.

THE WORD SUFFERING calls to mind pictures of emaciated bodies racked with pain; fly-covered, starving babies; or grieving parents who have lost a child. Perhaps your picture of suffering is of a personal experience when you have endured a loss, a betrayal, a rejection, or a physical illness or injury.

No matter the experience, the pain is all-consuming. Trying to change your mind or divert your thinking to another channel, or struggling to ignore it, is useless. The entire body sympathizes with the aching part. Daily routines are interrupted as mind, body, and emotions rush to support each other. Most disheartening is the feeling of separation from God—the excruciating loneliness when no one understands your heart or feels your feelings, and God is silent.

Not long ago my recovery from major back surgery, which was supposed to be simple, was complicated by severe, unrelenting pain. Days and nights blurred; the only relief came from heavy medication, which made alert and rational thinking nearly impossible. My plans to meet writing deadlines during recovery were being sabotaged by the pounding in my leg.

One sleepless night I sat wrapped in an afghan, sipping hot tea and crying. I had become depressed from the persistent attack, and was pleading with God for relief and resolve. Somehow I sensed the tension that had contracted my hands into fists and every body muscle into fighting position. The thought came that I should stop the fight and go with the flow—stop fighting the pain and relax into the experience.

The word rejoice came whispering to my mind. So I changed my focus and started that moment to praise God for the pain, for the suffering, for the privilege. And soon I was asleep!

Today the suffering is different—but nonetheless intense. And once again the remedy returns. I shall praise Him for the pain, and be pleased that I am given such a weighty trust and high honor.

Here's a quotation that is worth pondering: "Of all the gifts that Heaven can bestow upon men, fellowship with Christ in His sufferings is the most weighty trust and the highest honor" (Ellen G. White, *The Desire of Ages,* p. 225).

When you are in pain, praise God for this gift of fellowship with Christ in His suffering.   NANCY ROCKEY

Hardened Hearts

*We are the people he watches over, the sheep under his care. Oh, that you
would listen to his voice today! The Lord says, "Don't harden your hearts as
Israel did at Meribah, as they did at Massah in the wilderness. Ps. 95:7, 8, NLT.*

IN MY WORK at Weimar Institute and Lifestyle Center of America, I
have met many people with hardened hearts, well, hardened arteries at
least. They suffer with diabetes, obesity, arthritis, you name it. These
health guests learn the NEWSTART principles (nutrition, exercise, water,
sunlight, temperance, air, rest, trust in divine power), which have restored
thousands to health. One couple told me, "We are tired of getting sick,
taking medicine, then getting side effects from the medicine and having to
take even more medicine. We want to learn how to stay well naturally."

As guests struggle to break lifelong habits and recover from debilitating diseases, they often say, "I've known this stuff for years. I just haven't
been living it."

What about you? Do you, like Israel, whine for the fleshpots of Egypt
(Ex. 16:3), then wonder why you're not feeling good? God told Israel that
if they would listen and do what He said was right, obeying His laws—including the laws of health, then they would not suffer the diseases that the
Egyptians suffered (Ex. 15:26). But they didn't listen.

Neither did I. I knew God revealed more specific health information
to His messenger, Ellen White, who wrote that there would come a time
when it was best not to eat dairy products. But I was already a vegetarian.
Why be a fanatic and give up milk and cheese? Meanwhile, I carried an
extra 20 pounds, and endured an annoying congestion which medication
failed to cure. When I arrived at Weimar Institute to study massage, I tried
for myself the lifestyle I knew I should be living. Surprise! The extra
pounds slid off. My congestion disappeared. I learned to get well and stay
well by following God's laws of health.

Our son Elijah has gotten the healthy start that will save him from pain
and disease. Breast milk, whole plant food, a diet that's free of animal products, lots of water, fresh air, sunshine, and so on. Guess what? He doesn't
get colds, ear infections, and other "typical" childhood diseases.

Why not reexamine your health habits today? What have you known
for years, yet failed to practice? Don't harden your heart or your arteries
unnecessarily. It's not worth it.

*Lord, I want to live the lifestyle You designed for me. Strengthen my willpower
to do what I know I should.* HOLLY SUE JOERS

Where Has All the Time Gone?

Then he returned to his disciples and found them sleeping. "Could you men not keep watch with me for one hour?" he asked Peter. "Watch and pray so that you will not fall into temptation. The spirit is willing, but the body is weak." Matt. 26:40, 41, NIV.

THE FIRST TIME I was really hit by the value of time was when I received the call from my mother telling me my sister had been hit by a drunk driver and had died. Rebecca was gone. My soul mate, confidante, and debating opponent! Her day had not even lasted 24 hours. She had used up 22 years, 17 days, two hours, and 56 minutes of time— that was her allowance. Not a minute more and not a minute less.

In the front of the Bible she had given me three months before were inscribed the words: "To Tabitha on your 20th birthday. Love, Rebecca." This was followed by, "Come to me, all whose work is hard, whose load is heavy; and I will give you relief. Bend your necks to my yoke, and learn from me, for I am gentle and humble-hearted; and your souls will find relief. For my yoke is good to bear, my load is light" (Matt. 11:28-30, NEB).

In just 22 years Rebecca had learned a secret many of us are still trying to learn: to accept Jesus' invitation to come to Him, to learn of Him and find relief in Him.

How often we ignore His invitation and do our own thing because we're too busy! We schedule too many appointments and hurry our way through life. We struggle with our jobs and relationships, have sleepless nights over our children, run to meetings, shop, and then stop by church for a quick "rest" on Sabbath morning before starting the next week of rush and stress.

God must wonder at our intelligence. His instructions are simple and straightforward: "Come to me," but we seem to forget them in our hurry. A prayer in front of the bathroom mirror, with a toothbrush stuck in the mouth, may be our only time for God—until tragedy strikes.

God has given us an open invitation to decrease our stress level, get rid of our problems, and receive His peace. But it will never happen unless we turn off the television, click off the Internet, and cancel activities that build only ego instead of treasures in heaven.

Why not commit each moment of your life to Christ? Take time to turn your burdens over to Him and trust Him to see you through.

Have you accepted Christ's invitation to come to Him and give Him your burdens? TABITHA ABEL-COOPER

Whole-hearted

Create in me a clean heart, O God, and renew a steadfast spirit within me. Ps. 51:10, NKJV.

AN ALMOST EERIE quietness pervaded the operating room as each member of the surgical team proceeded with professional skill to make his or her assigned preoperative preparations. The hum of the respirator and the rhythmical pumping of the blood bypass machine were broken occasionally by the muffled voices of the doctors as John Doe's chest was opened for a triple bypass.

I was a critical care nurse, in training at the Baptist Hospital in Nashville, Tennessee, assigned to observe.

As a white-gowned surgeon approached the operating table, two other doctors stepped back, leaving just one doctor to assist. I was positioned at the patient's head so that I could have a clear view of the almost motionless organ. The head surgeon reached gently for the heart and held it quietly until it stopped beating. With a nod to the technician in charge of the blood machine, the doctor indicated that the clamp should be applied that would divert John Doe's blood to the machine.

It took only a short time to repair and replace the damaged vessels in the heart. Then as gently as the heart had been stopped, it was thumped to restart; and as we held our breath and waited, the heart slowly began to *lub-dub.* Another victorious nod and the clamp was released. The wonderful blood of life was again activated by its God-given pump. The operating room was no longer quiet. Cheers and congratulations marked the atmosphere.

That exhilarating moment reminded me of the master Creator, who so often reveals His spiritual lessons through the physical reactions of our "fearfully and wonderfully made" bodies.

Our sin-sick hearts have to be stopped, repaired, and restored by the Great Physician. As we open the clamp to our hearts, the blood of Jesus begins our new flow of spiritual life. We are then nursed by the tender love and care (TLC) of Jesus through His Holy Spirit.

Perhaps John Doe did not realize his serious condition until he could no longer control his life alone and needed surgical repair. Now I must question, am I allowing my spiritual life to drift carelessly along?

As I left the operating room that day, I could only pray, "Create in me a clean heart, O God, and renew a steadfast spirit within me."

How is the health of your heart? Ask God now to create in you a whole and healthy heart.   EVELYN R. CHISHOLM

The Power of Personal Religion

"The Lord bless you and keep you; the Lord make His face shine
upon you, and be gracious to you; the Lord lift up His
countenance upon you, and give you peace." Num. 6:24-26, NKJV.

RESEARCHERS HAVE SURPRISING evidence that people who believe in God as a heavenly parent who loves and cares for them, and who actively cultivate that faith, have one of the most effective resources available for managing stress in a crisis and achieving long-term health. Listen to what five famous people have to say on the power of personal religion to detoxify stress:

The "grandfather" of jogging for fitness, cardiologist George Sheehan, credits religion with an almost unequaled power to relieve stress by providing an inner sense of calm and tranquility, a sense that no defeat is final, and a sense of lasting security

During his three years as a prisoner of war at Auschwitz, Jewish psychiatrist Victor Frankl found that if he could help fellow prisoners believe that their experience, horrendous though it was, had some meaning, he could help them maintain the will to survive. He later wrote in his classic, *Man's Search for Meaning:* "There is nothing in the world, I venture to say, that would so effectively help one to survive even the worst condition, as the knowledge that there is a meaning in one's life. . . . Suffering ceases to be suffering in some way at the moment it finds a meaning." (See Romans 8:28.)

In his book *Stress/Unstress: How You Can Control Stress at Home and on the Job,* Dr. Keith Sehnert advocates finding a quiet time each day for prayer and reading the Bible or other devotional literature as a vital component of a well-rounded stress-management program.

Skip MacCarty, in his "Stress: Beyond Coping" seminar, tells of a time when five major stressors were impacting him, resulting in sleepless nights. One night he practiced a key principle from his seminar: he reviewed each problem thoroughly with God, then released them to God one by one. He reports that that night he was able to sleep peacefully for the first time in weeks.

Highly respected author and psychiatrist Paul Tournier said that he used to live a restless life, always racing the clock. But he reported that once he began to devote an hour a day to quiet reflection, devotional meditation, and prayer, he was happier, healthier, and better able to distinguish between priorities, and actually accomplished more.

Why not spend some extra time today with your forever Friend and discover just how powerful this relationship can be in detoxifying stress.   DWIGHT K. NELSON

Obedience or Abuse

Do you not know that you are the temple of God and that the Spirit of God dwells in you? If anyone defiles the temple of God, God will destroy him. For the temple of God is holy, which temple you are. 1 Cor. 3:16, 17, NKJV.

THE BRAIN FUNCTIONS at different levels. The highest is critical thinking or discretion. The second is voluntary motor function—the ability to balance, to breathe on purpose, to focus eyes on an object or touch a finger to the tip of your nose while your eyes are closed. The lowest level is involuntary motor function—the automatic actions of breathing or the beating of your heart.

If one abuses the body with harmful substances, deprives it of sleep, or overeats, the highest level goes first. Abuse it more vigorously and the next level quits working. Abuse it still more and the brain loses the ability to move the muscles of the heart or lungs—death is the result!

One abusive substance is alcohol. If the blood alcohol level begins to rise, the most sensitive or delicate work of the brain grinds to a halt. I often ask, "If you were a nondrinking observer at a party, what would be the first evidence that those imbibing have alcohol in their blood?" The most common answers are slurred speech, unstable walking, double vision. Wrong! The first evidence is loss of discretion—that wonderful sense of when to speak or not; what's appropriate and what's not. Discretion is a result of frontal lobe thinking; it's the part of the brain where the Holy Spirit speaks to you—it's the temple where the Spirit of God dwells!

Scripture says that God will destroy anyone who defiles His temple. This isn't an angry threat by a power-hungry God, but a loving warning. God is trying to save us, and the only way He can accomplish that is by His Holy Spirit living in us, molding us into Christ's likeness.

To maintain the power of discretion—to make the right choices—we must maintain our brains free from abuse. "In order to render to God perfect service, you must have clear conceptions of His requirements. You should . . . [work so that] the fine nerves of the brain be not weakened, benumbed, or paralyzed, making it impossible for you to discern sacred things, and to value the atonement, the cleansing blood of Christ, as of priceless worth" (Ellen G. White, *Testimonies for the Church*, vol. 2, p. 46?.

Lord, give me wisdom and self-control to not abuse Your temple in me!

JIM BRACKETT

Keeping the Commandment
With a Promise

Honor your father and your mother, that your days may be long
upon the land which the Lord your God is giving you. Ex. 20:12, NKJV.

I'M AMAZED AT the healing power of close relationships, especially family relationships. Many studies have shown that having close associations decreases your susceptibility to disease in general. But one of the most interesting studies began in 1952 when Dr. Stanley King and his associates randomly selected 126 healthy male Harvard students and asked them how close they knew their parents and whether or not they had a good relationship with them.

Thirty-five years later, medical records were obtained on these participants and a detailed medical and psychological history was conducted. Here's what they found: 91 percent who did not have a close relationship with their mothers had serious diseases in midlife, including coronary artery disease, hypertension, duodenal ulcer, and alcoholism, as compared to 45 percent who did have close relationships with their mothers. Similarly, 82 percent who did not have a close relationship with their father had diagnosed diseases in midlife as compared to 50 percent who had a close relationship with their fathers. The most incredible finding was that 100 percent of those who did not have close relationships with both their mothers and fathers, had disease diagnosed in midlife compared to 47 percent who had close relationships with both.

This significant correlation of good relationships with parents and future health was independent of a family history of illness, smoking, emotional stress, subsequent health or divorce of parents, and students' marital history.

The researchers concluded that just the fact that someone knows you closely and cares for you promotes immune function and healing.

God commanded that we maintain a healthy relationship with our parents when He wrote the fifth commandment. And isn't it interesting that this is the only commandment with the promise of long life attached? God, our Creator, obviously knew we needed this protective factor. What a different world this would be if we would take God at His Word.

Isn't it about time we obey God's commandment by forgiving and being kind to our parents, regardless of past hurts, and then begin to enjoy the health benefits?

KATHLEEN H. LIWIDJAJA-KUNTARAF

The Power of Intercessory Prayer

And the Lord restored Job's losses when he prayed for his friends. Indeed the Lord gave Job twice as much as he had before. Job 42:10, NKJV.

ALMOST EVERYONE knows someone, or has heard of someone, who miraculously recovered from an illness as a result of prayer. Yet it is one thing to believe prayer heals by pointing to a few cases, and quite another to prove it scientifically. But that's exactly what two researchers have done.

Dale Mathews, M.D., a professor and internist at Georgetown University School of Medicine, along with Sally Marlowe, R.N., a nurse practitioner, conducted a study on prayer, using the same design and controls that any scientist would use to evaluate a new drug.

Forty arthritis patients from the Arthritis/Pain Treatment Center in Clearwater, Florida, were treated with prayer during an intensive, hands-on healing session. The patients then were split into two groups. Half received booster doses of long-distance prayer without their knowledge, every day for six months, while the other half received no additional prayer. Of course, a control group received no prayer at all from beginning to end. All of the patients were monitored by trained clinical professionals who relied on standardized diagnostic measurements such as grip strength tests and blood analysis to monitor signs of progress.

Now that the results are in, there is no doubt that God is listening to the prayers of His people and granting their requests. Healing happens even though the person being prayed for doesn't know it! More studies on intercessory prayer are now being conducted—and so far the results are positive.

But there is another aspect of intercessory prayer—the positive effect that prayer has on the person who prays. Remember Job? He lost everything in one day! He literally went from riches to rags. Then came the incredible pain of boils from head to foot. But when others counseled him to curse God and die, he responded, "Though He slay me, yet will I trust Him," and he continued to pray. What faith! But when was it that God gave him everything back? Not when Job prayed for himself, although he was agonizing in pain. It was when he prayed for his friends! Apparently there is a throw-back blessing to those who pray for others. Job experienced it. And you can too!

Lord, give me a heart that weeps, rejoices, and prays for others, regardless of my own situation.   GERARD MCLANE

Light at the End of the Tunnel

When I was in distress, I sought the Lord; at night I stretched out untiring
hands and my soul refused to be comforted. I remembered you, O God,
and I groaned; I mused, and my spirit grew faint. You kept my eyes
from closing; I was too troubled to speak. Ps. 77:2-4, NIV.

CAROLYN OPENED HER eyes and sighed. She should get up but couldn't will her body to move. What was happening to her? The sun was shining outside, but she couldn't get the fog to lift in her mind. She had everything to live for—if you saw her life from the perspective of others; but from her own perspective—nothing!

The feelings of hopelessness and sleeplessness, guilt, and being far from God expressed by David are all symptoms of what we now know to be the illness of depression. This is a genetically determined disease caused by a decrease in certain chemicals in the brain. The sufferer feels that a heavy cloud is pressing on his or her shoulders. These feelings may be so intense as to lead to suicidal thoughts or actions!

Mild forms of this condition may be helped by exercise, but often the sufferer is too ill to initiate the activity. Even dedicated Christians may feel God has deserted them and say like David, "I remembered You, O God, and I groaned."

For these people, medication may be necessary and indeed life-saving. It is no more possible for the person with a true clinical depression to "smarten up and liven up" than it is for the young diabetic to reduce his blood sugar simply by thinking it is lower. Both are suffering from chemical disorders that need chemical treatment.

Christians often have a lot of guilt over feeling depressed. For these people the good news is that this is not their fault. They have an illness *and it is treatable*. In spite of some possible side effects, when antidepressant medications are used carefully and judiciously, they can be life changing and life-saving.

All depression sufferers should be treated with compassion and encouragement. They need to get their chemistry as near to normal as possible, and to remember that the same psalmist who wrote the depressing words of Psalm 77 also wrote Psalm 81:1, "Sing for joy to God our strength" (NIV).

O Lord, give me compassion for others who suffer from conditions I don't un-
derstand. And when my own life turns bleak, give me wisdom to seek the help I
need. Amen.   RUTH LENNOX

Getting Older and Getting Better

*You are worthy, O Lord, to receive glory and honor and power: for You created
all things, and by Your will they exist and were created. Rev. 4:11, NKJV.*

MOST OF US have learned that we'd better take care of ourselves because
our days are numbered. But we've also learned that even when our bodies have been neglected, if we start treating them right the improvement
can be astonishing.

Hulda Crooks lost her husband when she was about 60 years old. Her
own health was deteriorating and her doctor told her that if she didn't start
getting exercise she would soon follow her mate. She took him seriously
and began to walk, increasing the distance every day. Then she began hiking. She started following the trails of Mount San Gorgornio, near her
home in Southern California. Eventually she tackled Mount Whitney, the
highest mountain in the contiguous 48 states. By the time she was 91 she
had hiked to the top of Mount Whitney and back 23 times.

Then there's Jack Lalanne. Somewhere he heard that after 30 years of
age we lose two percent of our muscle mass every year; when we are about
70 or so we don't have the strength to get out of a chair. He was the first
exercise guru on television—more than 50 years ago. When he was 45
years old he completed 1,000 push-ups and 1,000 chin-ups in less than an
hour and a half. (I'm not sure I could do 1,000 chin-ups in a week. Maybe
someone reading this can't even do one!) At 60 years he shackled his wrists
behind him, tied his ankles together, and attached himself to a 1,000-
pound boat that he pulled, porpoise-like, from Alcatraz to Fisherman's
Wharf, a distance of about seven miles. At 70 years, hands and feet similarly shackled, he towed 70 boats with a person in each for almost two
miles across Long Beach Harbor. At 80 he was going to do the same thing
with 80 boats, but I've heard his wife put her foot down.

Our bodies are indeed wonderfully made! If you're growing older and
concerned about your health going downhill, why not start treating your
body right. Who knows what possibilities God has created within you!
And think about the glory and honor you will be showing to the God of
the universe for His marvelous creation.

God, give me the self-discipline to get better for You.   JIM BRACKETT

Trusted With Trials

*Then the Lord said to Satan, "Have you considered My servant Job,
that there is none like him on the earth, a blameless and upright
man, one who fears God and shuns evil?" Job 1:8, NKJV.*

WE THINK WE have trials! What would it be like to lose seven sons, three daughters, all your servants, and thousands of sheep, camels, and cattle in one day? Then before you have time to recover from the shock, you're notified that you have also lost every material possession! If that combination of events isn't enough of a heart-rending trial, you are now smitten with painful, oozing boils from the top of your head to the soles of your feet! Adding insult to injury, your spouse says, "Curse God and die!"

Thank God for the story of Job, who cries out in his pain, "Though He slay me, yet will I trust Him" (Job 13:15, NKJV). This story gives special insight into the controversy between Christ and Satan that is raging over every soul.

Satan made the accusation "Job serves You only because of what he gets from You." God had to set Job's record straight by allowing him to be tested to the nth degree. God proved that Job did not serve Him because of all of His blessings, but because he loved Him.

God proved that Job was trustworthy. How about you? Do you murmur and complain when you're tested with fiery trials?

Next time, remember that God is endeavoring to show that you are worthy of His trust. If you submit to the refining fire, all the dross will be burned away and your character will shine like the purest gold. You will become like Jesus, who is making you safe to be trusted in His sinless universe.

Here's a reassuring thought: "The Father's presence encircled Christ, and nothing befell Him but that which infinite love permitted for the blessing of the world. Here was His source of comfort, and it is for us. He who is imbued with the Spirit of Christ abides in Christ. The blow that is aimed at him falls upon the Savior, who surrounds him with His presence. Whatever comes to him comes from Christ. He has no need to resist evil, for Christ is his defense. Nothing can touch him except by our Lord's permission" (Ellen G. White, *Thoughts From the Mount of Blessing*, p. 71).

Regardless of what's happening in your life today, can you say as Job did, "Though He slay me, yet will I trust Him"? KAY COLLINS

Avoiding the Rotten Hole

Examine yourselves to see whether you are in the faith;
test yourselves. Do you not realize that Christ Jesus is in you
—unless, of course, you fail the test? 2 Cor. 13:5, NIV.

PATIENTS TELL ME, "My tooth just broke off, and I didn't even know anything was wrong!" How does that happen? The problem begins in a small way. Decay starts in a tooth when bacterial plaque releases acid onto the enamel, breaking down the enamel. Once the decay is through the enamel, the softer part of the tooth is undermined by bacterial acid and a small cavity has begun.

A cavity that looks small on the outside is actually much larger underneath. The tooth is being undermined by the decay; if the decay remains undetected, the enamel will break away, leaving a large hole in your tooth. That is why you need to have your teeth examined regularly by a dentist. The dentist has ways to detect cavities and their size. One is by examining the teeth directly. He can tell if the possible cavity is soft and needs filled. X-rays can also help detect decay.

Some people think a tiny black spot on their teeth is not a big enough reason to go to the dentist because it doesn't hurt yet! They are wrong to let that small spot fool them. Once the decay goes through the enamel, it will spread quickly. The rotten area will continue to enlarge and begin to affect the nerve. At first the tooth may be sensitive to cold and sweet. Then as the cavity grows closer to the nerve, it will become sensitive to heat as well, and may have episodes of sensitivity with no apparent cause. Eventually the decay will reach the nerve and severe pain sets in, and the bacteria will damage the nerve beyond repair. The bacteria enter the nerve chamber of the tooth, and the tooth becomes abscessed.

This problem can be prevented easily by simply filling the tooth before the decay reaches the nerve. If a person waits too long and lets the nerve become damaged, the dentist will have to remove the nerve and all the bacteria and fill in the nerve chamber with a filling material to prevent an abscess.

Satan is a destroyer and seeks to decay our relationship with Jesus—to create a vast rotten hole between us. Jesus is the restorer; He can stop Satan's decay in our life and bring healing to our soul.

What can you do today to make sure Satan doesn't create a rotten hole between you and Jesus?						EDDIE C. TOWLES

MARCH 25

Elevation From the Pit of Fear

I waited patiently for the Lord; he turned to me and heard my cry. He lifted me out of the slimy pit, out of the mud and mire; he set my feet on a rock and gave me a firm place to stand. He put a new song in my mouth, a hymn of praise to our God. Many will see and fear and put their trust in the Lord. Ps. 40:1-3, NIV.

ONCE I HAD a mole on my face. Every time I shaved it would bleed, so I had it surgically removed. The doctor said it was a common mole and not cancerous. I was thankful for the good news. Not everyone, however, is as fortunate.

Onecia had a mole on her leg and had it surgically removed. The test results were not good. The mole was the dreaded melanoma. The very word can send shock waves of terror through one's mind, as often it is a death sentence! A few days later, Onecia asked to be anointed.

That evening, the elders and I knelt around her and her husband. Tearfully we anointed her and pled with God to heal her according to His will. She had more extensive surgery and skin grafts. Here's the rest of the story, in her words:

"The pit of fear that engulfs one at a time like this cannot be described. It is worse than the illness. The ritual of anointing calls for repentance and submission to God, while God's gift back to us is *cleansing of spirit and elevation from the pit of fear.* In my case, my health was restored. But I also like to revisit the anointing service in my mind, and remember the merciful God who gave us hope at a time of despair. Satan is always ready to tempt us to doubt, but God is even more ready to help us in our time of need!"

But what if her experience had yielded a different outcome, as it did for Dr. Calvin Thrash? He was a saint of a man; with his wife, Agatha, he started the Uchee Pines Institute, a lifestyle center in Seale, Alabama. He too was diagnosed with melanoma. It was successfully removed, but later it returned. He was anointed, but the cancer took his life. But he, too, was delivered from the pit of fear; he died praising God for His love.

Regardless of the outcome, there is no reason to fear, and no reason for faith to waiver. God holds the whole world in His hands—and your life as well!

Are you anxious today? Trust God; you too can experience the miracle of being delivered from the pit of fear! JIM COX, with KAY KUZMA

94

A Helper's High

Let us not become weary in doing good, for at the proper time we will reap a harvest if we do not give up. Gal. 6:9, NIV.

CHRISTIANITY FOSTERS A "reach out and touch somebody" service philosophy. We do this because God said to. Here are a dozen admonitions that call for service:

1. Have mercy on the poor (Prov. 14:21). 2. Help your neighbor (Isa. 41:6). 3. Feed the hungry (Isa. 58:7). 4. Give a drink (Matt. 10:42). 5. If you have two coats, give one to someone who needs it (Luke 3:11). 6. Give, and it shall be given to you (Luke 6:38). 7. Care for others (1 Cor. 12:25). 8. Be kind and tenderhearted (Eph. 4:32). 9. Support the weak (1 Thess. 5:14). 10. Visit the fatherless and widows (James 1:27). 11. Clothe the naked (James 2:15, 16). 12. If our enemies are hungry, feed them (Prov. 25:21).

But what most don't realize is that we actually improve our own health, as well as the health of those around us, when we practice simple kindness, benevolence, and service to others.

Allan Luks, in his book *The Healing Power of Doing Good,* says that when people volunteer to help those around them, they get a rush of good feeling that he calls a "helper's high." This feeling can sharply reduce stress and release the body's natural painkillers, the endorphins. This initial "rush" is then followed by a longer-lasting period of improved emotional well-being.

Those who regularly visit in the hospitals to pray, to take flowers, and to sing can get this helper's high. Nearly eight out of ten volunteers said the good feelings of the helping syndrome returns, though in diminished intensity, when the helping act is remembered. Imagine, just thinking about it produces the helper's high!

Finding the time is the biggest obstacle to helping others. That's one of the reasons I believe God created a special day for healing and serving. It's the Sabbath.

Most Christians observe a special day for worship and reflection, but too many forget that Jesus said we should also do good on the Sabbath. "If any of you has a sheep and it falls into a pit on the Sabbath, will you not take hold of it and lift it out? How much more valuable is a man than a sheep! Therefore it is lawful to do good on the Sabbath" (Matt. 12:12, NIV).

Plan today what you can do to help someone this next Sabbath. In doing so, you'll experience the greater blessing—the helper's high!

DEWITT S. WILLIAMS

Love in the Twenty-first Century

Though I speak with the tongues of men and of angels, but have not love,
I have become sounding brass or a clanging cymbal. 1 Cor. 13:1, NKJV.

THE ABOVE LINES are so familiar it's easy to merely parrot them without considering the real meaning. Have you ever wondered what the apostle Paul would have said about love if he were writing today? Perhaps he would have said something like this:

If I speak with the confidence of Rush Limbaugh and sing with the ease of Celine Dion but don't have love, my words are like scraping fingernails on a frozen windshield.

If I can program NASA's mainframe computer and outsmart my chemistry professor, if I can memorize the Psalms and read Leviticus without dozing, or if I can even predict the future, but have not love, my value is equal to a pitcher of slime.

If I give my Tommy Hilfiger wardrobe to Goodwill and let my little sister rummage through my closet, if I go to the stake and die as a martyr, or if I donate a gallon of blood every hour, but don't have love, my offerings are useless.

Love is patient—even if it means skipping a trip to 31 Flavors in order to tutor an immigrant.

Love is kind—it doesn't stoop to ethnic slurs.

Love does not envy the basketball team captain, the National Merit finalist, the class president, or even the blond who sports the most even tan.

Love doesn't get a swelled head over straight A's or a scholarship to Princeton. Love isn't snooty about a new Corvette or a season pass to the world's premiere ski resort. Love never jeers at the overweight kid in PE.

Love smiles when getting cut off on the interstate. Love submits an honest tax return. Love doesn't whine about the referee's bad call. Love believes that God always provides the best stuff in life. Love hangs on to hope when the family is splitting apart.

Love does not change like hemlines and hairdos. Love is like the Energizer bunny. It lasts and lasts and keeps on going. In the end only three things will remain: faith, hope, and love. But the greatest of these is love.

God loves you supremely, and asks you to love others as He loves you. How would you rate yourself when it comes to truly loving others? What could you do to improve that rating? KARL HAFFNER

Making Lemonade

I tell you the truth, if you have faith as small as a mustard seed,
you can say to this mountain, "Move from here to there" and it
will move. Nothing will be impossible for you. Matt. 17:20, NIV.

THE DAY AFTER my father's funeral, I was surprised that instead of flowers, a package was delivered to my sorrowing mother. She opened it and found a basket with dry moss on top. A note explained that this was a spring garden, but it certainly didn't look like much. The directions said to place it where it would receive sunlight, water it, and in a short time she would have a basket of tulips, hyacinths, and daffodils.

When the basket bloomed, it was so beautiful that Mom decided to take it to church. Just as the service began the pastor asked Mom if she would give the children's story. She consented. As she began to walk down the aisle she was still trying to decide what she should tell. Then her eyes fell on the basket of spring flowers and she thought, *I'll tell the children how Grandpa Roy is in the "Waiting Place," waiting for Jesus to come, just like those bulbs were waiting to bloom.* The children sat spellbound as she explained to them this difficult subject. When she finished the story she asked, "And what will Grandpa be like when Jesus comes?"

McKenzie stretched out her arms and with a big smile said, "He'll be brand new."

After the service the pastor told Mom he'd never heard a more beautiful explanation of death and suggested she write a children' storybook. She did, and that was the start of her brand new life. With the encouragement of my sister, Margie, and friends, Mother wrote *The Waiting Place* and also a book about the universe. Along with the books, she has written songs and designed toys that are now being marketed.

You've heard it said, "If life gives you a lemon, make lemonade." I believe Mother has not only made lemonade but a lemon meringue pie as well! Now at 77 years of age Mom continues to praise the Lord and expect miracles. She is living the words to one of her latest songs,

"Set your course on high, for it's all up to you,
To choose the right course you wish to pursue.
Your life can be useful. Don't be left behind.
When the journey's over, you've had a great time."

Today is a brand-new day to begin to pursue your dream and to bloom for God.

RITA STEVENS

Restoring the Abundant Life

Worship the Lord your God, and his blessing
will be on your food and water. Ex. 23:25, NIV.

MELVIN REALLY WANTED to go to Rio de Janeiro. The president of his company and a number of delegates were going there to meet leaders from other countries. As head of security, his job was to arrange for their safety and protection, and oversee the operation once they arrived. It was an exciting assignment and also the chance of a lifetime to see one of the world's most beautiful cities.

But Melvin had serious health problems. He was overweight, his blood pressure was too high, and even daily injections of insulin were not controlling his diabetes. He'd had these problems for 17 years, but despite following all the doctors' orders he kept getting worse. As the time neared for the trip he felt so sick and discouraged he knew there was little chance he could go.

His boss urged him to attend Weimar Institute, a live-in health center in California that specialized in problems like his. "It's very biblically oriented," he said. Any ray of hope was welcome. Melvin, only 49, was determined to fight for his life.

At Weimar he ate a natural diet, whole plant foods that were not processed or refined. He learned that high-fiber foods stabilized blood sugar levels, a very low fat intake helped activate the body's natural insulin, and normalizing weight was an important factor in reversing this disease.

Exercise, he was told, helped the body use up its excess blood sugar. Soon he was walking up to 15 miles a day. This helped him lower his blood pressure, lose weight, reduce his insulin needs, banish depression, and condition his body.

At the end of the month he could hardly believe the results. He had lost 22 pounds, his blood pressure was normal without medication, and his blood sugar was staying within normal limits without any insulin injections. "I felt like a man out of prison," he told me. "I can't remember ever feeling better in my life."

And yes, he went to Rio, feeling great and functioning well.

When I talked to Melvin a couple years later, he assured me he was doing quite well and was busy planning a company trip to Costa Rica.

God has given principles for us to live by that can restore abundant health. Don't accept your condition as something you've got to endure, until you first try a healthy lifestyle change.

Lord, thank You for blessing my efforts to "get back on track" with Your principles.

AILEEN LUDINGTON

Doctor's Day

Luke the beloved physician and Demas greet you. Col. 4:14, NKJV.

IN THE UNITED STATES March 30 is Doctor's Day. Back in the 1930s Mrs. Charles Almond of Winder, Georgia, suggested that a day be observed annually to recognize and honor members of the medical profession. March 30 was chosen because it was on that date in 1842 that ether was first used as an anesthetic agent in surgery by Dr. Crawford Long, a Georgia physician. His contribution to painless surgery was indeed a medical milestone.

The first observance of Doctor's Day was in 1933; citizens of Barrow County, Georgia, placed red carnations on the graves of deceased physicians, including the grave of Dr. Long. But it wasn't until 1990 that Congress officially designated March 30 as national Doctor's Day.

A doctor's life in the United States can be frustrating. The physician's highest responsibility and honor is to be the patient's advocate. But the pressures of the public, government, employers, and insurance companies to decrease cost while improving quality create constant tension and ethical dilemmas unknown to physicians just a few short years ago. The hassles of managed care, mounting paperwork, reduced reimbursement, long hours, fear of law suits, fragmented family life, staggering educational debt, and loss of autonomy have driven many physicians to the brink. Many are opting for early retirement or entering nonclinical fields.

For those not in the medical field it's sometimes difficult to have much sympathy for the plight of today's physician, since they still enjoy a relatively comfortable lifestyle and considerable community prestige.

When Jesus healed the 10 lepers, only one came back to thank Him. Jesus said, "Were not all ten cleansed? Where are the other nine? Was no one found to return and give praise to God except this foreigner?" (Luke 17:17, 18, NIV). Even the Great Physician lamented such lack of gratitude.

Although you should never forget that God is the source of all healing, take a moment today to write a short note to your physicians expressing your thanks and appreciation. It will go a long way toward making their day—and it might even make them seem less hurried and harried at your next office visit.

Thank You, Lord, for Your servants, the physicians, who bring Your healing to so many. GREGORY R. WISE

Ask, Believe, and Receive!

Ask, and it will be given to you; seek, and you will find; knock, and it will be opened to you. Matt. 7:7, NKJV.

I WAS IN CHARGE of community health ministries for my church in Chino, California, and for the Portuguese community there. We decided to buy a machine that could measure cholesterol. The program was highly successful. Everyone was eager to get their test done.

One day a scared old woman came to me. "Doctor," she said, "my cholesterol is too high. I don't know what to do. It's more than 260 mg/dl and I am in real trouble."

I started to give her advice about the effect of diet and exercise on cholesterol. She explained she didn't need advice, just another test to see if the diet she had been on was working.

"How long has it been since you were tested?"

"Two weeks," she replied.

I told her that there had not been enough time for her cholesterol to drop significantly and tried to prepare her for bad news. She was so nervous about what the test might show that I tried to calm her down. Then as I prepared the machine, she started to pray. "Please, Lord," she pleaded, "Help me with this exam. Make it be normal, please."

I did the finger puncture, put the blood drop in the cassette, and while I waited for the result I attempted to give her some support. I told her she must first change her lifestyle. After time she would see the results in her blood test.

Then the machine *bipped* the result: 165 mg/dl. I was surprised, but she wasn't.

She told me, "Doctor, you didn't believe God would do a miracle for me, did you? Don't you trust Him?" I was speechless. I just congratulated her and continued my work.

Since then I've thought a lot about what happened that day. Why is it that we so often fail to mention prayer when we give lifestyle advice to someone suffering from an illness that could have been prevented? Prayer should really be at the top of our list. First, we should ask for the miracle of healing, as this woman did; and second, for the miracle of enough willpower to live a healthy lifestyle. God does say that if we ask, it will be given.

Have you claimed God's promise in Matthew 7:7 today?

HILDEMAR DOS SANTOS

How Healthy Is Your Frontal Lobe?*

*See that no one renders evil for evil to anyone, but always pursue
what is good both for yourselves and for all. 1 Thess. 5:15, NKJV.*

TWENTY-FIVE-YEAR-OLD Phineas Gage was in charge of blasting a railroad bed through a mountainous area. But what happened on September 13, 1848, destroyed the person his family, friends, and employers knew, and sent into society a man who looked like Phineas but wasn't.

As Phineas was preparing for blasting, he drilled a hole in the rock and poured in explosive powder. But instead of adding sand on top of the powder and then pounding it down with a tamping iron, he started pounding directly on the powder. A spark ignited the powder, and the blast drove the tamping iron up the hole and through Phineas' head. It entered under his left cheekbone, went behind his left eye, through his frontal lobe, and out again, landing several yards away.

Amazingly, Phineas didn't die. Within a short time he regained consciousness and was able to talk, and even walk with the aid of his coworkers. He lost the use of his left eye, but other than that he made a nearly complete recovery—physically. But he was no longer the same man.

Before the accident he was a well-loved, responsible, and intelligent husband and worker. Employee records referred to him as a capable foreman. He had high morals and was a pious churchgoer.

Although his movement, speech, and memory were not affected by the accident, his moral decline was immediate. He became irreverent and prone to excessive profanity. He lost all respect for social customs and became totally irresponsible. He ended up losing his job, leaving his wife and family, and joining a traveling circus.

Are you interested in developing a character with integrity and the capacity for making wholesome decisions? Then don't do anything to compromise the function of your frontal lobe!

Start by eating a good brain-food diet and avoiding drugs. Why does alcohol, caffeine, and nicotine affect behavior in such a marked degree? Because they attack the frontal lobe, causing loss of control and fuzzy thinking. Why are coffee and gossiping so often related? It's suggested that the caffeine loosens the tongue! Illicit drugs kill brain cells; but even certain prescription drugs can be harmful, especially those that restrict the flow of blood.

Remember, how you treat your body today affects your thinking tomorrow!

KAY KUZMA

---

*Niel Nedley. *Proof Positive,* "Story of Phineas Gage."

APRIL 2

Mountaintop Experience

*Hear me, O Lord, hear me, that this people may know that You are the Lord
God, and that You have turned their hearts back to You again. 1 Kings 18:37, NKJV.*

MOUNT LASSEN LOOMED ahead—breathtaking in its grandeur. Even
the July sun had not melted all the snow. What a challenge it offered to
our multifamily group: parents, aunts, uncles, and cousins. It must be
climbed! To Robert and me it would be a new experience.

We were informed of the rigorous climb, the steep winding paths and
the snow fields to be crossed. That did not discourage us. After a hefty
camp breakfast, the family caravan was on its way to the base starting point.

The description was correct. As we climbed, tiredness slowed us down
while others forged ahead. We could not stop, for our goal was nothing
less than the mountain crest. Near the top, the ascent was slower, one step
at a time, one foot ahead of the other. We would not be deterred! Others
were ahead, expecting us, which was an encouragement.

As the first group rounded the large boulders to the summit, they were
filled with awe and praise at the beauty and vastness, the wonders of God's
creation. They began singing "How Great Thou Art." Their voices
echoed from the peak. Soon we too joined the others in songs of praise.
What a mountaintop experience!

It reminds me of Elijah's mountaintop experience. God had manifested
His power and majesty in a mighty way. When Elijah prayed, "Hear me,
O Lord," fire came down from heaven and consumed his sacrifice. God
was alive—and the prophets of Baal were put to rout. Elijah worked all day
without food. His courage was strong despite the stress. Then God answered again. Rain came, and with it a psychological high that gave Elijah
energy to run more than 25 miles in front of Ahab's chariot to Jezreel.

Then Jezebel's threat! Elijah's body craved rest, but fear for his life
drove him to the desert—running without food or sleep for another 120
miles. Exhausted, he became depressed and despondent. Only after he was
restored by food, rest, and communion with God was he able to resume
his divinely-assigned work.

Elijah had temporarily forgotten that the same things that lead to a
mountaintop experience keep one from the valley of discouragement:
meeting physical needs and communing with God.

May you have a mountaintop experience communing with God today.

LENNA LEE CHASE DAVIDSON

102

God's Sexual Software

You have heard that it was said, "Do not commit adultery." But I tell you that anyone who looks at a woman lustfully has already committed adultery with her in his heart. Matt. 5:27, 28, NIV.

THEY WERE FRIENDS and colleagues. He was the CEO, someone who made her feel important. She was the director of community relations and made him look good. They seemed to bring out the creativity in each other. When he invited her to lunch—on her day off—red flags began to fly. She asked, "Why?" He was truthful, "I was lonely for a good conversation—and we've been so busy we haven't had time to talk."

Innocent? Yes . . . but!

God has put certain software into our brains to keep our marriages stimulating and need-fulfilling. If used properly, it leads to long, meaningful marriages. But if we aren't aware of the exclusive nature of this software, it can easily lead to an affair.

Here's how the software is programmed: Men's greatest need is sexual fulfillment (companionship); women—emotional fulfillment (communication). When a man meets a woman's emotional needs there is a built-in tendency for him to expect a sexual payoff, and a woman is more ready to give it since her needs are met. This is the key to a vibrant marriage.

But here's the problem: even if a woman is happily married, if she begins to feel her emotional needs are being met by another man she will feel drawn to that man sexually. And having met her emotional needs, it is natural for him to expect a payoff. A woman can't safely take a companionship role with a man without him eventually expecting sex. A man can't safely take the role of a good listener without eventually breaking down a woman's resistance to say no.

Keeping these needs met in marriage is one way to avoid an affair. But it's not enough. A woman must be careful working so closely with a man that she becomes his needed companion—for his own creativity, career, or self-esteem. And a man must not linger in conversation with a woman so long that she becomes addicted to having her emotional needs met by him.

Here's the question: Is it healthy for a married man or woman to work with a person of the opposite sex? The answer: No, not exclusively or for long periods of time where companionship and emotional needs are being met by someone other than the spouse.

Wise God, help me to live a Christlike life at home and in the workplace.

KAY KUZMA

God's Natural Remedies

Now the Lord God had planted a garden in the east, in Eden; and there he put the man he had formed. And the Lord God made all kinds of trees grow out of the ground— trees that were pleasing to the eye and good for food. In the middle of the garden were the tree of life and the tree of the knowledge of good and evil. Gen. 2:8, 9, NIV.

IN GOD'S BEGINNING garden everything was perfect. There were no thorns, decay, or poisonous substances. But Satan changed all that. The amazing thing is that God, even in nature, was a step ahead of Satan, and created remedies for bad things.

Just imagine: The air is filled with the sweet smells and sounds of spring. As you walk through your garden to stop and smell your newly blooming roses, you notice that another of God's creatures has found that same flower. You watch the creature buzz around, then make its way into the bud to collect the nutritious nectar. Suddenly, as you are watching the little worker, you feel a sharp sting on your arm. Looking down, you see your creature's little friend leaving your arm, and a red dot now begins to appear on it. Bee sting! Quickly your brain thinks of all the remedies that you have heard of to help this very common problem: Charcoal, baking soda, mud, raw potato. . . .

Across the yard you spot your vegetable garden and see the little onion shoots sprouting out of the ground. This reminds you of a remedy that you heard about: A cut onion on a bee sting will draw out the poison. Running to the garden, you dig up an onion and take it inside to slice it up and place it on the large red spot on your arm. Within a few minutes the poison is drawn out and the stinger floats easily to the surface. This decreases your sense of pain, and you begin to feel better.

The more we learn about nature, the more we appreciate a wonderful, all-wise God who has provided for our health needs. We praise Him for the remedies within nature—and for the remedies available through modern medicine when no natural remedy is available.

Discovering nature's remedies can be as beneficial to your body as when you study God's Word and find its remedies for the soul. If you study the Bible, God's messages of comfort can be triggered in your mind to help you find peace. Just as Jesus cleanses us and pulls out the "stings" in our lives, there is something good in God's nature that can fix the evil Satan has engineered. That's the way our loving Creator God planned it.

Is Satan trying to poison your life? Open your Bible and find God's remedy. It's there!   MELINDA WORDEN

Pushing Your Pause Button

Remember the Sabbath day, to keep in holy. Six days you shall labor and do all your work, but the seventh day is the Sabbath of the Lord your God. In it you shall do no work. Ex. 20:8-10, NKJV.

WE LIVE IN AN "I'm too busy" world. Fast foods; 15-minute oil changes; one-hour photo development. Even surgery is done on an outpatient basis—you're on your way home before you've had a chance to rest! Modern society is stuck in the fast-forwarding mode. But even the VCR has a pause button. And if we want to find ultimate health and live longer, we've got to find the lost rhythm between action and rest. That healthy ratio between work and play. That balance between doing it our way and doing it God's way.

There is an answer to the "I'm too busy" refrain. It's found in God's commandment to "Remember the Sabbath day, to keep it holy." It's the winning formula of six days for us and one for God, or calculated in hours: 144 for us and 24 for God. But to get the benefits, it can't be sprinkled a little here and there. Just as catnapping can't take the place of a good night's sleep, so mini-vacations cannot take the place of the 24-hour pause that God has commanded we observe.

Wayne Muller writes in his book *Sabbath: Remembering the Sacred Rhythm of Rest and Delight*, "Sabbath is more than the absence of work; it is a day when we partake of the wisdom, peace and delight that grow only in the soil of time—time consecrated specifically for play, refreshment, and renewal."

How can you step off the "I'm too busy" merry-go-round and keep God's Sabbath day holy? How can you celebrate this pause in time so you'll come away refreshed and revived?

Celebrate the beginning of the Sabbath. The Jews and many Bible-believing Christians observe Sabbath on the seventh day, from sundown Friday night until sundown Saturday night. Put away the ritual things you do during the week, such as newspapers and TV, and create Sabbath rituals. Light candles, set the table with the aroma of fresh flowers and the sparkle of your very best china. Fix some special food, something that week after week becomes associated with God's time. As you taste it you remember God and all that He has done for you. Worship Him. When your mind is focused on God, you can't think about yourself and all you have to do.

Are you experiencing the rest and delight God wants you to enjoy? Press the pause button and celebrate God's holy Sabbath. JAN W. KUZMA

Solving Insomnia

But as they sailed He fell asleep. And a windstorm came down on the lake, and they were filling with water, and were in jeopardy. Luke 8:23, NKJV.

FATIGUE IS ONE of the 10 most common reasons people go to the doctor. The remedy should be simple. Get more sleep. But amazingly, a significant percentage of tired people can't fall asleep—or they wake up after a few hours. Although 34 percent of older people complain of insomnia, sleep problems are common in all ages.

King Saul suffered from insomnia. I'm sure it didn't help that he had turned away from God. Guilt has a way of keeping us up at night. Contrast Saul's palace insomnia to Peter's ability to sleep even when imprisoned unjustly. He had to be awakened by an angel before being set free. The best illustration of a sound sleeper, however, is Jesus, asleep in the boat in the midst of the fury of a storm. How did He do that?

Troublesome emotions can keep us up walking the floor at night. Guilt, anger, fear, anxiety, bitterness. But your lifestyle can do the same. It all has to do with the production of the hormone melatonin. In 1933 melatonin was discovered to be a natural sleep aid. It decreases the time to fall asleep by 14 minutes; improves sleep efficiency—but not total sleep time; helps travelers overcome jet lag; and is especially helpful in solving sleep problems of the elderly. In two years after its discovery it was so popular that 24 companies in the United States were marketing it. Everyone was popping pills. But the body's own production of melatonin can be enhanced with the proper lifestyle.

One of the best things you can do to increase melatonin at night is to expose yourself to bright outdoor light early in the day. At the same time, if you want to fall asleep quickly, avoid bright artificial lights. Sleep in total darkness. And try to get to sleep before midnight. Two hours of good sleep before midnight is worth more than four hours after 12:00.

Exercise also boosts melatonin. And you get it in your diet. Melatonin is high in oats, corn, rice, barley, tomatoes, and bananas. Foods high in tryptophan and vitamin B_6 tend to increase melatonin levels. So eat nuts, sesame and pumpkin seeds, and bell peppers. Fasting tends to stimulate melatonin production, especially during the evening hours. Be sure to get enough calcium and avoid anti-inflammatory drugs, antidepressants, and sleep aids.

Jesus' lifestyle allowed Him to sleep through a storm. What aspects of His lifestyle might we emulate? KAY KUZMA

Dejunk Your Life

*You still lack one thing. Sell all that you have and distribute to the poor,
and you will have treasure in heaven; and come, follow Me. Luke 18: 22, NKJV.*

HOW MUCH TIME do you spend picking up and putting things away,
looking for something you just had, or digging through your dresser draw-
ers searching for a missing sock? Is your desk piled high with junk mail?
And does your closet look like a thrift shop filled with outgrown stuff?

Don Aslett, author of *Clutter's Last Stand,* estimates that the average
family in America has 75 percent more toys and 25 percent more furniture
than it really needs. In addition, garages, originally designed for automobiles, now store old refrigerators and burned-out dryers, and are graveyards
for unused sports and camping equipment. We have become a generation
rich in possessions! But the question is, Are possessions controlling you, or
are you controlling them?

Maybe the answer is to follow Christ's advice to the rich young ruler
to give his possessions to the poor and begin to dejunk your life. Try these
dejunking ideas:

• Every time you purchase a new garment, dispose of an old one. If
you can't part with a particular garment, store it for six months. If you
haven't worn it in that time, send it to a thrift shop.

• Sort your mail while standing next to the wastebasket. Open the important mail and organize it into categories such as bills to be paid or correspondence to be answered. Reduce the piles of old magazines by tearing
out the articles or recipes you wish to keep and file them. Then take what's
left to the recycling center.

• Find some poor families in your community with children younger
than yours who would enjoy the toys and clothing that your children have
outgrown. And give them away.

• Have an annual garage sale and turn your trash into cash. It will
amaze you what people will buy if the price is right.

Does your personal life need to be dejunked? Too many Christians store
up negative emotions of guilt and vindictiveness. Others hold on to unhealthy
habits. Like Christian in John Bunyan's classic, *Pilgrim's Progress,* you may need
to come to the cross and let the burdensome knapsack of sin fall off your back.
Determine that from this day forward, whether it be emotions, habits, or possessions that are cluttering and controlling you, you will dejunk your life.

*Do you have something cluttering your life that Jesus may be asking you to get
rid of?*   GORDON BOTTING

Delivering Delight

Delight yourself also in the Lord, and He shall
give you the desires of your heart. Ps. 37:4, NKJV.

WHEN MY CD player jammed last summer, I panicked. A part of my soul died. Music was my life support system. The words found in a German opera house expressed my feelings, "Bach gave us God's word, Mozart gave us God's laughter, Beethoven gave us God's fire." I believe God gave us music that we might pray without words. And my line to God had been jammed.

I'd always liked music. As a kid, if I wasn't listening to a hockey game I was listening to music. I'd even put a little transistor radio under my pillow to listen to when I was supposed to be sleeping.

After a serious car accident landed me in the hospital for eight months, friends and classmates came to the rescue with a cassette player and an AM-FM radio. It was the best medicine I ever had—with no ill side effects! When, for my fifteenth birthday, Mom and Dad topped it off with speakers, I was a happy camper.

In time, things changed, but my love for music remained. I was always asking my roommates to put it on. Paralyzed from my neck down, I'm dependent on others for some very simple things.

Soon, however, I learned to live on my own. I enjoyed my independence, but I could listen to music only when someone was around (only six hours a day).

Then on my thirty-seventh birthday my family gave me a stereo shelf system complete with radio, receiver, dual-cassette deck, five-disc CD player, and the most important part (for me at least)—a remote control. I could listen to music any time I wanted! I was ecstatic!

The day the music died, I knew I had to get that stereo fixed immediately. I could not go back to hours of silence. But the only person I knew who could help me was leaving that day on a week's trip. I was devastated. But she arranged for someone to pick up the system and take it for repair, and she promised that her son would reinstall it for me!

In Matthew 25 the King says "Come, you blessed, . . . inherit the kingdom" to those who had fed the hungry, gave the thirsty some water, clothed the naked, and visited the sick and those in prison. I'd add, "And those who restored music to the soul of a quadriplegic."

God wants to give everyone the desires of his or her heart—but He may need
you to be the delivery person! Who might need you today? THERESE ALLEN

Balancing Your Mary and Your Martha Sides

As Jesus and his disciples were on their way, he came to a village where a woman named Martha opened her home to him. Luke 10:38, NIV.

I PERSONALLY FEEL that Martha has been much maligned. There are two sides to us all, a harmony—an equanimity—to our natures that includes the Martha-side as well as the Mary-side. It takes the oars of both faith and works to row our ship through earth's uneven waters and to live a healthy, balanced lifestyle.

The Martha in us takes care of the practical in life: the everyday cleaning and toiling and taking care of our families and the necessary duties; the Mary in us takes care of our spiritual health by joining Jesus in the Garden each morning to have Him hold us close while we love Him and thank Him and bring before Him in prayer our loved ones and our everyday concerns.

The Mary in us studies to do well; the Martha in us does well. We need both. Perhaps there is a lesson here that we have not before considered. Martha worked very hard to feed at least 13 extra people that day. She was the angel for this hungry and tired group. While Mary had the privilege of sitting at the feet of Jesus and absorbing wisdom, Martha was busy preparing the meal. We are told, "But Martha was distracted by all the preparations that had to be made" (Luke 10:40, NIV). Years ago we had five sons to feed every day so I can understand why Martha was distracted!

Let us remember that God is a God of the hearth-keeper as well as the heart-keeper. It was Martha who unwittingly fulfilled the hospitality call: "Do not forget to entertain strangers, for by so doing some people have entertained angels without knowing it" (Heb. 13:2, NIV).

Also, when their brother Lazarus died, it was Martha who went out to meet Jesus while Mary stayed home (John 11:20). Both were needed! Some of us are the meeters and greeters and some of us are the quiet ones who wait at home. Neither should be criticized.

My dear friend Joyce called one day and told me she had finally figured out why we were such good friends: she was Martha and I was Mary! Bless her dear heart, she is the one who brings the food to church and then cleans up afterward. Me? I eat her wonderful food, thank her, and pray that God grants her many more years!

What could you do today to bring your Mary and your Martha sides into a healthy balance? PAT NORDMAN

109

Has Your Spring Sprung?

*The poor and needy seek water, but there is none, their tongues fail for thirst. I,
the Lord, will hear them; I, the God of Israel, will not forsake them. I will open rivers
in desolate heights, and fountains in the midst of the valleys; I will make the
wilderness a pool of water, and the dry land springs of water. Isa. 41:17, 18, NKJV.*

WHEN YOU HEAR the word "spring," what comes to mind? Daffodils,
cherry blossoms, green grass, and sunshine; rebirth as the rhythm of nature
springs to life once again? Spring is a wonderful time of the year.

But there's another kind of spring—a tightly coiled wire that after
being stretched or depressed, springs back into shape. Bed mattresses have
them, and so do trampolines and cars. We sometimes think of that bounce-
back effect when we comment, "Look at the spring in his step!" Or,
"She'll spring back in a few days!"

When your soul is stretched out of shape, do you have what it takes
to spring back?

You might not think you do—but God does! His promise is found in
the third meaning of the word "spring." Since moving to Tennessee I've
become fascinated with icy cold springs of water that gush out from
between layers of rock. There's one just below our house in Cleveland.
For decades—maybe centuries—it has run strong, forming a good-sized
creek that meanders through the grassy fields. Before the convenience of
indoor refrigeration people used to store milk and other perishables in its
cold water. We used this spring to chill watermelons for my daughter's
wedding when we ran out of refrigerator space. And I thought then, what
a blessing to have a spring!

If you've never seen the source of a gushing spring, drunk from its clear
water, or dipped your toes in it on a scorching hot day and felt instantly re-
vitalized, it may be more difficult for you to understand the intensity of
hope and healing that my stretched-out soul feels when I read the promise
in Isaiah 41:17, 18: "I will make . . . the dry land springs of water."

God is in the business of putting "spring" back into our lives. Not little trickles of spring. Not a drop here and there. No, if you feel your plight
is rather desolate, He can open rivers in your life; if you're in a bewilder-
ing wilderness, He can create a calming pool of water to refresh you; if
your life has become dry and barren, He promises you not just a spring of
water—but *springs of water.*

Lord, flood my soul with Your springs of life.   KAY KUZMA

The Weight Loss Paradox

The counsel of the Lord stands forever, the plans of
His heart to all generations. Ps. 33:11, NKJV.

JESUS SURE MADE some paradoxical statements that left many people scratching their heads.

Such as: "Lose your life to find it" (Matt. 10:39). "The least is the greatest" (Luke 9:48). "The first will be last, and the last first" (Mark 10:31). "Love your enemies, bless them that curse you" (Matt. 5:44).

If obesity were a problem in those days, I'm sure He would have said something just as paradoxical: "If you want to lose weight, you must gain it." Sound preposterous? Let me explain.

"Losing weight" is the number one New Year's resolution made—and broken—each year. Everywhere you turn—TV commercials, printed ads, signs on telephone poles, e-mail—you can find advertising for the latest quick way to lose weight.

Americans spend as much as $33 billion dollars on an obsession to lose weight. While many try to lose weight for aesthetic reasons, there are sound medical reasons why obese people need to lose weight. Many chronic diseases such as type 2 diabetes, hypertension, heart disease, and even cancer are related to obesity.

Then why do I believe Jesus would say we need to gain weight in order to lose weight? Because He knows that when you lose weight quickly through gimmicks, starvation, and fad diets, you end up losing the wrong weight, i.e., muscle and water, while you set your body up to gain fat.

Instead, a focus on preserving and even gaining muscle will help you choose healthy weight-loss behaviors. Choices can be evaluated by asking the question "Will this cause me to gain muscle and lose fat or vice versa?"

A healthy weight-loss approach would consist of a balance between cardiovascular (aerobic) exercise, strength training, stretching, proper nutrition, and most of all, not obsessing about your weight on the scale. Monitor your progress by improvements in your body fat percentage or by how your clothes fit.

"Gaining muscle weight to lose fat weight" may sound like a radical idea, but once we understand the physiology behind how our bodies work, we can see why His way is a plan for all generations (Ps. 33:11).

Lord, help me to remember that Your counsel is true, even though it may seem paradoxical. ERNIE MEDINA, JR.

It's Time to Celebrate Traditions

You shall keep it [the feast of Tabernacles] as a feast to the Lord for seven days in the year. It shall be a statute forever in your generations. Lev. 23:41, NKJV.

TRADITIONS ARE BUILT when beliefs, rituals, customs, songs, and stories are handed down from one generation to another. And traditions build strong meaningful relationships. I'm told that ancient Israel celebrated various traditions and feast days 91 times a year. These celebrations were characterized by music, food, banners, rituals, laughter, and rejoicing. Can't you see the families coming together—children jumping, romping, and squealing in delight, teens chatting together in small groups, parents greeting others and getting caught up on the news since the last celebration, and grandparents sitting back in pride and delight. What a fun way to build healthy family relationships.

Just as God asked the Israelites to celebrate events, tradition-making should be a part of every couple's life. When two people marry, they bring with them some of the family traditions from their own homes. Sometimes these will fit together nicely, and other times there may be conflict. One of the challenging tasks of a newly married couple is to create rituals and traditions that will be a unique blend of their own. That's what makes families unique. And that's what builds memories.

Start with daily and weekly rituals you'd like to establish. Perhaps it's holding hands during prayer or kissing afterward. Singing a blessing or a goodnight prayer. The ritual of a goodbye kiss; the honk of the horn as the car turns out into the street; or the mid-morning call just to say, "I love you." Celebrate Sabbath: wake up to the soft strains of a Sabbath CD, read a spiritual story, recite a text, sing "Day Is Dying in the West."

Never let a special day go by without some kind of ritual celebration: a blueberry waffle breakfast or some other treat, a card or gift, a song sung, or an evening out. Celebrate anniversaries. One couple, reluctant to wait for a whole year to celebrate their marriage, inaugurated "month-aversaries," which they celebrate the eighteenth day of every month, because they were married on July 18.

Birthdays should be special, as well as Valentine's Day, St. Patrick's, Easter, and Thanksgiving. You can even celebrate Groundhog Day! Whatever helps couples build a lasting memory will add to the togetherness and intimacy that most deeply desire.

Make a list of the traditions that your family celebrates. Begin today to build a new tradition. ALBERTA MAZAT

Blessings in Sickness

*I will praise You, for I am fearfully and wonderfully made; marvelous are
Your works, and that my soul knows very well. My frame was not hidden
from You, when I was made in secret, and skillfully wrought
in the lowest parts of the earth. Ps. 139:14, 15, NKJV.*

I WOKE UP ONE morning with a head that felt 50 pounds heavier than
normal and a disturbing feeling in my stomach that notified me that work
was not an option this particular day.

I called in to inform my secretary of my situation—and spent the
whole day sleeping, waking for one to two minute intervals in between.
During these intervals I would try to get up because I felt that I was wasting time in bed just thinking of all the housework I could do, projects I
could complete, letters I could write. I'm used to always going, going,
going. . . . I couldn't afford to be sick.

To my disappointment, I'd get up, feel awful, and have to lay back
down and go back to sleep. About midday I thought about eating something, but only managed a few oranges and crackers. Mentally I was not
satisfied but physically I was. I tried a couple more crackers and symptoms
of nausea threatened to rid me of the little nourishment I just received.

Not being able to work or eat, I settled on reading a little, then it was
back to bed until the next morning. Twenty-four hours later, I felt well
enough for work and was thankful to be out of bed.

When I reflected back over my seemingly unproductive day, the Holy
Spirit enabled me to see the blessings in it all. "You see," He said, "I have
placed within your body innate functions that will allow you to heal.
Without these symptoms, you would be left to your own demise. If you
hadn't had the 50-pound weight on your head that forced you to sleep,
your body would not have had the increased energy and vital force that it
needed to fight off the disease agents that were invading your body.
Without the feeling of nausea that prevented you from eating more than a
very small portion, your body would have had to put off the job of fighting off invaders in order to digest large portions of food, thus prolonging
your illness.

"You rested all day as a result of my innate designs, placed there to
help you."

My response was, "Lord, I am truly fearfully and wonderfully made!"

*The next time the flu or a virus makes you feel miserable, remember it's all part
of God's wonderful plan of healing! Praise Him!*   TABASURI CHAPMAN

Reframing With Consideration

For He knows our frame; He remembers that we are dust. Ps. 103:14, NKJV.

KIDS PRIZE FAIRNESS long before they study the judicial system. Watch school children monitoring their own behavior in play; they're quick to warn, "not fair." They'll admonish each other to "take turns." They end debates with the agreement to "repeat the play." There's something comforting about being treated fairly.

In his play *King Lear* Shakespeare presents an example that is worthy of modeling: reframing our view of a person based on his/her extenuating circumstances. Let me explain:

At first the king plans to divide his kingdom among his three daughters with the understanding that they maintain him and his 100 knights. But when his daughter Cordelia refuses to flatter him as her sisters have, Lear leaves his estate to the other daughters. Cordelia is left without lands or dowry.

But instead of receiving generous treatment from his ruling daughters and their husbands, Lear is thrown out of their houses and abandoned in a storm. Later the two wily daughters rival for the affections of wicked Edmund; one sister poisons the other and eventually takes her own life.

In the end, debilitated by rage and ill-treatment, the broken old man again meets his disenfranchised daughter, Cordelia. Aware that he has sorely mistreated her, Lear says, "If you have poison for me I will drink it. . . . You have some cause, they [the sisters] have not."

Cordelia responds in a surprising manner: "No cause, No cause," she says. Of course she has cause! She merely overlooks it because she considers his dazed, frail, weak frame.

This godlike willingness to reframe others with consideration for their frailty has been credited with strengthening human relationships in remarkable ways. Putting the most favorable "frame" on another's behavior, even a mistaken one, can smooth the relationship.

Consider a typical frame placed on a tardy spouse. "Inconsiderate! Disorganized!" This frame is likely to create conflict. But suppose the tardy behavior is framed as "what to expect of a confirmed extrovert." Or "the likely result of wanting to please the boss." Or "unwillingness to cut off a needy person who monopolizes a phone conversation."

Reframing others in the best possible light, with consideration for their circumstances, eases relationships. Today's text underscores the godlike nature of such an act.

Thank You, Lord, for considering my "frame"—and treating me accordingly.

EDNA MAYE LOVELESS

Let the Owner Take Charge

I know how to live on almost nothing or with everything. I have learned the secret of living in every situation, whether it is with a full stomach or empty, with plenty or little. For I can do everything with the help of Christ who gives me the strength I need. Phil. 4:12, 13, NLT.

IF YOU'VE EVER felt stress, compare your life with the apostle Paul's: "I have worked harder, been put in jail more often, been whipped times without number, and faced death again and again. Five different times the Jews gave me thirty-nine lashes. Three times I was beaten with rods. Once I was stoned. Three times I was shipwrecked. Once I spent a whole night and a day adrift at sea. I have traveled many weary miles. I have faced danger from flooded rivers and from robbers. I have faced danger from my own people, the Jews, as well as from the Gentiles. I have faced danger in the cities, in the deserts, and on the stormy seas. And I have faced danger from men who claim to be Christians but are not. I have lived with weariness and pain and sleepless nights. Often I have been hungry and thirsty and have gone without food. Often I have shivered with cold, without enough clothing to keep me warm. Then, besides all this, I have the daily burden of how the churches are getting along" (2 Cor. 11:23-28, NLT). How was Paul able to handle all this? He didn't. He let God do it! (Phil. 4:12, 13).

Pretend you are an employee of a large business owned by a single proprietor. You're working on a multimillion-dollar deal that will either make or break the company. Every decision and action is critical. But you don't have to worry about it because the owner is in control. You trust that he knows what he's doing. Everything is in his hands, not yours.

You can have that same peace every day by relying on the infinite power, strength, and wisdom of your Savior. You don't have to be stressed out and sink under the load of your trials and responsibilities—let the Owner take charge!

"When we can . . . rest confidingly in His love and shut ourselves in with Him, resting peacefully in His love, the sense of His presence will inspire a deep, tranquil joy. This experience gains for us a faith that enables us not to fret, not to worry, but to depend upon a power that is infinite. We shall have the power of the Highest with us. . . . Jesus stands by our side. . . . As the trials come, the power of God will come with them"(Ellen G. White, *My Life Today*, p. 184).

Exercise those trust muscles and let God carry the load.   RISË RAFFERTY

Keys to Physical and Spiritual Health

All Scripture is inspired by God and is useful to teach us what is true and to make us realize what is wrong in our lives. . . . It is God's way of preparing us in every way, fully equipped for every good thing God wants us to do. 2 Tim. 3:16, 17, NLT.

MOST OF MY physical therapy patients have some sort of physical disability. To help them regain as much function as possible, I challenge them to build *strength, flexibility,* and *endurance.*

Strength: When muscles aren't used, they atrophy—they become smaller and weaker. Body strength is not static—it's either going up or down. We strengthen our bodies by challenging them, pushing bit by bit. If you're not challenging your body by moving and lifting, you're weakening it. And when muscles weaken, body functions start declining, and you're more prone to injury.

Flexibility: Another problem with inactivity is that the body tends to become stiff. Injuries occur when muscles are tense and not stretched. Flexibility is maintained by activity.

Endurance: Aerobic/cardiovascular training works the heart and lungs, causing them to become stronger and more efficient. Endurance exercise will give you energy during the day.

Physical exercise has some direct parallels to spiritual health. Without spiritual exercise we become morally weak. Start with strength training. How? The Bible says the Lord is our strength. You can't be spiritually strong by yourself. Instead, you've got to plug into His strength. You've got to grow closer to Him. How? "Be diligent to present yourself approved to God, a worker who does not need to be ashamed, rightly dividing the word of truth." We've got to do some vigorous Bible study to get to really know its Author. We can't just sit around daydreaming and vegetating and still expect to strengthen our characters!

What about *flexibility?* The closer we get to God the more our actions will be motivated by love and not good works. Love is fluid; it meets needs. It bends to reach others where they are. Legalism is rigid and causes injuries. Love heals.

And *endurance?* The more we study God's Word, the more we'll want to study. It's like training for a marathon: start a little at a time, and before you know it your mind is ready to handle more complex concepts and truths.

Lord, help me remember that strength, flexibility, and endurance are the keys to health—physically and spiritually.

JEANNINE CHOBOTAR, with KAY KUZMA

What I Learned on Flight 847

But I say to you, love your enemies, bless those who curse you, do good to those who hate you, and pray for those who spitefully use you and persecute you. Matt. 5:44, NKJV.

MY FATHER HAS always been my mentor, spiritually and in other aspects of life. Growing up, I can remember him complimenting people on the fine work that they did. I especially noticed that he did this for those who worked service-type jobs that people so often take for granted. One time Dad complimented a flight attendant who was having to deal with some passengers who were treating her rudely. She was so thankful that she arranged for my dad to sit in first class! I've tried to follow my dad's example and treat others with courtesy and respect.

Last year my husband and I were fortunate to be able to fly to a vacation spot. On one of the longest legs of our flight, which was about four hours, I sat between my husband and an over-sized woman with a persistent cough. Now this cough wasn't an ordinary cough but one that sounded like she was going to wretch up her stomach. In intervals of 15 seconds she coughed and coughed. I became physically ill.

When I realized this woman was not only making me sick but angry, I started to pray, *Lord, please make this woman stop coughing.* But the coughing persisted.

Then a thought came to me. This poor woman must be miserable herself. So I changed my prayer: *Lord, this woman is not doing well. For* her *sake help her stop so she can get some relief and feel better.* Not too much later the coughing let up a bit, and my tolerance improved.

Throughout the flight the attendant could tell I must be uncomfortable sitting next to this woman, but I was always polite and always smiled. At the end of the flight I had fallen asleep with my head on my husband's shoulder when I felt something being placed in my lap. When I opened my eyes, to my surprise, there was a bottle of champagne with a cloth napkin wrapped around it. Written on the napkin was the message "Thanks for your smile and manners, from American Airlines, Flight 847."

To this date the unopened champaign bottle reminds me to always treat people with respect, and to pray for those who are making people miserable, because they themselves are probably even more miserable.

Can you think of someone who bugs you? Maybe it's prayer time!

KARI ST. CLAIR

Use It or Lose It

I praise you, for this body is incredibly and wonderfully made.
Your whole creation is amazing. Ps. 139:14, Clear Word.

THERE IS AN old adage that says "If you don't use it you lose it." This is especially true with the human body.

A study was done recently at Harvard University Medical Center on the appearance of brains during autopsy evaluation. The brains of people who had spent a lot of time playing Bingo, which takes no intellectual ability, had a completely different appearance from the brains of people who were often involved in intellectual endeavors. We may have 100 billion brain cells, but they need to be used or we'll lose them.

When a baby is born with a deviated eye, if it is not surgically corrected in a timely manner the baby will never see out of that eye. To keep functional, the retina of the eye has to be used.

Our muscles and joints have to be used; otherwise, contraction deformities will develop and we will never be able to use these muscles and joints again.

To keep healthy, the heart also has to be used—for more than just sitting. Exercise is very beneficial for the cardiovascular mechanism. Dr. Kenneth Cooper has been exercising people for decades at his aerobic clinic in Dallas, Texas. These people have less morbidity, greater longevity, and best of all they have a better quality of life.

As a physician, I have to say over and over that we are "wonderfully and marvelously made." I am continuously amazed at the intricacies of the human body, anatomically and physiologically. But we weren't created to sit on the shelf. To keep all of these functions working correctly we need to use them.

There is an amazing amount of information in the Bible, but this information will not have the power to change our lives unless we work with the Holy Spirit. *We must let the Holy Spirit use us* or our intimate connection with God will be lost. Just as a battery corrodes when it is not used for a long period of time, if we do not maintain our connection with the Holy Spirit worldly things will corrode our connection with God. We've got to use it, or we'll lose it!

Lord, teach me how to be used by Your Holy Spirit to keep my relationship with God in good condition. M. C. HOLLINGSEAD

Come on Over

Share with God's people who are in need. Practice hospitality. Rom. 12:13, NIV.

IT WAS A LOT of hard work. I spent hours cleaning the house, cooking the meal, baking, and laying out a starched tablecloth on the dining room table, topped with china place settings flanked by beautiful ornate silverware. I went the extra mile to ensure that everything was arranged to perfection. All of this effort for a few quickly passing hours when guests came to our home and dined. And now that it is all over, I feel terrific!

Few things are as rewarding to me as cooking a lovely meal for people. Figuring out the menu with my guest's likes and dislikes in mind is a special challenge that I relish. I've been known to serve a proper English breakfast in bed to two giggling teenage girls, on a beautiful tray laden with floral dishes, linen napkins, and tiny presents wrapped in tissue with silky bows.

My husband's boss enjoys tart tastes, so I remember to sprinkle a few cranberries over his salad. A light pasta salad on a bed of bibb lettuce with a steaming cup of herbal tea, set on a gingham cloth, made a beautiful Monday afternoon lunch with my cousin.

As I think about the surprised and expectant faces of my guests when they receive the first course of their meal, I can't help but smile. Indeed, everyone at the table is made to feel special. Forget phoning for a pizza delivery; my friends and family are worth the effort of an attentively prepared meal. I value them enough to expend the energy; and somehow in the effort of giving, I feel renewed. After all, this isn't the "dress rehearsal"; our lives, right now, are the one go around that we get.

Owning beautiful dishes and cooking like Julia Child isn't necessary; as long as your recipes include a healthy portion of love, you'll get along just fine. With that in mind, what could be a better use of time than breaking bread together, encouraging one another, and consuming nutritious fare that not only nourishes the body but the spirits as well?

Ready to receive a special blessing in your life? Want to feel fantastic after a few hours of hard work? Then it's time to give something away. Invite some folks over; you warm their hearts, and they'll warm your home.

Whom could you invite over this week so you can practice your hospitality?

MICHELE DEPPE

Isaiah's Fast

Is not this the kind of fasting I have chosen. . . . Is it not to share your food with the hungry and to provide the poor wanderer with shelter—when you see the naked, to clothe him, and not to turn away from your own flesh and blood? Isa. 58:6, 7, NIV.

EVEN BEFORE I LEARNED the health principles of the Bible, I was a veteran "juicer." Apples, carrots, and celery made a quick "ACC" cocktail in my Champion juicer. Fresh pineapple and comfrey leaves became a blended "green drink." Whenever I felt a flu bug coming on or just a general case of the blaahs, I could count on a short juice fast to put the pep back into my step.

Some years ago I was battling the grandaddy of flu bugs, a particularly resistant old rascal that refused to buzz off after its allotted 24 hours. I flushed that bug with "ACC" cocktail. No luck. I assaulted it with acid-packed "green drinks." Still no change. Finally, I concocted an evil-tasting brew heavy on horseradish juice. It didn't kill the bug but it almost killed me to swallow it!

At last I lay down, aching, congested, and feeling done in, and opened my Bible to see what it had to say about fasting. That's when I found Isaiah's fast about doing good to others, along with the promise "Your healing will quickly appear. . . . Then you will call, and the Lord will answer; you will cry for help, and he will say: Here am I" Isa. 58:8, 9, NIV).

Miserable though I was, I couldn't wait to put this unlikely "fast" to the test. Since I didn't know anyone on my block who was truly hungry, I sat down and wrote a $20 check to ADRA's relief fund. As I pictured my check putting an extra ladle of porridge in the bowl of many hungry little South American niños, I felt a surprising warmth in my heart. The chills from my flu were beginning to melt. How to "cover the naked" had me stumped until I remembered a friend—a single mother with a broken washing machine. A phone call later, she and her mountain of laundry were on their way over to visit my washing machine. Her gratitude for my thoughtfulness was so sincere that I could almost feel my health returning.

Since that day, fasting has taken on a new meaning for me. I still enjoy my "ACC" cocktails and "green drink" juice fasts, but I try not to let an illness pass without doing a kind deed for someone less fortunate. In this way I can help them and myself at the same time.

The next time you can't seem to shake that flu bug, try Isaiah's fast—along with some fresh, nutritious juice!   CAROL KIMURA

Noise, Noise, Everywhere

Then He arose and rebuked the wind, and said to the sea, "Peace, be still!"
And the wind ceased and there was a great calm. Mark 4:39, NKJV.

I AM AN APOSTLE of silence. I work in a library where quiet is important. But even in the library there is the noise of the copy machine, doors
closing, muffled whispers, and computer keys clicking. Friends tell me that
I am becoming a fanatic about noise. It assaults us on every side. There's
no way we can ignore it! Even our cars talk to us—or buzz and ding to get
our attention!

Several years ago I decided to peruse a back issue of *The Congressional
Record,* a most interesting document that we get daily. Dr. Lloyd John
Ogilvie was the Chaplain of the Senate. His prayer spoke to my soul—and
I'd like to share it with you:

"Dear Father, our lives are polluted with noise. The blaring sounds of
a noisy society bombard our ears and agitate our souls. The television set
is seldom turned off. We turn on our car radio at the same time we turn
the ignition key. Music is piped into everywhere we go, from the grocery
to the gym. On the streets horns blare, tires screech and tempers flare.
Meanwhile, people around us talk constantly trying to find out what they
want to say in the welter of words. It's so easy to lose the art of being quiet.

"Even in this quiet moment, our minds are racing, our nervous systems are on red alert, and we're like sprinters waiting for the starter's gun
to go off. Calm us down, Lord, so we can work creatively today.

"Lord, we hear Your voice saying, 'Peace, be still.' We want the miracle of that stillness and accept it as Your gift. We breathe out the tension
and breathe in the breath of Your spirit. In this time of prayer speak to us
the whisper of Your love and assurance, grace, and guidance. Get us ready
for a day in which we can be still inside while living in a noisy world. In
the name of our Lord and Savior. Amen."

Isaiah 30:15 tells us that "in quietness and in confidence shall be your
strength." There is no way we can enter the heart of God unless we go to
the "mountaintop" with Jesus! That means shutting off the computers,
TVs, radios, telephones, and all the other paraphernalia that shout at us.

*Lord, may my life respond with the same calm as the wind and the waves when
You commanded, "Peace, be still."* PAT NORDMAN

Been There, Done That. Now What?

I know the best thing we can do is to always enjoy life, because
God's gift to us is the happiness we get from our food and
drink and from the work we do. Eccl. 3:12, 13, CEV.

MY COLLEAGUE HAS a passionate love for golf. He's been to Scotland, England, Palm Desert, and other areas famous for their golf courses, to play and revel in their beauty and challenge. He even has had the pleasure of achieving a "hole-in-one." *Been there, done that. Now what?*

Mr. B enjoys traveling to "out-of-the-way" places: Sudan, Morocco, Pacific Islands, Greenland, Antarctica. He and his wife bring back fascinating stories of their adventures and travels. *Been there, done that. Now what?*

Dr. J has achieved national recognition in her medical specialty, and has been invited to speak and put on conferences from Hawaii to Miami. *Been there, done that. Now what?*

Mr. K has achieved financial independence so that his only fiscal worry is how to keep from losing it! *Been there, done that. Now what?*

Solomon was well acquainted with the five "W's": Work, Wisdom, Wealth, Women, and Worship. Here's what he learned:

• Work: It doesn't make sense to work just because we're jealous of each other (Eccl. 4:4).

• Wisdom: Discovering wisdom is as senseless as chasing the wind (Eccl. 1:17).

• Wealth: It's unfair to work so hard for things only to have someone else enjoy them (Eccl. 6:2).

• Women: Life is short, so love and enjoy your wife (Eccl. 9:9).

• Worship: When you worship God, think before making promises (Eccl. 5:1, 2).

Life is a journey and it is the travel along that journey that we are to enjoy. We should not sacrifice the enjoyment of that travel in order to reach the goals of wealth, wisdom (education), the fame of work, illicit sexual pleasures, or pride in our worship of God.

Solomon's advice is simple. Work hard, enjoy the fruits of your work, share your knowledge and wisdom with others, love your mate, and honor God in everything you do. When we look back on our lives, will we see that we have been chasing the wind or can we say, "I'm ready for God to bring every deed into judgment because I have loved Him and kept His commandments" (see Eccl. 12:13, 14)?

What could you do to enjoy to the fullest your journey through this day?

BURTON A. BRIGGS

Emotional Paralysis

When Jesus saw their faith, he said to the paralytic, "Son, your sins are forgiven. . . . I tell you, get up, take your mat and go home." Mark 2:5-11, NIV.

RUTH WAS EMOTIONALLY paralyzed by her feelings of being alone. As a child, she watched as her mother fought a losing battle with cancer. Her feelings of abandonment escalated when her father's job demanded that he be away from home days at a time.

As a young pregnant wife with a 2-year-old daughter, Ruth again felt abandoned as her physician husband served his country in New Guinea during World War II. Then at 55 she was widowed when her dearly loved mate suffered a fatal heart attack.

From childhood Ruth had been told, "Be a big girl; don't cry!" and she never did. She never was able to go through a healthy grieving process. Instead she continued to stifle her emotions.

At the age of 82 my mom (Ruth) lay dying from malnutrition and dehydration, physically paralyzed by a disease she had been struggling with for 10 years—PSP or progressive supranuclear palsy. Her body slowly quit working. First she had trouble walking, then she couldn't turn her head. Slowly paralysis took the rest of her body. Although her mind remained sharp, she lost her ability to speak and finally she couldn't swallow. She refused the slow torture of a feeding tube and chose to die as she had lived—with grace and dignity.

Often we are paralyzed by feelings of aloneness. We feel abandoned and rejected. Deep inside we feel like we're not good enough to be loved by anyone! But Jesus says to us, just as He did to that paralytic 2,000 years ago, "My child, your sins are forgiven." And then, "I tell you, get up, take your mat and go home."

Jesus wants to say to you, "I love you! I accept you! You can trust Me! You don't have to stay paralyzed by feelings of separateness! Get up—and come Home!"

My mom's friendship with God had been her lifeline since childhood, and her service for others had been her life's work. Her last days and hours were spent at home in the arms of her children. Finally, as she breathed her last soft breath I knew my mother truly was sleeping in Jesus until He comes. And I plan to be there to hear Him say to her, "Get up—it's time to come Home!"

Do you sometimes feel paralyzed by rejection and loneliness? Jesus is able to heal emotional paralysis as well as physical paralysis. Why not ask Him?

PATRICIA YINGLING MUNCY

The Fidget Factor

*You comprehend my path and my lying down, and are
acquainted with all my ways. Ps. 139:3, NKJV.*

I CAN STILL HEAR my mother's voice saying to me when I was small,
"Just sit still. Stop fidgeting." Obediently I'd force myself to sit still. Before
long, I'd forget and scratch my arm, wiggle my toes, or squirm in the chair.
She must have admonished me hundreds of times.

When I was about 8, I watched elderly Mr. Lampson walk down the
street. His hands shook badly as he walked. My mother told me he had St.
Vitus' Dance, and couldn't help it. Would I end up like Mr. Lampson? I
decided that if I could keep perfectly still for five minutes then I didn't
have Mr. Lampson's disease. I survived the five-minute ordeal, proving I
wasn't sick, but it was one of the most difficult things I've ever done.

Over the years I've felt something must be wrong with me.
Comments such as "Don't you ever quit wiggling?" have even made me
feel guilty that I can't sit still like others—so in order to fit in, I try harder.

But no more! At last, I have found approval for my fidgeting.
According to the results of a 1998 study at the Mayo clinic, fidgeting is definitely a weight-loss factor. For eight days, 16 volunteers stuffed themselves
with a thousand extra calories. They all gained weight; the highest was 16
pounds, but others added as little as two pounds. Dr. Michael Jensen, who
conducted the experiment, said the difference was the fidget factor! Those
who were natural fidgeters gained less weight. What an affirmation for me.
Being restless, squirming, and moving not only has Mayo Clinic approval,
but now I've learned it's a wonderful, built-in weight reducer.

"Every motion counts," Jensen said. "It's not just big motions such as
climbing stairs that made the difference, but getting up often, stretching,
tapping a foot, or wiggling." He was talking my lifestyle!

The fidget factor made me realize how easily we take on guilt. As soon
as anyone frowns and disapproves of what we do, we assume they're correct.
We change behavior, or try to change. If we continue with our old ways, as
I did, blips of guilt permeate our lives. Now I have scientific approval to
move around when I pray, stand when I read, and pace while I think!

Wise God, thank You for making me the way I am. Amen.

CECIL MURPHEY

Energized at Play

It's true that there are different gifts, but they all come from the same Holy Spirit. There are different ministries, but we all serve the same Lord. 1 Cor. 12:4, 5, Clear Word.

I'M PLAYING WITH my class of college students, taking a gamble that the particular video clip I'm showing them of Carreras, Domingo, and Pavarotti in concert in Rome will help make my point about the importance of play in student-centered learning.

I point out some of the signals the singers are using that are part of co-operative play. "The audience wants another encore, and the tenors are going to try something they've never done before," I explain. "First, they plan what they're going to do. Now watch them cue each other in."

We get caught up in the electricity of the moment, as if we are in the audience at Terme di Caracalla, thrilling with collective joy in the creative spontaneity of the music. Then it's over, and I as teacher don't know quite what to do next. Will I overkill my point with more words?

But in order to understand how important play is to children's learning, my students need to see how important it is to *their* development as teachers. So I hazard one final comment.

"Like these tenors, some of your greatest teaching happens when you play, trying out new ideas just for fun! I'm experimenting on you, too!"

We laugh, and my students get up to go. Did they get the idea? I don't know. I'm still trying to grasp it myself! But at this moment, I feel the miracle of teaching for me. Though I have put heart and soul into this class, I'm walking out of my classroom with more energy than I walked in with. It's a God-given exhilaration that comes at special moments when I'm doing my best at teaching! I enjoy many other activities—but I get this unique surge of vitality only from teaching.

Eric Liddell, winner of Olympic gold in 1924 and dramatized in the movie *Chariots of Fire,* said it this way, "I believe God made me for a purpose. But He also made me fast, and when I run I feel His pleasure." You can almost see God's pleasure beaming down on his joyful face, his head thrown back, blond hair streaming behind him, as he flies down the track. What a God, who loves us this way!

What is it that you do when you feel most keenly the touch of God and are energized? What is your gift?   CHERYL WOOLSEY DESJARLAIS

Two Are Better Than One

Two are better than one, because they have a good reward for their labor. For if they fall, one will lift up his companion. But woe to him who is alone when he falls, for he has no one to help him up. Eccl. 4:9, 10, NKJV.

WHEN YOUR FINGER gets cut, it automatically bleeds. The blood vessel will suddenly constrict to slow down the blood flow so that clotting can start to take place. At the same time the hematoma, the accumulating pool of blood outside the blood vessel, will press against the blood vessel to prevent further bleeding. Then a series of reactions takes place that activates the platelets so that they can stick to the injured area, along with the collagen and other proteins—particularly thrombin. They form a mesh that plugs the injury. Then a series of reactions take place involving at least 10 blood-clotting factors. Finally, the fibroblast will come to the destroyed epithelium and rebuild the tissue to make it look as normal as it used to be—a healed wound.

Wouldn't it be great if church members could react to wounded souls like the blood vessel, platelets, and plasma cooperatively impacting the injured area to heal the wound?

Dr. Thomas Oxman and his colleagues at the University of Texas Medical School examined the relationship of social support and religion to the mortality of men and women six months after undergoing elective open heart surgery. Here is what they found:

Those who lacked participation in an organized social group such as a club, church, or synagogue had a fourfold increase in chance of dying six months post surgery, even after controlling the medical factors that might have influenced survival, such as severity of heart disease, age, or previous cardiac surgery.

Those who did not draw strength and comfort from their religion were three times more likely to die six months post surgery. Those without regular group participation and not having comfort from religion were more than seven times more likely to die six months post surgery.

Imagine, combining religion and social support in the church setting is a factor in medicine that causes a sevenfold difference in mortality six months after the open heart surgery. If there were an approved drug that reduced mortality by seven fold, virtually every physician in the country would be recommending it to their patients. In fact, it would be malpractice not to.

Lord, help me to always be a healing agent to the wounded souls around me.

KATHLEEN H. LIWIDJAJA-KUNTARAF

Hate, the Devil's Worst Weapon

Whoever hates his brother is a murderer, and you know that no murderer has eternal life abiding in him. 1 John 3:15, NKJV.

"DEAR 'MOTHER.'" (This was how Jules addressed his e-mail to me.) "I am from Rwanda. In April 1994 I lost my mother, my elder sister, and many of my relatives during the genocide in my country. My father had been murdered before by the same army. Our murderers were very well organized and their aim was to kill everybody in my ethnic group.

"When my mother realized that our murderers were near, she divided us into groups and sent us in different directions so hopefully some could escape. I was in a group of three children.

"After only 20 minutes I saw the group with my mother, sister, and many neighbors lying on the road with blood on their faces and clothes. They had already been murdered. We had to continue our own way because the enemy was near us, killing other people. None of us wept at that moment. Our lives were in danger, and we had to prove strong in character, without which we would have been too discouraged to run away and would have been caught and killed, too.

"No one in my group died, but it is not easy to forget what happened to us and our dear family, and to forget the people who ran after us to kill us.

"Sometimes I do not understand the meaning of this life on Earth, because I don't understand the reason for hate and how it can result in genocide and so many evil actions.

"I remember very often what happened to me. I am afraid of a future explosion if I do not do something for my life now. I know I must pray for forgiveness, but to forgive is not easy.

"Your 'son,' Jules"

(I replied.) "Dear Jules, Hate is the devil's most cruel weapon, because it destroys both the one who hates (no murderer has eternal life) and the victim. Forgiveness is the undeserved gift you must give to the killers. The gift you are to give yourself is a Bible promise such as Psalm 119:165, 'Great peace have they which love thy law: and nothing shall offend them.' When a bad memory comes, exchange gifts. Remember the forgiveness you gave, and repeat the Bible promise. Over time, you'll find that God's love within you is stronger than hate."

Are you being troubled by a negative emotion? Exchange gifts and see if God's Word hidden in your heart doesn't make a difference. KAY KUZMA

No Man Is an Island

For none of us lives to himself, and no one dies to himself. For if we live,
we live to the Lord; and if we die, we die to the Lord.
Therefore, whether we live or die, we are the Lord's. Rom. 14:7, 8, NKJV.

HAVE YOU HEARD about the "Ni-Hon-San" study (Nippon [Japan]-Honolulu-San Francisco)? Researchers selected 11,900 Japanese and compared the health of those who lived in Japan to those who had migrated to Honolulu and San Francisco, respectively.

The incidence of heart disease was the lowest in Japan, intermediate in Hawaii, and highest in California. This difference was not explained by differences in diet, blood pressure, or cholesterol level. They found the incidence of smoking was higher in Japan, even though the prevalence of heart disease was lower there.

At first it appeared that the closer the Japanese came to the American mainland, the sicker they became. However, this was a wrong conclusion. The researchers then classified the Japanese-Americans in California according to the degree to which they retained their traditional Japanese culture, socializing with one another as a closely knit community. Here is what they discovered: The most traditional group of Japanese-Americans, who maintained their social networks and family ties, just as they used to have in Japan, had a prevalence of heart disease as low as those living in Japan. In contrast, the group that was most Westernized in the sense of living a very individualistic life, had a three- to five-fold increase in heart disease. In other words, social networks and close family ties protect against disease and premature death.

Romans 14:7 says: "None of us lives to himself, and no one dies to himself." The text is referring to God's constant presence, but based on the research it would be just as appropriate to use this phrase when talking about human relationships!

Where can you find close associations and fellowship? Try church. Weekdays are so busy. So when Sabbath comes, oh, what a welcome day of rest! Because we are commanded by God to stop cleaning house, stop gardening, and stop working, it gives us time to enjoy fellowshipping with the Lord and others.

No man is an island. We all need one another. And it's good for our health!

What can you do today to strengthen your relationship with a neighbor or friend?

KATHLEEN H. LIWIDJAJA-KUNTARAF

The Trend-setter's Diet

*Unless you . . . become as little children, you will by
no means enter the kingdom of heaven. Matt. 18:3, NKJV.*

"GRANDMA, IS THIS a real hot dog?" Megan asked when she saw the
corn dog on her plate. We were in the Loma Linda University cafeteria,
and I assured her that no meat was served in that place.

But Megan was cautious. She looked at her salad. "Grandma, are you
sure these aren't real bacon bits?" I again reassured her, but perhaps there
was a touch of impatience in my voice.

Megan lifted her serious 4-year-old eyes and looked straight into mine. "I
need to be careful, Grandma," she said solemnly. "I have never eaten any meat
in my life, and I don't ever want to. So when I'm not home, I need to ask."

Megan was right. Nutritional research confirms that people who don't
eat animal products have greater longevity, fewer heart attacks and strokes,
fewer weight problems, lower cholesterol, lower blood pressure, and less
diabetes. They have less cancer of the breast, prostate, and colon, and fewer
hemorrhoids. They also have fewer stones of the kidney and gall bladder,
less kidney disease, and less gouty arthritis. Their bones are stronger; they
have less osteoporosis.

An editorial in the *Journal of the American Medical Association* states: "A
total vegetarian diet could prevent up to 97 percent of our heart attacks."

Although the human body can nourish itself on animal foods, it lacks
the protection against large amounts of fat and cholesterol that carnivorous
animals have. Therefore, excessive fat and cholesterol stack up in the bloodstream. Arteries thicken and narrow, and plaque forms. Blood supplies to
vital organs diminish. The stage is set for many of our killer diseases.

In a lifetime, the average American meateater subsidizes the killing of
a thousand chickens and turkeys, dozens of pigs, sheep, and cows, plus
thousands of sea creatures.

Today the Eden diet is "in." On every side we are urged to eat more
fruits, vegetables, and grains because they contain phytochemicals, antioxidants, and fiber—substances that the body needs to protect itself from cancer and other health threats.

The food fanatics of yesteryear have now become today's trend-setters.
Whether they are a CEO, lawyer, tennis champion, or housewife, vege-
tarians are widely respected. Today, vegetarianism is increasingly viewed as
smart, healthy, caring, and a responsible choice.

Lord, help me to be willing to make sacrifices for my ultimate well-being.

AILEEN LUDINGTON

The Faith Factor

Be of good cheer . . . ; your faith has made you well. Matt. 9:22, NKJV.

IF YOUR HEALTH club membership and your latest diet haven't rewarded you with the vibrant life you're seeking, perhaps you need a spiritual checkup. Scientific data is rapidly confirming that Christians are healthier than the general population and that there is a definite relationship between spiritual faith and physical health. It's called "the faith factor!"

At Purdue University, medical sociologist Kenneth F. Ferraro gathered responses from 1,473 people nationwide on health-influencing factors such as age, income, and education. They were asked how often they prayed, whether they considered themselves strong in faith, how often they attended synagogue or church services, and whether they read religious literature.

Twice as many non-practicing subjects reported health problems. Nine percent of those in the non-practicing category reported poor health, compared to only three percent in the practicing category. Also, while 26 percent of those who never attended worship reported excellent health, 36 percent of the weekly attenders reported excellent health. "Whether or not people are actively involved in their religion makes the biggest difference in health status," Ferraro says.

A 1995 study at Dartmouth-Hitchcock Medical Center found that one of the best predictors of survival among 232 heart surgery patients was the degree to which the patients drew comfort and strength from religious faith. Those who didn't, had a death rate three times higher.

A 1996 study of 4,000 elderly persons found that those who attend religious services are less depressed and are physically healthier than those who don't attend or who worship at home. Numerous studies have shown that nonchurchgoers have a suicide rate four times higher than that of those who attend church regularly.

So what makes "the faith factor" good medicine? First, people who nurture their faith by attending religious services tend to have strong networks of friends who make sure they get proper medical care. The Christian community is a caring, loving, ever-present family.

Second, Bible principles are healthy ones. Not only are we told what to eat (Lev. 11), but we are reminded of the benefits of such things as a positive attitude: A merry heart is good medicine. And finally, the best "medicine" of all: God answers prayer!

By being involved with a spiritual growth group you can bolster your immune system!　　　　　　　　　　　　　　　　　　　　　　DeWITT S. WILLIAMS

Choices

Train up a child in the way he should go, and when
he is old he will not depart from it. Prov. 22:6, NKJV.

RECENTLY A NURSE educator came to our youngest son's elementary school with a variety of body parts in jars—hearts, lungs, livers, kidneys, and brains. For more than an hour she kept adolescent students and teachers alike in rapt attention as she told the story of each organ.

• The enlarged heart of a father who died early with congestive heart failure. His high-blood pressure, because of too much stress, lack of exercise, and a high-fatty diet took him from his family before his time.

• A lung of a non-smoking woman who died of lung cancer before she was a grandma, because of the smoke from her husband's cigarettes. Breathing second-hand smoke for two hours equals smoking approximately one pack of cigarettes. Another tarred lung was from a man who smoked three packs of cigarettes a day. His lung was black and mangled from the poison he had inhaled. The nurse educator said that each cigarette takes about seven minutes off a smoker's life and that nicotine kills our respiratory organ. Long-time smokers breathe through these half-dead lungs. Their breath smells like a dead cow. That really made an impact upon the students.

• The enlarged liver of a man who started drinking at a young age. The liver is vital for the health of the body; if alcohol damages the liver beyond repair the body cannot get rid of its waste.

• A shriveled-up kidney of a man who was overweight, had diabetes, and untreated high-blood pressure. Without the aid of kidneys to filter the toxins from your body, you would need to be hooked up to a dialysis machine, which cleanses your blood.

• The immature brain of a baby who's mother drank during pregnancy. Just as heat cooks an egg, an immature brain is 'scrambled' by too much alcohol. Children and youth, especially, need to be careful about drinking alcohol because brains not fully mature are more susceptible to damage and may not have full capacity as an adult.

These elementary students will never forget the lessons learned that day. If we educate our children in healthy living when they are young, then they will live to grow old!

Creator God, forgive me for the damage that I have done to the organs You created in me. Give me strength to make healthy choices.

KEVIN and SANDRA CLAY

The Bible and *Hugiés*

*Jesus answered them, "Healthy people don't need a doctor—sick people do.
I have come to call sinners to turn from their sins, not to spend my time
with those who think they are already good enough." Luke 5:31, 32, NLT.*

WHEN JESUS INVITED Matthew the tax collector to "follow Me," Matthew responded joyfully by organizing a great banquet for his friends, including Jesus. When the Pharisees complained to His disciples, Jesus responded by saying, "It is not the healthy *[hugiaino]* who need a doctor, but the sick. I have not come to call the righteous, but sinners to repentance" (Luke 5:31, NIV).

The Greek word *hugiaino* comes from *hugiés,* a Greek term for health, soundness, and wholeness. Paul repeatedly uses the word, as in "sound doctrine" (1 Tim. 1:10), sound words (2 Tim. 1:13), and being "sound" in the faith (Titus 1:13). Perhaps the most popular use of the term in the Bible is found in 3 John 2: "Beloved, I pray that you may prosper in all things and be in health, just as your soul prospers" (NKJV).

Throughout Scripture health is intimately tied to both mental and spiritual well-being. This is most evident in the Psalms. For example, in Psalm 6, often thought to express David's anguish over his son Absalom, we read, "O Lord, heal me, for my bones are in agony. My soul is in anguish" (verses 2, 3, NIV). The psalm of the cross, Psalm 22, graphically portrays this theme, as does Psalm 31: "Be merciful to me, O Lord, for I am in distress; my eyes grow weak with sorrow, my soul and my body with grief. My life is consumed by anguish and my years by groaning; my strength fails because of my affliction, and my bones grow weak" (verses 9, 10, NIV).

In Proverbs, Solomon repeatedly delineates the health advantages that come through knowing and loving God. "Do not be wise in your own eyes; fear the Lord and shun evil. This will bring health to your body and nourishment to your bones" (Prov. 3:7, 8, NIV).

In *The Ministry of Healing,* the health classic by Ellen G. White, a constant theme is the deep-seated relationship between physical, mental, and spiritual health. "The relation that exists between the mind and the body is very intimate. When one is affected, the other sympathizes. . . . Courage, hope, faith, sympathy, love, promote health and prolong life" (p. 241).

Lord, I want to be healthy, spiritually and physically. Impress upon me what I should do this day to reach Your goal for me. DAVID C. NIEMAN

Prayer Works

And it happened that the father of Publius lay sick of a fever and dysentery. Paul went in to him and prayed, and he laid his hands on him and healed him. Acts 28:8, NKJV.

PRAYING FOR HEALING is a fundamental concept in most cultures. Here at the Lifestyle Center of America we continue that tradition—praying to God, our Creator; asking Him to re-create health in our patients and give them willpower to continue living a healthy lifestyle.

And God is answering prayers. We've seen incredible miracles happen in just a few weeks. Many leave with significant improvements and reversals in their physiology and biochemistry. Some come to us able to walk only a few steps and leave walking a mile a day. Others bring a suitcaseful of medications and are overwhelmed with joy when they realize they don't need them anymore.

What we are doing in terms of lifestyle change is highly scientific—but what's exciting to me is that the benefits of prayer have also been scientifically proven!

One of my favorite studies concerning the power of prayer began in 1987 with Randolph C. Byrd, M.D., a man of faith and science. He yearned to do more for his patients. Dr. Byrd knew prayer could be effective. He wondered, *Could the effectiveness of prayer be measured?*

Dr. Byrd planned and implemented a scientific study to determine if persons who were prayed for during their illness (or following surgery) would recover more completely, more painlessly, and more effectively than similar patients who did not receive intercessory prayer. For 10 months Dr. Byrd and his colleagues followed the progress of 392 patients in the coronary care unit of a San Francisco hospital. The results of this study were reported in *Southern Medical Journal,* July 1988. Patients were randomly assigned either to receive or not to receive intercessory prayer. This was a well-designed study; neither patients nor caregivers knew who was in which group.

Analysis of Dr. Byrd's data showed that after entry into the study the prayer group had less congestive heart failure, required less diuretic and antibiotic therapy, had fewer episodes of pneumonia, had fewer cardiac arrests, and were less frequently intubated and ventilated. In 20 of the 26 categories studied, the patients who had intercessory prayer as part of their treatment fared better than those who where not prayed for.

Isn't it exciting to realize that prayer works today just as it did in Bible times? *Is there someone you know who needs your prayers?*   GERARD MCLANE

Trick Yourself Into Good Health

Now when the tempter came to Him, he said, "If You are the Son of God, command that these stones become bread." But He answered and said. "It is written, 'Man shall not live by bread alone, but by every word that proceeds from the mouth of God.' " Matt. 4:3, 4, NKJV.

DO CRAVINGS SOMETIMES grab you and push you to do what you vowed you wouldn't do? You give up French fries and shakes. Suddenly, *bang!* The craving hits. What do you do?

Wendy Sullivan found a way to trick herself into eating a better diet and dealing with those troublesome cravings. Her strategy has merit. For six days Wendy eats healthy foods in reasonable portions. But on the seventh day she eats whatever she wants. It's a day of rest from her diet. She calls it a "cheat day."

This "cheat day" tricks Wendy into controlling her cravings instead of allowing them to control her. She explains: "When I was grocery shopping I saw a dark chocolate bar I really wanted, so I told myself, 'I'm going to have this on Sunday.' I bought it and left it sitting on our kitchen counter all week, knowing I was going to have it on Sunday. But a funny thing happened. By Sunday, I didn't want it. The desire for it had just been an impulse of the moment. There was something comforting, though, about knowing that I could eat it on Sunday if I wanted."

Wendy goes on to explain, "To some people the idea of having a cheat day may sound like a cop out, especially when you are trying to make a complete lifestyle change and eat more healthfully. It's a strategy that's quite effective. Let's say that on Monday I suddenly have a craving for pizza. Of course the craving is all in my head. But if I tell myself I can never have pizza again my body feels rebellious and I want to cheat right then and there. So instead, I tell myself that I can have some pizza—just not today. I can have it on Sunday, my cheat day. Then my body and mind don't rebel so much. But this funny thing happens. By the time Sunday rolls around, I usually don't feel like eating pizza anymore. Problem solved! It doesn't always work that way. Sometimes I indulge, but what I imagined was better than the real thing!"

Sin is like that. It tempts you and creates a craving for the forbidden. If you don't have a strategy to overcome you'll likely fall. And when you do, you'll discover it just wasn't worth it!

What strategies do you have? What about using the strategy Jesus used in today's text? KAY KUZMA

The Breath of Life

*And God said, Let there be a firmament [the expanse of the sky]
in the midst of the waters, and let it separate the waters
[below] from the waters [above]. Gen. 1:6, Amplified.*

IN ORDER TO HAVE good blood, we must breathe well. Full, deep inspirations of pure air, which fill the lungs with oxygen, purify the blood. They impart to it a bright color and send it, a life-giving current, to every part of the body. A good respiration soothes the nerves; it stimulates the appetite and renders digestion more perfect; and it induces sound, refreshing sleep.

The lungs should be allowed the greatest freedom possible. Their capacity is developed by free action; it diminishes if they are cramped and compressed. Hence the ill effects of the practice so common, especially in sedentary pursuits, of stooping at one's work. In this position it is impossible to breathe deeply. Superficial breathing soon becomes a habit, and the lungs lose their power to expand. . . .

Thus an insufficient supply of oxygen is received. The blood moves sluggishly. The waste, poisonous matter, which should be thrown off in the exhalations from the lungs, is retained, and the blood becomes impure. Not only the lungs, but the stomach, liver, and brain are affected. The skin becomes sallow, digestion is retarded; the heart is depressed; the brain is clouded; the thoughts are confused; gloom settles upon the spirits; the whole system becomes depressed and inactive, and peculiarly susceptible to disease.

The lungs are constantly throwing off impurities, and they need to be constantly supplied with fresh air. Impure air does not afford the necessary supply of oxygen, and the blood passes to the brain and other organs without being vitalized. Hence the necessity of thorough ventilation. To live in close ill-ventilated rooms, where the air is dead and vitiated, weakens the entire system. It becomes peculiarly sensitive to the influence of cold, and a slight exposure induces disease.

Vigor declines as years advance, leaving less vitality with which to resist unhealthful influences; hence the greater necessity for the aged to have plenty of sunlight, and fresh, pure air.

Let there be a current of air and an abundance of light in every room in the house.

Throw open the window, take five deep slow breaths of fresh air by expanding your diaphragm, not just lifting your chest . . . and praise the Lord! Wow! It feels good, doesn't it? ELLEN G. WHITE—*The Ministry of Healing,* pp. 272-275.

From Battered to Blessed

I am crucified with Christ: nevertheless I live; yet not I, but Christ liveth in me: and the life which I now live in the flesh I live by the faith of the Son of God, who loved me, and gave himself for me. Gal. 2:20.

IT WAS 3:00 A.M. when I was jerked out of bed. Insanely furious, my inebriated husband threw our infant daughter into the crib. As I raced to see if Becky was OK, I felt my head being pulled backward by my hair, and I was literally flying across the room. I could hear her screaming, while I felt the impact of his boot, first in my face, then in my stomach, arms and legs, until the pain was so intense I could no longer detect where on my body I was being hit. I heard someone call. That must have sobered him up a bit because with one more kick from his boot, he was gone. I didn't move from my fetal position on the floor as I heard the back door slam and his car drive away. I just wanted to die there on the floor, but my daughter needed me. I knew I had to get out of the house before my husband returned.

Suddenly I heard the back door close. Thinking he'd come back, I panicked, but my legs refused to move. Then my terror turned to tears at the sight of my sister, Linda, standing there in her robe and slippers. God had awakened her and impressed her to check on me. A miracle!

Glancing first at me and then at the room, she burst into tears. "This is enough!" She marched to the phone, and made reservations, and then called our parents in Texas to say we'd be on the next plane. And that's how I escaped from the man who almost destroyed me.

Yes, in my first marriage I was one of 3 to 4 million women in the U.S. each year who are the victims of domestic abuse. Why did I stay so long? I was embarrassed to leave; wasn't marriage a lifelong commitment? And I believed his lie that it was my fault. I had no money. And although I was scared to stay, I was even more afraid of leaving. I thought he would kill me.

Now, I know God does not want anyone living in a situation where they are verbally threatened, demeaned, and insulted, or physically abused. If that's happening to you, God can make a way of escape—and restore you, for you are the daughter of the King—His precious treasure whom He died to redeem. Read yourself into Scripture: "For the Lord has chosen you, [your name], for Himself—*you* for His special treasure" (Ps. 135:4, my own paraphrase).

Father God, thank You for rescuing me, restoring me, and blessing me abundantly.

BRENDA WALSH

Tuberculosis Still Kills Today

And don't let us yield to temptation, but deliver us from the evil one. Matt. 6:13, NLT.

I HADN'T SEEN Tina for a while. Then I learned she had tuberculosis. I couldn't believe it. I thought that disease died out years ago with the discovery of antibiotics. I was wrong!

Tuberculosis (TB) is a killer with impressive credentials. It was described thousands of years ago in ancient writings. Evidence of tubercular decay has been found in the spines of Egyptian mummies, and the disease was common both in ancient Greece and Imperial Rome. In more recent times, TB led to the deaths of John Keats, Robert Louis Stevenson, and Frederick Chopin.

For millennia, it was not known that bacteria was the cause of this disease. The infection spreads through the lymph nodes and bloodstream and can cause tissue death in any organ in the body, but the lungs are most vulnerable. Over the past two centuries it has killed 1 billion people.

TB is currently the leading cause of mortality from a single infectious agent—accounting for 26 percent of preventable adult deaths in the developing world. There are an estimated eight million new cases of tuberculosis and three million deaths attributable to TB per year. Here's the bad news: A new and highly resistant form of the bacteria that causes TB has emerged, creating a public-health hazard in poverty areas of many large cities. Tuberculosis is also increasing rapidly in countries with high rates of HIV infection. In fact, half of HIV patients will likely develop TB.

What can be done? Don't panic, it is nearly impossible to catch TB simply by passing an infected person on the street. To be at risk, you must be exposed to the organisms constantly, by living or working in close quarters with someone who has the active disease. Even then, because the bacteria generally stay dormant after they invade the body, only 10 percent of people infected will come down with the active disease.

How can you protect yourself from this dreaded infection? By keeping your immune system healthy. It's people who are malnourished or have compromised immune systems because of AIDS or blood cancers (such as leukemia) who are most at risk.

Just as I thought TB was no longer a problem, Satan wants us to believe that sin is no longer a problem for you. He wants you to hang around with sinners, thinking you're immune to temptation, and then, when your resistance has been compromised, *bang!* He'll getcha!

Lord, help me to make wise choices to keep my spiritual and physical immune system healthy. KAY KUZMA and ELMAR SAKALA

The Lord Has Restored My Soul

*The Lord is my shepherd; I shall not want. He maketh me to lie down
in green pastures: he leadeth me beside the still waters. He restoreth my soul:
he leadeth me in the paths of righteousness for his name's sake. Ps. 23:1-3.*

"YOU MUST COME. Mother has fallen and broken her hip," my sister
Norma urged me. "She will be having surgery today!" I immediately made
arrangements and flew from Tulsa, Oklahoma, to Bozeman, Montana.

When I arrived at the hospital, Mother was already out of surgery. She
looked up drowsily and smiled at me. Norma was a supervising nurse in
the hospital, and Mother rejoiced that both of her daughters could be with
her in this dark experience.

I sang a song to my mother about how God restores our souls in the
valley experiences of life. Then she shared with me something that just
wrung my heart! She has suffered with palsy of her hands and head for
many years. She said that she felt all alone in her church family, for when
she tried to be friendly she seemed to shake more. It seemed to her that
the members were uncomfortable and withdrew from her. Tears came to
my eyes as she told me how lonesome she felt.

God purposed that something good should come out of the pain of breaking her hip, for "all things work together for good to those who love God"
(Rom. 8:28, NKJV). All of the hospital personnel who cared for Mother came
to love her and treated her with the utmost dignity and kindness.

Norma and her husband, Dave, were so highly thought of by the
members of their church that many came to visit Mother. She actually
came to enjoy her valley experience. These people brought the sunshine
of God's healing love into her room—and it warmed her heart once again.

One night as I was sleeping on the cot in her room, I awakened to the
sound of my precious mother's voice, singing, "You may have all this
world, but give me Jesus." I listened quietly and joyfully as she continued
to sing and to talk to her Savior.

As I prepared to fly back to Tulsa, Mother said, "You know, honey,
through this trial God has restored my soul. If I feel others are cool toward
me, I'll just reach out and warm them up with God's love."

*Is there someone in your church family who doesn't seem to have friends?
Maybe their soul needs to be restored with the love you can give!*

KAY COLLINS

Seasoning the World

*You are the world's seasoning, to make it tolerable. If you lose
your flavor, what will happen to the world? Matt. 5:13, TLB.*

WE WERE LOOKING forward to meeting the new family who had
moved in next door. Seeing the husband, Ron approached him with his
hand extended. "Hi, I'm Ron Flowers," he said. "Welcome to our—"
Ignoring the greeting, the newcomer lengthened the lead on his two
Dobermans, turned on his heel, and strode away.

Though baffled, Ron recovered, but this first encounter marked the
tenor of our relationship with this man as long as he lived next door. We
did visit from time to time over the backyard fence with his shy wife, who
seemed to want friendship, but it is their little boy who lingers in our
memory. His young age and strange habits isolated him in our neighborhood of teenagers. Whenever our sons came home from academy he
would hang around, hoping to play with them or to be invited in.

One day Karen was startled to find the little boy sitting on our living
room couch by himself. He had obviously let himself in the through the
front door without a sound. "Why, Darron, I didn't know you were
here!" she exclaimed, as her pulse quieted a little.

"Oh, please, Mrs. Flowers, let me stay," he pleaded. "I like to sit in
here because it's pretty, and nobody's fighting." Karen sat beside him, as-
suring him he could stay as long as he liked, and pondered the times she
had been quick to send him home because he seemed to be in the way.

Darron and his family simply left one day. No one knows where they
went. The house got new owners again, and it would be easy to just forget. But somehow we think of Darron from time to time. We keep hoping that because he witnessed at our house a man and a woman who love
each other, two boys who laughed and played and knew they could take
their parents' love for granted, that because he has seen it once, it could be
true for him in the home he will one day establish.

Countless Darrons around us long for affection and love. They search
for models of what it means to be a caring family. They hunger for the
warmth of our touch, our embrace. Through us, God wants to show His
love to the world. Perhaps for Darron, even if love wasn't happening very
well at his house, being near it in ours will count for something.

What could you do today that would season your neighbors with God's love?

KAREN and RON FLOWERS

Desiring the Milk of His Word

As newborn babes, desire the sincere milk of the
word, that ye may grow thereby. 1 Peter 2:2.

I REMEMBER SO vividly my three babies and how anxious they were when they knew they were going to have breakfast, lunch, dinner, or a midnight snack at my breast. Their plump little bodies, pumping arms and legs, their tiny hands bursting with activity, their baby faces full of anticipation, their mouths wide open, and that familiar panting noise as if this were to be the only meal of their lives. Static, then, for a moment as they started sucking, and then a tremendous peace as if all their troubles were gone, as if they knew with certainty that everything was now going to be alright. Then the wonderful sleep, no tension at all in their beautiful baby faces, waiting for the next cycle, in complete trust that the meal will be provided again and again.

I've thought of that a lot in connection with our feeding on the Word of God. It's interesting that Peter talks about how our desire for God's Word should be like a newborn's desire for milk. Why is it we're sometimes so reluctant to open our Bibles? Why is it so easy to let other things crowd into our busy lives? Why do we feed on radio and television programs rather than reading the Book that was written by God Himself.

Babies don't question whether their mother's milk is good for them. They just eagerly drink. We don't have to tell them that they will be able to absorb vital elements such as zinc and iron, or that they will be getting anti-inflammatory properties from their mother's milk, or that babies on mother's milk seem to have fewer difficulties with low self-esteem and learning problems such as dyslexia. They just trust that what we give them is good for them.

Shouldn't we trust our heavenly Father with the same baby-like trust, and eagerly drink deeply from the milk of His Word? Or do we need to be told the benefits: that His Word tucked into our brains will help us avoid harmful temptations; that His Word offers encouragement, love, understanding, and forgiveness; that His Word strengthens our thinking and decision-making processes, and that once we drink there comes the tremendous peace and certainty that with God everything is going to be alright.

Lord, help me to be like a newborn baby—eager to drink the milk of Your Word.

MARTHA A. LEE

Eating for Healthy Teeth and Gums

For I command you today to love the Lord your God, to walk in his ways, and to keep his commands, decrees and laws; then you will live and increase, and the Lord your God will bless you in the land you are entering to possess. Deut. 30:16, NIV.

RIGHT NOW, EVEN if you've just brushed your teeth, you have a mouth full of bacteria. That's why bacterial plaque is constantly forming on your teeth and gum tissues. Just as people need to eat to stay alive, so does the bacteria. It feeds on the sugars that are found in the food you eat. The more sugar, the more bacteria, the more plaque, the more acid, and the more dental disease!

When I ask children if they will quit eating sugar to protect their teeth from decay, they all raise their hands. Then I ask them if they will stop drinking soft drinks, eating candy bars or cookies, and chewing gum, and their hands go down very quickly. They do not realize that all those "foods" contain large amounts of sugar.

Most adults have no idea how much hidden sugar they are pouring into their bodies. They drink orange juice instead of eating a whole orange. Oops! Extra sugar! Pasta's good for you, right? Well, not as good as whole grain! And for desert they unroll a strawberry fruit roll-up and enjoy the sweet sticky taste, not realizing that the concentrated sugars are feeding an army of harmful bacteria, while a couple fresh strawberries would satisfy their sweet tooth, add important nutrients to their diet, and supply natural sugars—which aren't nearly as satisfying to bacteria as refined sugars! As a dentist, I see small children with their two front teeth eaten away because they've been put to bed with a bottle of milk! Children fall asleep with their teeth coated with sweet milk, and while they sleep the acid in the milk causes severe tooth decay. It's called the nursing bottle syndrome.

I also see a lot of decay in teenagers. Their teeth are more susceptible to these acids than adults; their diet of soft drinks and candy bars results in increased decay during the teen years.

God's original plant-based diet is best suited to the needs of our bodies. Satan has taken God's foods and shown us how to process them—to our harm. Jesus does not want us to have unhealthy teeth and gums. If we follow God's original diet as closely as we can, we can be protected from many of the diseases falling on us as sinful human beings.

Lord, give me the willpower to choose God's original foods.

EDDIE C. TOWLES

A Fresh, New Beginning

Create in me a clean heart, O God; and renew a right spirit within me. . . . Restore unto me the joy of thy salvation; and uphold me with thy free spirit. Ps. 51:10-12.

THE WEIGHT OF regret can sometimes be enormous. Even though others' words and actions toward me can be a source of pain, it is the pain I have caused others through my mistakes and insensitivities that leaves a heaviness in my heart that truly defines regret.

How do I deal with my mistakes and sins? How do I manage the pain that my mistakes have caused? Can I find joy and peace in my daily living?

My sins toward others have caused irreparable damage! How do I right the wrongs? I begin by asking God's forgiveness. I must accept this forgiveness and believe with all my heart that God is able and willing to forgive. The Bible says that I am then to seek forgiveness from the one I have hurt. Making things right may seem impossible but I am to seek forgiveness and to do all I can to make it right. Then I must put the "mess" in God's trustworthy hands.

What happens to my faith when forgiveness from the offended person and God has been asked and received, yet the pain remains? Seeking of forgiveness from God and from the one whom we have hurt does not always erase the financial, emotional, or physical scars that the sin has caused. I must trust that God will bring blessings and healing to the circumstance. God will be there for the one I have hurt, and He will be there for me as I ask for His mercy and seek His forgiveness.

Every day I place the brokenness of my life in God's hands and ask for joy and a confidence for living. It seems to me that to live a joyous and victorious life is within the grasp of one who daily beholds the One that can bring victory out of defeat and peace and joy out of sadness. It is the simple process of laying my life at His feet; knowing with assurance that His grace is sufficient.

I do believe that by beholding Christ and His love for me, I can walk in newness of life. Each day I choose to place my life and the lives of those I have hurt in His care and know with absolute assurance that one day God will graciously give to His children a fresh, new beginning.

If you are feeling regret about something you have done, perhaps today is the day to ask forgiveness and experience the joy of a "clean heart." HERMAN HARP

The Measure of Success

Whatever your hand finds to do, do it with your might; for there is no work or device or knowledge or wisdom in the grave where you are going. Eccl. 9:10, NKJV.

GOD CAN WORK miracles through the hands of gifted surgeons who dedicate their talents to His service. One of those is Dr. Benjamin Carson, head of pediatric neurosurgery at Johns Hopkins Hospital in Baltimore, Maryland. He's renowned for the separation of Siamese, or conjoined, twins.

In 1997, at the request of neurosurgeon Sam Mokgokong, Dr. Carson led a medical team of more than two dozen physicians from the Medical University of Southern Africa (the only major black teaching hospital in South Africa) in one of these separations. "This was not only a medical challenge," Dr. Carson said, "but a social one. Always a stepchild throughout apartheid, they knew that if this operation could be performed at this hospital, they could stand shoulder to shoulder with other major medical universities."

These 11-month-old twin boys were joined at the top of their heads, facing opposite directions. There were 13 previous separation attempts and none were successful. Dr. Carson requested a stereo unit so they could hear inspirational music throughout the surgery. After 19 hours they were only three fourths of the way done, but the arteries were so entangled that it was feared they wouldn't have enough blood in all of South Africa to do the job. He suggested stopping and then resuming the operation in a couple of months. Dr. Mokgokong replied, "We don't have the equipment to do that here." So they kept going.

Dr. Carson commented, "I had none of my fancy equipment, just my scalpel and faith in God. Some of those blood vessels were thinner than a sheet of paper. When I made that final cut 28 hours later, the "Hallelujah Chorus" came over the stereo system. Everyone had goose bumps. Within three weeks the boys were crawling around normally, and we only used three units of blood. As far as we know, this is the first time anybody's been able to completely separate conjoined at the head twins in one operation—not only with both surviving, but apparently with no deficits. The self-esteem of everyone went through the roof; people were dancing in the streets. Now that is what success is, it's taking your God-given talent and developing it in order to elevate others—and never being ashamed of God."

God wants to work miracles with your hands, too. Will you dedicate them to His service? LAVERNE HENDERSON

Light in the Dungeon

For this is the Eternal's promise: "Those who survive the sword shall find grace in the dungeon." Jer. 31:2, Moffatt.

HOW DO WE find grace—God's divine love and protection—in our dungeons of despair, fatigue, or pain? What grace can there be in the dark night of our souls? Can we really sing songs in the strange land of affliction as did Paul and Silas at midnight in the Philippian prison (Acts 16:25)?

It seems impossible. But it's when we are most broken and crushed that God is the closest. He dwells with those that have broken hearts. He says, "I live in a high and holy place, but also with him who is contrite [crushed] and lowly in spirit" (Isa. 57:15, NIV).

God has promised that it is when we are in the dungeon that we will find Him and His compassion. Remember the story of Daniel's three companions who were thrown into a fiery furnace? Three were thrown in but when the king looked in, he saw four people. He commented, "The form of the fourth is like the Son of God" (Dan. 3:25). Why? Because it was God!

The "form of the fourth" is with us in our anguish, too. God says: "I will turn their mourning into joy and I will comfort them and make them rejoice, for their captivity with all its sorrows will be behind them" (Jer. 31:13, TLB).

We complain of our circumstances; we think it is impossible to live a believing life in the environment and situation that makes knots in our hearts. But frustration can become fruitfulness, and resistance can become resourcefulness. Corrie ten Boom found grace in her dungeon. She shares the horror of her and her sister Betsie's imprisonment in a Nazi concentration camp, Ravensbruck, in her book *The Hiding Place*. Corrie survived the camp, her private and terrible dungeon, and found strength and grace to bring comfort to millions worldwide.

Regardless of what may come our way, we have no excuse to languish in our dungeons. All things are possible with God—even serenity in the midst of a hopeless situation, humanly speaking.

How is it possible? Reinforcement against a dungeon experience is made beforehand, while we are in the Light, in prayer and study of God's precious Word. One doesn't learn to swim when one is drowning, and the anchor must be secured before the storm.

How are you preparing today to so live in the Light that you'll be ready for any dungeon that life may throw you into? PAT NORDMAN

Leaning on Him

Therefore I will boast all the more gladly about my weaknesses,
so that Christ's power may rest on me. 2 Cor. 12:9, NIV.

I WAS DIAGNOSED with lupus just before my junior year of high school. In those days little was known about the disease—and that hasn't greatly changed! I was told to be careful about being in the sunlight and getting too tired. But as an active adolescent I pretty much ignored the doctor's advice. I spent hours outdoors working on my tan and doing anything I wanted to do. I put the disease out of my mind, other than the frequent rash on my face that I attributed to "allergies."

I always said that I wouldn't let lupus interfere with my "real life." For many years I didn't. I camped, hiked, backpacked, rode horses, and about everything else I wanted to. I also raised a family of little girls and several foster children, taught elementary school, and worked in the church in a variety of capacities. I thought that my health and energy would go on forever.

Once my girls were on their own my life slowed down a little. I slept more and found it difficult to get out of bed because my joints were so stiff and sore. I began running fevers, and had other physical symptoms. The medications prescribed by my rheumatologist were not very helpful, so I tried to ignore the worsening pain. I began to limp, but decided that I was stronger than any ailment. When my doctor suggested that I use a cane, I fought the idea. I wouldn't allow myself to be dependent on anything but my will power.

Finally the day came when I had to surrender my pride and buy a cane, something I saw as a symbol of weakness. As I leaned on it when I walked, I discovered that I could walk faster and with less pain. By depending on it, I became stronger and could walk farther and for longer than before.

I always considered myself to be strong and in need of no one. I could handle everything myself. God was an important part of my life, but I didn't really depend on Him. With lupus, I was faced with something I couldn't handle by myself. I had to lean on my Lord, and in doing that, I discovered His strength. I have found, as the apostle Paul said, that God's grace is sufficient for me, for His power is made perfect in my weakness.

Are you stressed out trying to live on your own willpower and self-sufficiency? Perhaps it's time to let the Lord take over the driver's seat in your life, and enjoy the contentment that is available in Him. DONNA ENGBERTSON

How to Stop Brain Cell Death

You shall come to the grave at a full age, as a
sheaf of grain ripens in its season. Job 5:26, NKJV.

BEGINNING SHORTLY AFTER birth, when the number of brain cells that we possess are probably at their maximum, those cells begin to die at a frightening rate—perhaps as many as 50,000 per day! Multiply that by the number of days you have lived and you get some staggering figures. That's about 18,250,000 cells every year!

In spite of this brain drain, brain performance in healthy people does not significantly change over a 50-year period. For some, performance actually improves even into the mid-70s and older.

The principle of *redundancy* holds that we have so many more brain cells than we could possibly use that we can afford to lose a tremendous number. The principle "use it or lose it" may be directing this massive extermination of brain cells. Is it possible that we are not providing our brains with the enrichment of fascinating opportunities that our brains are capable of handling?

In spite of this death of brain cells, undamaged brain cells in the elderly can grow more dendrites, providing more communication sites. That is the principle of *plasticity*. Those fewer brain cells are more active and search out new connections if they are called upon to perform, even in advancing years. The more experience, learning, and practice, the greater the number of connections.

Decreases in memory span and in the ability to process information rapidly and to integrate incoming information become frightening or discouraging to many who are aging. But you can be encouraged: recent studies show that even the physical loss or deterioration of thousands of brain cells does not necessarily reduce the functioning potential of an aging person. It may take a little longer to process some tasks, but the lack of speed can be more than offset by the wisdom born of experience.

It is also possible that most of these "losses" in function can be halted or even reversed by use. For maximum brain health, exercise all your different thinking centers—logical thinking, analytical problem solving, artistic expression, creative thinking, memorization, sensory stimulation, language and motor skills.

The plasticity of the brain can continue even into the oldest years, but you've got to use it, if you don't want to lose it!

Dear God, thank You for creating me with enough brain cells for eternity. Help me to use them so I won't lose them. ELDEN M. CHALMERS

Currency of Activity

*The Lord God took the man and put him in the Garden of
Eden to work it and take care of it. Gen. 2:15, NIV.*

HAVE YOU EVER wondered what it might be like to live in a perfect
land, a place of perfect health, perfect happiness, and perfect peace? Such
a place once existed here on Planet Earth. We call it the Garden of Eden,
the original home of Adam and Eve.

Can you picture what life might have been like in the Garden of Eden?
Swimming with the dolphins at dawn. Leisurely walking alongside a brook
at sunset. Sipping coconut juice under a shady palm. Working in the rose-
bushes . . . What? Wait a minute. Working in Paradise? Can that be?
Apparently so. Though Adam and Eve likely had plenty of time for rest
and relaxation, meditation, and play, they also had work to do. God did
not want His children to be idle. He wanted them to stay active. So He
gave them the job tending and caring for their garden home.

Working helped Adam and Eve maintain strong, healthy bodies. They
experienced the mental satisfaction and pride of watching the garden flourish under their care. They enjoyed the social benefits of working together
for a common goal. As they assisted with the amazing process of life, they
gained a deeper sense of spiritual connection to their Creator.

The benefits Adam and Eve experienced in Eden can be ours today.
When you begin a regular routine of exercise, you will see many dramatic
results. Physically you will grow stronger, sleep better, and be less susceptible to injury. Mentally you will have less stress, be able to think more
clearly, and have a more positive outlook on life. Socially you will sense
more confidence in yourself because you feel better and look better.
Spiritually you will find a deeper connection to your Creator who made
you for a life of health, happiness, and peace.

But the benefits of activity come only when action is consistent.
Baseball great Cal Thomas once said, "Life is like a bank. You can't take
more out than you put in." Every day that we continue to be physically active is like putting money into a bank. Of course, nothing in life is certain.
But if you continue to deposit the currency of activity on a regular basis,
you can reasonably expect the payoff of a longer, healthier, happier life.

*What do you plan to do today that will give you the exercise necessary to enjoy
a longer, healthier, happier life?*   TODD CHOBOTAR

Healing Waters

*And he showed me a pure river of water of life, clear as crystal,
proceeding from the throne of God and of the Lamb. Rev. 22:1, NKJV.*

ONE OF THE JOYS of my childhood was wading in Beaver Creek,
which flowed by the sand-hills ranch of friends. To take off shoes and
socks, pull on an old dress, and race for the cool freshness of the crystal-
clear stream was my idea of delight on a hot summer Sabbath afternoon.
Ahhh, the soothing, refreshing feel of gently flowing water!

One forenoon in early spring my husband and I sat on the banks of the
Crow Wing River in northern Minnesota. We had come away from the
bustling city to the old family farm, now unoccupied. The Crow Wing
was a deep river, hurrying with the surge of spring thaws on its way to the
mighty Mississippi. As we watched the fast-flowing water swirling along
and listened to the voices of its song, the stresses of a busy life seemed to
be carried along with the current.

Not long ago at the home of friends in Oklahoma, I strolled under
lofty trees to a miniature spring-fed creek. There I found a seat in just the
right place to hear the gentle murmur of the water rippling over the peb-
bles and watch the bits of leaves and sticks being carried along with the
flow. What a soothing, restful place to relax and meditate!

Contrast the healing energy one finds sitting next to a gently flowing
stream to the destructive power of angry flood waters out of control. The
first is a symbol of God's kingdom, with the pure, crystal-clear Water of
Life flowing from God's throne. The brown murky torrent that rushes
down the valley, carrying its burden of rocks and soil, illustrates the devastation of Satan's kingdom of sin and sorrow.

If we don't follow Jesus' instruction to "Come aside by yourselves to
a deserted place and rest a while" (Mark 6:31, NKJV), it's easy to get swept
away by the flood of temptation and overcommitment. When that happens we need to remember who's in control. Just as Jesus stilled the angry
waves on stormy Galilee, He can still the waters of our life.

I am looking forward to a time of quiet reflection beside the river of
life in the New Jerusalem, aren't you? What a thrill it will be when we can
drink of the gentle water of life, after every trace of sin and distress has
been removed.

*Dear Lord, still the raging waters of my life with Your healing Water of Life.
Amen.*   VELDA NELSON

Commandments for Healthy Living

The law of the wise is a fountain of life, to turn one
away from the snares of death. Prov. 13:14, NKJV.

GOD MAKES THINGS simple! He didn't give us 2,457 rules to live by. He simply chose 10 absolutely essential commandments for healthy, moral living. The first four have to do with connecting with the God of the universe—our Creator. Number 1 says to worship only God. Number 2 clarifies the first: God wants such an intimate relationship with us that we should never worship pictures or statues of Him. Number 3: Worship means speaking respectfully of God—never using His name in any other way than worshipfully. Number 4 tells us when to worship and gives us time off to do it. Keep the seventh day as Sabbath—24 hours during which we are not to work. I can't think of a better way to insure good spiritual health than to keep these first four commandments.

The next six commandments have to do with connecting with each other. Keep these and you'll be socially healthy; you'll save yourself a lot of heartache and keep from hurting others. Number 5 addresses the relationship of parents and child. God says to respect your parents. Honor them. To do so will be good for your physical health—and you'll likely live longer than if you carry around a load of bitterness. Number 6: Don't murder—physically or psychologically. Yes, we can kill others with our words if we're not careful. Number 7: Respect the marriage covenant. Respect and be true to your own spouse, and respect the sacred bond of other married couples. Specifically, don't commit adultery. Can you imagine how much healthier our lives would be if we wouldn't even allow our minds to think about improper behavior with those of the opposite sex! Number 8: Don't steal. Respect other people's property. Number 9: Don't lie. Be truthful in everything you do, and you'll be safe to be around. Finally, Number 10: Be happy for what other people have; don't covet their possessions.

God's Word also contains principles that can keep us physically healthy. But they're not as organized as the 10 commandments found in Exodus 20:1-17. So I've turned to scientific research. Here are the top five commandments that will do more than anything else to decrease your risk of getting a chronic disease: Number 1: Don't smoke. Number 2: Avoid a sedentary lifestyle—exercise. Number 3: Eat a variety of fruits and vegetables and avoid high-fat foods. Number 4: Avoid pushing yourself beyond the limits—rest. Number 5: Avoid the intake of alcohol.

God, give me the willpower to be a commandment keeper!   KAY KUZMA

The Push for Power

"Not by might nor by power, but by My Spirit,"
says the Lord of hosts. Zech. 4:6, NKJV.

FROM THE WHITE HOUSE to corporate America to who gets to be first down the playground slide, a common, almost worshiped trait of human existence is *power*. Power to manipulate. Power to control. Power to make things happen. Power to get what I want. Power to get you to do what I want. We all dance to its music, if but for a little while. But today, the push for power has come to shove. There's power lingo, power plays, power wardrobe; even power table manners, such as "Never stoop to retrieve dropped silver."

The overall guide to power could probably be summed up in that phrase, *"Never stoop."* Never put yourself down. Never admit mistakes. Never loosen your grip on your rung of the ladder. But where does this push for power lead?

One afternoon while attending Andrews University in Berrien Springs, Michigan, I rode my bike to boxing champion Muhammad Ali's sprawling farm on the shores of the St. Joseph River. The entrance to the farm was barred by a splintered, rusted gate. Tall weeds grew along the drive where immaculate flowers once had been. There were cracks in the asphalt and garbage littered the entryway. Faded, peeling buildings house the place where the once "great one" still spends some time.

In 1988 sportswriter Gary Smith interviewed Ali at his farm. Ali escorted Smith out to the barn. On the floor, leaning against the walls, were mementos of Ali in his prime. Photos and portraits of the champ, punching and dancing. Sculpted body. Fists beating the air. Championship belt held high in triumph. But on the pictures were white streaks—bird droppings. Ali looked into the rafters at the pigeons who had made his gym their home. And then he did something significant. Perhaps it was a gesture of closure. Maybe despair. Whatever the reason, he walked over to the row of pictures and turned them, one by one, toward the wall. He then walked out the door, mumbling. "I had the world. I—and it—wasn't nothin'. Look now!"

Look now at your life. What do you see? Are you living the life of the power-hungry, or a life like Christ's? Christ stooped to wash His disciples' feet—and by His power He was raised from the dead. That's something to think about!

Instead of pushing for power, glorify your heavenly Father. With His power you can successfully complete the destiny that God has for you. STEVEN L. HALEY

For Heaven's and Health's Sake—Pray!

*These things I have spoken to you, that in Me you
may have peace. In the world you will have tribulation; but be
of good cheer, I have overcome the world. John 16:33, NKJV.*

I WAS RAISED in a church where there were congregants known as "prayer warriors." They were the "old saints" (probably my present age) who came to understand through the years that serious prayers get results. They prayed through an issue; they prayed until the Lord said, "Done. . . . Next?"

Talking about things can relieve a person, but genuine prayer can bring the miracle of a cure. Most of the really important miracles cannot be seen right away—especially in health.

Prayer may promote health through a special form of stress relief, according to Harvard researcher Herbert Benson, M.D., who pioneered the "relaxation response." Prayer elicits the relaxation response by regularly reducing blood pressure in people with hypertension, and blood sugar among diabetics. It may also ease anxiety, depression, insomnia, and headaches. Research now suggests that prayer can benefit sick people by easing chronic pain, and controlling nausea from chemotherapy. Scientists have proven that people who pray heal faster than those who don't.

As Christians we don't need scientific evidence to assure us that prayer can make a difference. We've known about that for a while. The most important thing is to understand that prayer is not an end in itself, as many New Agers contend. Jesus Christ, the object of our prayer, has the capability of performing miracles seen and unseen. As an example, prayer affects our immune system. Prayer affects dispositions and attitudes. Sincere prayers of repentance can help resolve deep feelings of guilt and shame that sap health, vitality, and life itself.

Our loving Lord knows us better than any counselor could after eight hours of daily counseling for many years. He is ready to demonstrate that He is the Lord of life, the Lord of relief, the Lord of peace, the Lord of joy, and the Lord of wholeness. He can change things as fast as we can exhale if we earnestly seek Him and let Him lead.

What an advantage we have over the rest of the world. Shouldn't we Christians be the healthiest people on this planet? Are we appropriating through faith these precious blessings that are available to us? Are you? If not, why not?

Here's a challenge: Become a prayer warrior for someone who needs life, relief, peace, joy, or wholeness. Keep praying until the Lord says, "Done. . . . Next?"

E. JOHN REINHOLD

Forgive Your Hecklers

Be kind to one another, tenderhearted, forgiving one another,
even as God in Christ forgave you. Eph. 4:32, NKJV.

TOO OFTEN, WHEN bad things happen to us, and we feel like a failure, we want to blame someone. We want to make someone else hurt. What we need to do is look for a solution. We must stop the blame game and start taking responsibility for our own emotions and behavior.

In His sermon on the mount Jesus commented about people with a compulsion to criticize others: "First remove the plank from your own eye, and then you will see clearly to remove the speck from your brother's eye" (Matt. 7:5, NKJV). Look for the good in others; learn to forgive, and take responsibility for the solution.

Herdan Harding tells a story of a baseball player in the Los Angeles Dodgers' minor league system. When something went wrong the athlete would break or throw bats, apparently as a way to forestall other people from criticizing him. Such behavior, though, made him somewhat of a target, especially to two fans who heckled him on a routine and rigorous basis.

Once, after the batter had struck out, the two young men again began taunting him. The player strode over to the fence near where they sat and gestured to them to come down. They weren't so sure they wanted to, but they gathered their courage and went. Instead of being furious, which would have been his typical reaction, he chose to respond differently. Grabbing his bat by the barrel, he extended the handle to the two men and said, "Do you guys want a Dodgers' bat?"

After that, they never badgered him again. They attended almost every game and supported and encouraged him just as loudly as previously they had heckled him. It was one of the things that changed the baseball player's life, because he realized that he could choose to do things differently. Not only did it alter his outlook, but it actually had an advantageous transformation on his environment as well.

He may or may not have known it, but this baseball player followed Paul's advice in Ephesians 4:32 when he forgave the two hecklers. You see, if we hold grudges and hurts, then our hearts sicken, our souls shrivel, and eventually our bodies will suffer physically as well.

The next time someone makes fun of you, take control of your outlook. Return evil with good and see what a difference it makes. DES CUMMINGS, JR.

Go-Go Juice

*Listen to counsel and receive instruction, that you
may be wise in your latter days. Prov. 19:20, NKJV.*

I USED TO DRINK a lot of coffee. By the time I went to university I was accustomed to drinking four pots every day—something like 24 cups! While not everyone puts away 24 cups of coffee, North Americans consume a total of more than 35 million pounds every year. Add to this the millions of cans of caffeinated soda consumed a day and you begin to realize that North America is facing a major public health problem—caffeine addiction!

Doctors are beginning to tell patients to kick the caffeine habit, and for good reason. Caffeine has no nutritional value but it's linked to sleep disorders, headaches, high blood pressure and tension, irregular heartbeat, memory loss, tremors, and convulsions. Some studies seem to indicate that it acts as a catalyst for carcinogens, increasing the odds of getting cancer.

Dr. Jan W. Kuzma, in his book *Live Ten Healthy Years Longer,* mentions an interesting study done on typists. A group of typists was set up who had used no caffeine for two weeks. Their typing was accurate, and they correctly estimated their speed. Then each participant drank two cups of coffee. Their accuracy decreased considerably. However, in their self-evaluations they thought they were doing much better in speed and accuracy then when they had not used caffeine.

So much for the idea that caffeine improves one's performance! On a construction site where I once worked, we used to call coffee "go-go juice," because everybody assumed that it improved our ability to get things done. It turns out that the only thing it improved was our self estimate.

Satan is eager to tempt us with all kinds of "go-go juices" that mask our real sinful condition and make us think we're better than we are. Caffeinated drinks are not the only substances on his illusionary buffet table. There's also alcohol, tobacco, and drugs that alter moods and dull perceptions. When we're under the illusion that our performance is improved, there is no reason to repent, no reason to turn from evil, and no sense of need for the saving grace of God.

Say goodbye "go-go juice"; kick the habit—even if you're going to have to endure a few days of painful withdrawal symptoms—and say hello to the best drink on earth: a cool, clear cup of water.

Lord, help me avoid any substance that clouds my thinking, so that I may perceive accurately what your Holy Spirit is trying to communicate to me.

SHAWN BOONSTRA

Season Your Words With Salt

But encourage one another daily, as long as it is called Today, so that none of you may be hardened by sin's deceitfulness. Heb. 3:13, NIV.

HEBREWS 3:13 MAKES it clear that discouraging words break down a person's spiritual immune system. But did you know they also weaken the physical immune system?

In 1996 Drs. Janice Kiecolt Glazer and Ronald Glazer reported a study on couples who had been married for an average of 42 years but were constantly arguing and saying words of discouragement to one another. They found that the more they argued and criticized, the weaker their immune systems were. You might think heated arguments would have less impact on older couples because after all their years together they would have gotten used to put downs, or would have learned to deal with them. Unfortunately, discouraging words always have a negative impact.

The Glazers also studied 90 newlywed couples who agreed to spend their honeymoon in a hospital research unit for 24 hours. They were asked to have a 30-minute discussion on their marital problems. It was found that those who exhibited more negative and hostile behaviors during that 30-minute discussion showed greater decreases over 24 hours on four functional immunological assays. In other words, they found that the immune system is less effective when there is conflict and discouraging words thrown at each other—even though the couple had just gotten married and they were otherwise happy. Words have the power to weaken or strengthen the immune system!

Without words of encouragement, life can be meaningless. I once read about a millionaire who prided himself for never offering a tip for any service. On New Year's Day he got word that his chief accountant had committed suicide. Immediately he rushed over to the man's place. All the books were in perfect order. He had done his job well. Why had he taken his own life? After a thorough search this note was found: "In 30 years I have never had one word of encouragement. I am fed up."

Paul understood the power of speech when he advised, "Let no corrupt word proceed out of your mouth, but what is good for necessary edification, that it may impart grace to the hearers" (Eph. 4:29, NKJV). In other words, say only that which will be a blessing to others.

The next time you're tempted to tell someone off, remember to "let your speech always be with grace, seasoned with salt" (Col. 4:6, NKJV). By doing so, you will be boosting their spiritual and physical immune systems—and yours!

KATHLEEN H. LIWIDJAJA-KUNTARAF

Secondhand Drinking

Wine is a mocker, strong drink is a brawler, and whoever is led astray by it is not wise. Prov. 20:1, NKJV.

WE'VE ALL HEARD about the deadly effects of secondhand smoking, but did you know alcohol has a secondhand effect, too? Parental drinking hurts children. Alcohol causes drunkenness and disinhibition, so it's associated with unintended pregnancy, marital disruption, child abuse, incest, automobile accidents, career disruptions, educational underachievement, extramarital sexual affairs, cheating, stealing, dishonesty, employment underachievement, and the transmission of sexually transmitted diseases, including AIDS. The list could go on and on.

Parents might counter, "But I'm a social drinker. I don't get drunk. How can this possibly hurt my children?" In a study conducted among students who attended 69 parochial schools in North America during the 1994-1995 school year, students were asked if either of their parents used alcohol and whether or not the students had ever used alcohol. They were also asked about their sexual habits.

The results were striking. Only three and a half percent of the students who had never used alcohol and whose parents did not use alcohol were sexually experienced. However, if the student had tried alcohol and at least one of their parents was a user, the percentage of those who were experienced sexually increased tenfold to more than 30 percent. Since unprotected sexual intercourse is a strong AIDS risk factor, alcohol use in the home is a cofactor for these students' risk of transmitting or contracting the virus that causes AIDS.

Other data from that same research showed that if alcohol was not used by either parent, 37.6 percent of the students had tried alcohol. However, if a parent did use alcohol, the rate of alcohol use by the student jumped to 71.7 percent.

There was even a strong effect of the parents' alcohol use on the student's history of the use of many other drugs. If a parent was an alcohol user, the student's rate of tobacco use increased from 24.4 percent to 47.3 percent, marijuana use increased from 11.5 percent to 27.1 percent, cocaine use jumped from 2.2 percent to 6.7 percent, and use of other hard drugs increased from 4.9 percent to 14.6 percent. Parents who drink must seriously reflect on what they are doing to their children's health!

Is there some area of your life that is causing a negative effect on your children? If so, ask God to give you the strength to overcome. GARY HOPKINS

Surviving Shocks of Pain and Stress

As one whom his mother comforts, so I will comfort you. Isa. 66:13, NKJV.

A FEW YEARS AGO several medical researchers were studying the effect of the shocks of life on the central nervous system. They took a lamb and placed it in its pen alone. They then hooked up electric shock devices around the pen. As the lamb wandered to one side of the pen, the researchers threw a switch and the lamb was shocked. Immediately it twitched and scampered to another part of the pen. Soon the researchers shocked the lamb again. Again he ran.

As the research continued, the scientists discovered that the lamb would never return to a place where he had been previously shocked. After a series of shocks, the little lamb just stood in the center of his pen quivering. He had no place to run, and no place to hide. The shocks were everywhere. Completely overcome emotionally, filled with anxiety and stress, his nerves gave way.

The researchers then took this lamb's twin and placed it in a pen. This time, they put the lamb's mother in with him. Presently, they shocked him. Again the lamb ran, but this time he ran to his mother and snuggled up to her closely. Evidently she reassured him, because he left her side to begin eating again. The researchers threw the switch again, and once again the lamb ran to his mother. Reassuringly she consoled him again.

The researchers noticed a remarkable difference in the two lambs. The second lamb had no fear of returning to the spot where he received the shock. To the utter amazement of the researchers, further shocks no longer disturbed him. He showed none of the symptoms of nervousness, stress, and anxiety that his twin showed under the same circumstances.

What made this remarkable difference? He had the reassurance of someone to flee to in stress. He had confidence and power in someone outside of himself to cope with the stress.

We're the same way. When we have to face pain and anxiety alone, we can easily become overwhelmed. Satan knows this. That's why he's working so hard to make people feel alienated from family and friends.

Just as the lamb found reassurance in the presence of his mother, true rest for God's children is found in a loving, trust relationship with their Creator. Snuggled safe in the arms of Jesus we can withstand whatever shocks this world may inflict upon us.

Precious Lord, lead me safely through the land mines of pain, worry, and stress. Amen. MARK FINLEY

Death in the Pot

The sting of death is sin. . . . But thanks be to God, who gives us
the victory through our Lord Jesus Christ. 1 Cor. 15:56, 57, NKJV.

FOOD WAS SCARCE because of famine. The prophet Elisha had his servant prepare a great pot of stew to feed all his students. One student went out
into the field to gather herbs, found a wild gourd vine, picked a lapful, and
sliced them into the stew—having no idea they were poisonous. The students
must have been ravenously hungry, but when they tasted the soup they cried
out, "Man of God, there is death in the pot!" Elisha asked for some flour. He
put it into the pot and said, "'Serve it to the people, that they may eat.' And
there was nothing harmful in the pot" (2 Kings 4:40, 41, NKJV.)

Wouldn't it be wonderful if today a little flour could turn good-tasting
but harmful ingredients into harmless ones? Unfortunately, that miracle happened only to Elisha. It becomes our responsibility to watch carefully the
substances that flavor our foods, because some excitotoxins, such as MSG
(monosodium glutamate) and aspartame (the main ingredient in NutraSweet
or Equal and in diet drinks/foods), can be poisonous to certain people.

According to Russell Blaylock, M.D., author of *Excitotoxins: The Taste
That Kills,* excitotoxins are common neurotransmitters in the brain and behave as chemical messengers between neurons. The problem arises when
they accumulate in concentrations higher than needed, such as when MSG
or aspartame (NutraSweet) is added to the pot. They then act like poison
to the neurons. They overexcite neurons, causing them to fire their impulses very rapidly until they reach a state of extreme exhaustion. The destructive effects of these substances have been linked to Alzheimer's,
Parkinson's, AIDS, dementia, and other neuro-degenerative diseases.

There is a barrier that should prevent harmful substances from entering the brain, but weak spots exist and since it's not fully developed at
birth, babies and children are most vulnerable. Even in the adult brain the
barrier weakens under certain conditions that include head injury, stroke,
brain tumors, infections, hypoglycemia, low-calorie diets, and excessive
physical stress. To keep the barrier healthy requires a lot of cellular energy
and a good supply of antioxidants—especially vitamins C and E, and minerals such as magnesium. Whether or not MSG or aspartame will be poisonous to an individual depends on many variables, including a genetic
susceptibility to excitotoxins.

*Lord, give me self-control to put health before taste buds so I won't add "death
to the pot."*   RISÉ RAFFERTY

Walking Is Good for the Soul

Cause me to hear Your lovingkindness in the morning, for in You do I trust; cause me to know the way in which I should walk, for I lift up my soul to You. Ps. 143:8, NKJV.

GOD CREATED HUMANS to be active. Without regular exercise our bodies build up toxins, fat accumulates in tissues and arteries, our heart has to work harder and is less effective, we get depressed easier, and we age faster.

Exercise is one of the most valuable therapies ever invented! One scientist said that if a pharmaceutical company developed a pill that would do for us what exercise does, it would probably win a Nobel Prize in medicine and make a fortune for its shareholders.

"Why exercise?" some people ask. "The Bible doesn't say we should." No, but the Bible does describe the way the people of Bible times lived. What was the predominant transportation system? Walking. Even with all our scientific inventions, no one has been able to come up with an exercise that does more for the body.

Today, we think carefully about walking somewhere if it's more than a couple blocks, but consider this: Mary, Jesus' mother, walked almost a hundred miles from her home in Galilee to Judea when she was pregnant. In fact, she did it twice: once to visit Elizabeth and again to go to Bethlehem for the census.

It wasn't until I visited the Holy Land that I began to get an idea of how much walking the people had to do to get anyplace. It was an hour bus ride from Nazareth to the shores of Galilee where Jesus spent so much of His time ministering. I would have thought twice even hiking from the Sea of Galilee up to the closest hill, where it's likely that Christ gave His sermon on the mount. I was thankful I made the trip in an air conditioned bus! I can't imagine walking from Jericho to Jerusalem, now that I've been there. It was an uphill, rough, winding trail all the way. It took our bus more than an hour! I now realize why God didn't have to instruct His people to get exercise—they got it naturally.

All I have to do when I'm tempted to cheat on my exercise is to remember how much walking Jesus did, and I get up and put on my walking shoes. I want to be like Christ. As I walk each morning and evening I meditate and pray. And in the process, I've discovered that walking is not only good for the body, but it's also good for the soul.

Have you had your walk with Christ yet today?   JAN W. KUZMA

Learning About Praise and Priorities

Why are you cast down, O my soul, and why are you disquieted within me? Hope in God; for I shall again praise him, my help and my God. Ps. 42:11, NRSV.

ONE DAY AS I was racing to get some household tasks done so that I could get to sleep and zip into another day, I cried out a prayer to my heavenly Father, "My life is too busy! I don't even have enough time to stop and think, let alone time to pray and study my Bible. Lord, is there any way You could change my situation so I can have more time with You?"

Within a few weeks I was struck with a reoccurrence of an acute infection, which ended up turning into a chronic illness that left me unable to work for more than a year. Although I did not want to slow down that much, nor stop working altogether, I see God's hand of love even in this.

The first week that I was seriously ill, I listened to a radio talk show regarding the importance of slowing down, analyzing one's priorities in life, simplifying everything possible, and spending time according to carefully thought-out priorities.

You would think that because I'm not working and can't do what I used to do, that I'd have lots of time. But it takes time to cope with a chronic illness. Now my time is filled with doctor's appointments and therapies! So simplifying and carefully choosing what I do with my time (according to thought-out priorities) has become absolutely necessary for my survival.

I have learned other lessons as well. I have found that careful attention to a healthy lifestyle is imperative—*especially in illness.* The health habits of good nutrition, moderate exercise, abstention from harmful substances, scrupulous personal hygiene, drinking plenty of pure water, taking small sun baths, breathing deeply of fresh air, taking time for good sleep, rejuvenating recreation and relaxation time, and a deep, abiding trust in God and His power, may not be curative in my illness, yet they seem to make a profound difference in my symptoms and in my mental attitude.

I have learned every day, whether it's a relatively good day or not, to list at least five blessings from my loving heavenly Father. It's hard to be down when you're looking up and praising God for His great faithfulness, mercy, and goodness!

My prayer now is that the lessons I've learned through this illness will stay with me even if God blesses me with complete healing.

Dear Father, help me to be willing to learn the lessons You want me to learn.

JEAN MARIE HAMETZ

A Nineteenth-century Testimony

I delight to do Your will, O my God, and Your law is within my heart. Ps. 40:8, NKJV.

AN EPIDEMIC OF DIPHTHERIA was raging. Children were dying like flies. There was anxiety in every home. Prescribing drugs, such as arsenic, was common. The *Farmers' and Miners' Journal* published this so-called cure: "Take Spanish flies, pound and mix with Venice turpentine, spread it on a piece of soft cloth, and bind it over the throat, which will raise a blister, and soon remove the disease from the throat." The year: 1862.

In February 1863 two of James and Ellen White's sons were struck by this dreaded disease. Call it an incredible coincidence—or a miracle—but at this very time the Whites came across an article by Dr. James C. Jackson of Dansville, New York, reporting the success he had in treating diphtheria with water treatments. Since this made more sense to them than poisonous drugs or Spanish flies, they scrupulously followed Dr. Jackson's directions, and the children recovered.

Sadly, even though the Whites had successfully used water to treat diphtheria, 10 months later they relied on common medical practice when their oldest son, Henry, got pneumonia. Eight days later he died. They had ordered Dr. Jackson's books, which described the use of rational methods, but the Whites had been too busy traveling, writing, and speaking to unwrap and read them.

In February 1864 their son, Willie, got pneumonia. He was so sick he was delirious. The Whites were faced with a dilemma that could mean life or death to their child. They decided to treat him themselves, with water—and prayer. For seven days and nights, they continued using water freely on his head and changing compresses on his lungs, and praying unceasingly. On the fifth day he coughed blood. That night the parents were so exhausted they got someone else to continue the treatments while they tried to sleep. But Ellen was so anxious she couldn't sleep. Since she felt pressed for breath, she opened the door into a large hall and was at once relieved and went to sleep. She dreamed that an experienced physician stood by her son's bed and said, "That which gave you relief will also relieve your child. He needs air. You have kept him too warm."

After she applied this new information, Willie's fever broke; he recovered rapidly and had better health than he had had for several years.

Dear Lord, thank You for pure water and fresh air and the knowledge we have today about how to use them to fight disease.   KAY KUZMA

I See Death Coming

What shall we say then? Is there unrighteousness with God? Certainly not!
For He says to Moses, "I will have mercy on whomever I will have mercy, and I
will have compassion on whomever I will have compassion." Rom. 9:14, 15, NKJV.

IN AUGUST 1998 I was diagnosed with amyotrophic lateral sclerosis (ALS), more commonly known in the United States as Lou Gehrig's disease. I had only two or, at the most, five years to live.

ALS is a fatal neuromuscular disease that attacks the motor neurons (cells) that carry signals from the brain to the voluntary muscles. When the motor neurons die, the muscles no longer receive signals from the brain and begin to atrophy and die. From tripping to dropping things to slurred speech, ALS will eventually cause complete paralysis, then death. The mind is not affected and will remain quite sharp, regardless of the deteriorating condition of the body. There is no known cure.

When I heard the verdict, a trickle of a tear ran down my cheek, but it was more because I was thinking of being without my family and what would happen to them. About the only question I had was what was the Lord's purpose in my life now? Was He pulling a biblical "Job" on me and not giving me a lot of details?

Why do bad things happen to good people? It's a popular question—but a bad one! The Bible says, "No one is good—except God alone" (Mark 10:18, NIV). Therefore, a better question would be Why do bad things happen to some people and not to others? You are now left with two choices: randomness without God or control with God. You cannot look at one thing in this world and not see God (Rom. 1:20). So if God is "God" (i.e., all-knowing, all-powerful), then *He must be in control,* and I have nothing to worry about. I may be just one pixel in God's panoramic picture, but without my one dot of color that picture is incomplete. God finishes what He starts.

No, I still do not believe that death is an entity; and yes, I know that Satan brought sin into this universe, with all its subsequent suffering. But God will eradicate it all. Trust Him. He knows what He's doing. How He chooses to use this instrument is His business, not mine. Ellen White says, "So long as I live, I desire to keep Christ in view. This is my life purpose. This is what I am living for—to glorify Christ and to make sure of life eternal. This is the great purpose that should inspire everyone" (*Sermons and Talks,* vol. 2, p. 214). Sounds like pretty good advice to me.

Lord, I'm ready to walk the journey You have for me to walk, with unwavering trust in You.   THOMAS L. BROOKS

Uniquely Complementary

And the Lord God said, "It is not good that man should be alone;
I will make him a helper comparable to him." Gen. 2:18, NKJV.

WHAT MAKES A healthy marriage? Beyond the physical, is there really a difference between men and women? The feminist view has tried to tell us that a woman can do anything a man does. That may be partially true in the job market, but what would truly meet the deepest needs of a man to be masculine and a woman to be feminine?

In her intriguing research *In a Different Voice* Carol Gilligan reports that a man sees himself as competent and mature when he can move into his world as a complete and separate individual, free to make his own decisions and feel a sense of security within himself. In contrast, a woman is most concerned with nurturing close relationships, seen in intimate bonding with family and friends. For her, being a complete and fulfilled woman depends on warm attachments to others.

Differences between men and women can be traced to the Garden of Eden. Larry Crabb, in his book *Men and Women: Enjoying the Differences,* writes, "God's judgment of Eve was on both her uniquely feminine capacity to give birth and her relationship with Adam. In other words, her physical attachment to Adam would lead to moments of excruciating pain (in childbirth) and her personal attachment would involve heartache and battle.

"Adam's judgment was different. God required him to endure previously unknown difficulties as he sought to subdue his world. He would now have to work in a hostile environment where he would often fail and to live with a woman who would now be more concerned with her own needs than with his" (pp. 134, 135).

God's judgment on Adam focused on his work—it would be more difficult. But Eve's judgment focused on her need for relating deeply with her husband. God created man to meet his wife's deepest need for relationship. And God created woman to meet her husband's deepest need for affirmation as he moves purposefully into his world. In God's design, they fit together beautifully. Each supplies what the other needs. They are complementary. And because we are all different in special ways, each couple has a unique "fit" that is suitable only for them.

Thank You, Lord, for creating men and women different—and uniquely complementary. Give me the wisdom to glorify You by meeting my mate's deepest needs.

BEVERLY CHILSON BRANDSTATER

God Cleaned Up My Life

Behold, You desire truth in the inward parts, and in the hidden part You will make me to know wisdom. Ps. 51:6, NKJV.

EVEN THOUGH MY family was poor, I grew up in a home where Pepsi Cola was the preferred choice of drink. And I loved meat! My philosophy was that if the Bible allows me to have colas and clean meats, no one should tell me I shouldn't.

Over a period of time, however, we just had less meat in our home, until I became a vegetarian. But that didn't cure my addiction to sweets. When I'd travel, I loved eating a Mrs. Field's cookie or a cinnamon bun. At potluck meals or parties, I'd feast on desserts.

I've always had a lot of faith in the power of God. But I never asked God to change my taste buds. I liked eating what I ate! God, however, worked a miracle and changed me anyway—in spite of myself! Here's how it happened:

One day I began earnestly praying for spiritual discernment so that I wouldn't be confused by subtle error. I asked God to give me a clear mind. I didn't want anything I did to keep Three Angels Broadcasting Network (3ABN) from being a channel that God could use to spread His message to the world.

That same day, I went on a juice fast. When my fast was over and breakfast time came, my regular cold cereal didn't look good. Instead, I had some fruit. I went to Wendy's for lunch for a baked potato. I started to order cheese and broccoli, but I said, "Just give it to me plain." When I started eating it, I commented, "How do they make these things taste so good?" Suppertime came and all I wanted was a salad. Milk didn't even look good. A number of weeks went by before I realized that all this time, I hadn't eaten anything with eggs, milk, cheese, or sugar in it. I began to feel better, and my cholesterol went down.

There are many interested in spiritual health who don't realize that physical health habits, including what we eat, affect our ability to discern subtle differences between truth and error!

I realize my journey to better health is unique. I wasn't praying, "Lord, change my diet." I was praying that God would keep me from error or anything that would prevent God from being able to use 3ABN in spreading the Bible truth to the world. His answer was to change my diet.

Is there anything in your life that may be keeping you from good spiritual health?

DANNY SHELTON

Fresh Air of the Spirit

*Jesus said to them again, "Peace be with you. As the Father
has sent me, so I send you." When he had said this, he breathed on
them and said to them, "Receive the Holy Spirit." John 20:21, 22, NRSV.*

EVER SINCE GOD breathed into the nostrils of Adam the breath of life and Adam became a living being (Gen. 2:7), humans have sustained life with an important gas we call oxygen. Every day this Eden-like experience is repeated millions of times as babies enter the world and take their first breath. Without oxygen, life would cease in a matter of minutes.

God gave us lungs containing millions of tiny air sacs (alveoli) covered with intricate blood-filled capillaries. We breathe the oxygen into our lungs. Blood filled with carbon dioxide flows to the lungs; there the carbon dioxide is exchanged for oxygen. Millions of red blood cells then carry away the oxygen-filled blood to nourish the brain and other body organs, tissues, and cells. The exchange in the lungs takes milliseconds; a complete circuit of the body requires about one minute.

God designed this ingenious recycling process. The earth's plant life absorbs and uses the carbon dioxide we breathe out and gives off oxygen (90 percent from ocean algae). We breathe in the oxygen, and the process begins again. The purest air is found near moving waterfalls, bubbling rivers, and oceans. It is also present after electrical storms, in buildings with lots of plants, in mountains and forests. Pure air can slow our breathing rate, relieve allergies, lower blood pressure, and help us think more clearly. Obviously, it's especially needed during prayer and Bible study!

The Holy Spirit impresses our minds, so it's important to keep our brains healthy and well oxygenated. But it's in our own home where we might be getting the worst air—especially if it's a well-insulated, energy-efficient home with tight doors and windows! Toxins come from smoke, street and garage exhaust, gas stoves, appliances, radon, furnishings, personal and cleaning chemicals, dust, animal dander, pesticides, chlorinated water, and even air fresheners. The best solution is to use chemical products sparingly and open the windows for some fresh air and sunshine!

Jesus compares His breath to the Holy Spirit. As oxygen supports physical life, the Holy Spirit sustains spiritual life. Breathe deeply, stand erect with holy assurance, and always keep your mental windows open for the fresh air of the Spirit.

Have you been outside yet to be energized by God's free gift of life—pure, fresh air?   ELLA M. RYDZEWSKI

Still Grumpy?

The Lord has done great things for us, and we are glad. Ps. 126:3, NKJV.

THERE'S A STRONG connection between joy and life expectancy. A study was conducted on 660 people over age 50 in Oxford, Ohio. In 1975 they answered questions having to do with several things, including their attitudes about aging. Researchers checked to see which participants were still alive in 1998, and they noted when the others had died. It turned out that those who viewed aging as a positive experience lived, on average, 7.5 years longer.

That is an advantage far greater than what can be gained from lowering blood pressure or reducing cholesterol, each of which can add four years to your life. It also beats exercise, not smoking, and maintaining a healthy weight, strategies that can add one to three years.

If you wake up this morning with more health than illness, you are more blessed than the million who will not survive the week. If you have never experienced the danger of battle, the loneliness of imprisonment, the agony of torture, or the pangs of starvation, you are ahead of 500 million people in the world. If you can attend a church without fear of harassment, arrest, torture, or death, you are more blessed than three billion people in the world. If you have money in the bank and in your wallet and spare change in a dish, you are among the top eight percent of the world's wealthy. I hope you're not still grumpy!

Maybe it's time to write down some of the things for which you can be thankful. I wrote down the following: 1. For the taxes I pay, because it means I am employed. 2. For the mess to clean after a party, because it means I have been surrounded by friends. 3. For the clothes that fit a little too snugly, because it means I have enough to eat. 4. For a lawn that needs mowing, windows that need cleaning, and gutters that need fixing, because it means I have a home. 5. For all the complaining I hear about the government, because it means we have freedom of speech. 6. For the parking spot I find at the far end of the parking lot, because it means I have been blessed with transportation. 7. For the person behind me in church who sings off key, because it means I can hear. 8. For the pile of laundry and ironing, because it means I have clothes to wear. 9. For weariness and aching muscles at the end of the day, because it means I am capable of working.

See how many more things you can add to this "thankful for" list. And then say thank You to the Lord. TOM MOSTERT

"Sound" Medicine

Serve the Lord with gladness: come before His presence with singing. Ps. 100:2, NKJV.

I LOVE TO SING praises to the Lord, but I've learned that worship is not the only time we should sing.

A number of years ago while we were holding an evangelistic crusade in Northern California, a friend called and said that he was extremely discouraged. His wife had left him, his children had shunned him, he had stopped attending church, and his health was failing.

In his despair, he cried to us for help. We prayed together on the phone and then suggested that he take a 400-mile trip to meet with us for a spiritual lift. He agreed to come. Just before hanging up, the Lord impressed us to ask him to sing on the long drive—to sing anything, just *sing*.

When he arrived at our motor home, we could see that a miracle had taken place. He was a changed man; beaming with happiness! God had given him His counseling through singing as he drove those 400 miles. From that day on this man's attitude was changed from gloom to joy, all because he practiced God's "sound" therapy—singing.

At a recent crusade in Lincoln, Nebraska, a woman related to us how the therapy of singing had helped her and many other young women. Here is her testimony: "I was attending a LaLeche Club meeting with several other nursing mothers. We were comparing notes on the stress in our lives with new babies, other children, husbands, meals to prepare, laundry, and shopping. One of the mothers mentioned she wasn't having as much stress since her doctor had told her to sing when she began to feel stressed out—at any time, anywhere. Sing anything—just sing! She did and it really helped. The rest of us decided to try it. At the next monthly meeting we all agreed that singing decreased stress! I still sing when I'm upset, discouraged, sad, or under stress. It works! This was more than 20 years ago and I'll keep singing!"

Many years ago Ellen White wrote, "Song is a weapon that we can always use against discouragement" (*The Ministry of Healing*, p. 254). I think that's why the psalmist says, "Let the saints . . . sing aloud on their beds" (Ps. 149:5, NKJV). When do you go to bed? When you're tired, sick, or depressed. Isn't it interesting that the advice is to sing at that time, and not just to yourself, but aloud!

May the Lord help us to remember His goodness and great love—and to keep singing!   NANCY NEUHARTH

To Love Is to Forgive

Love never fails. 1 Cor. 13:8, NKJV.

I'M CONVINCED THAT our mental and physical health depends on our attitude toward others and how we treat them. Included in this is forgiveness. In fact, if I could choose the one gift from God that I personally need to have and to give, it would be the gift of forgiveness, both for others and for me.

Maltbie Babcock wrote years ago: "How sure we are of our own forgiveness from God. How certain we are that we are made in His image, when we forgive heartily and out of hand one who has wronged us. Sentimentally we may feel, and lightly we may say, 'To err is human, to forgive divine;' but we never taste the nobility and divinity of forgiving till we forgive and know the victory of forgiveness over our sense of being wronged, over mortified pride and wounded sensibilities. Here we are in living touch with Him who treats us as though nothing had happened—who turns His back upon the past, and bids us journey with Him into goodness and gladness, into newness of life." Well, God asks that we do the same for others and ourselves.

We all know someone whom we are reluctant to forgive, for whatever reasons. There's that bit of pride that hides in the corner of our heart and flashes out to bite us when that certain person digs in with sarcasm and corrodes our self-esteem. After being bitten royally one day—again—I asked myself if it would have bothered me so much if someone else had said this same thing. What a surprise to realize that I wouldn't have thought once, much less twice, about it. But it was *this person!* Why? I still haven't figured it out!

But it was at that moment I realized that *my* attitude was wrong, and that I was only hurting myself, not the other person, who probably wasn't even aware of what was happening. So I forgave, and now I'm learning to treat this person as though nothing had happened. In fact, I truly love this person now!

If there is one certainty in life it is this: "love *never* fails"—to give the gift of forgiveness. And it's God's gift of love that gets the process going. What a revelation and relief to finally put aside how I *feel* and to *will* a love that only God can give.

Forgiving Father, give me love for the person who corrodes my self-esteem; enough love to forgive—and enough willpower to love.　　　　　　PAT NORDMAN

I Was Lost but Now I'm Found

A thorn in the flesh was given to me. . . . And He said to me, "My grace is sufficient for you, for My strength is made perfect in weakness." 2 Cor. 12:7-9, NKJV.

I DIDN'T CARE much about school while growing up in Louisiana. My passion was riding my motorcycle. At 9 years of age I was racing Moto-Cross. Every weekend our family traveled all over the south, going from track to track. Racing was my life, but it all came to an end on June 7, 1980. I had a premonition something bad was going to happen but quickly brushed it away, even forgetting to pray as I usually did. The gate dropped. I was the first one around the first curve. Several laps later I came off a jump that threw me 20 feet into the air. The back end of the bike came over my head. I thought I could ride it out so I held on. My head hit first. The bike landed on top of me and broke my back in the lumbar area. I knew it the second I hit the ground. I was only 15 and paralyzed from the waist down.

Six months later, wheelchair-bound, I was in two auto accidents only five days apart. Traveling close to 100 mph, both cars were totaled. Scuba diving in 1996, I lost my air at 49 feet and nearly drowned. Again and again, God spared my life. I praise Him for being so patient with someone as stubborn as I, not allowing me to die in an unsaved condition.

In October 1997 I hit rock bottom. I cried and prayed as never before: "God, take control of my life; give me strength, knowledge, courage, wisdom—whatever I need. Mold me, shape me. Do anything to show people that You are the true and living God." It wasn't until then that I understood that I needed to die to myself and give up the ways of the world if I were to live for Christ.

Just four months later, the Lord blessed me with a lovely wife and step-daughter. Together we found Bible truth. I was privileged to nurse my wife through a long illness, but lost her in June 2002. Without Christ in my life, I wouldn't have been able to share all this. We serve a loving God. He tells us He will not put on us more than we can handle. I believe that with all my heart.

If God will accept me, He will accept anyone. He had to dig deep down and knock me around a little to get me to wake up. I know that God is real, because I see the changes He has made in my life. I was a bitter person, but now I see my disability as a gift. I understand that "it is not I, but Christ who lives in me." The weaker I get, the stronger He becomes. My life is so full of happiness, joy, and peace that it surpasses any words. To sum it up, it is amazing grace.

Thank You, Lord, for the thorns of the flesh that keep us humble and dead to self!

BUDDY IVEY

Reaping the Consequences of Foolishness

Forsake foolishness and live, and go in the way of understanding. Prov. 9:6, NKJV.

I HAD JUST gotten a four-wheel-drive Explorer and could hardly wait to head with it and a friend down to a deserted surf break in Baja, Mexico. After driving three hours south of the border, we turned off the highway onto a dirt road. About a mile from the coast the road crossed a little creek, maybe 30 feet across and about eight to 10 inches deep. I jammed through it as I had done on previous trips. Water sprayed everywhere. *Yeeehaw!* It was big-time fun!

After two days of good surfing, we started home. When we neared the creek I got this great idea. If I went fast enough, water would shoot really high and wash the dust off my car. So I speeded up. Water covered the car. But then the engine died.

I tried to restart the engine. *Click.* Nothing. Thinking it was water on the spark plugs, we waited for them to dry, tried again then waited some more. Nothing. I prayed. A man drove by, gave us some advice and some stuff to spray on the engine. We tried it, but it didn't work.

We figured if we could get the car 100 yards up to the main drag, maybe someone could help us. We began to push. After we struggled an hour, a fellow in a big pickup towed us up the hill.

There we stopped about 10 cars, but nobody could figure out what was wrong. Finally someone loaned us a 30-foot cable and a guy in a big rig towed us the 19 miles to town. Everyone who knew something about cars tried to help. We finally gave up and called a friend in California to come and tow us back to a dealership in the States. It was about dawn as we neared the border—almost 24 hours after trying to wash my car in the stream!

How could I have done such a dumb thing?

Why do we make foolish choices when we know better? Why do people disobey the laws of health—smoking, drinking, caffeine, alcohol, burning the midnight oil, or overeating, when they know the consequences?

I ruined the engine of my car for the pleasure of the moment—for an exhilarating high. About $3,000 fixed the engine. When we ruin our bodies, we're seldom so lucky! That's why the proverb "forsake foolishness and live" is worth remembering!

Lord, give me understanding to avoid doing foolish things today.

KEVIN KUZMA

Need an Extra Scoop of Christ's Salt?

Salt is good, but if the salt loses its flavor, how will you season it? Have salt in yourselves, and have peace with one another. Mark 9:50, NKJV.

A LITTLE SALT is essential in our diet. I discovered that when I went on a fruit diet for a few days and began to have leg cramps. My good friend Dr. Bernell Baldwin smiled and said, "Try a pinch of salt!" It worked! The whole electrolyte system of our bodies depends on the right mixture of salts. But in developed countries the problem is seldom too little salt!

Salt causes the retention of fluids—which raises blood pressure, and that can be a killer! One third of the population has high blood pressure, and it's no wonder, since we consume 20 times more salt than we need! Natural foods are low in sodium (salt) and high in potassium, which helps control blood pressure. But processed foods send salt intake off the charts. (Three teaspoons of ketchup has 1,000 mg. of salt; a dill pickle, 3,000; one teaspoon of pure salt has 5,000 mg.) Processed foods that we think of as sweet are loaded with salt. One cup of Jell-O chocolate pudding contains 1,200 mg., and a piece of cake can easily exceed 1,000 mg. Almost all commercially canned vegetables and soups are "salt mines."

If you're at risk for high blood pressure, you could live 15 years longer if you just stopped salting your food. And when you do, surprise! Your taste buds awaken and you'll begin to enjoy the natural flavors of foods and the exotic taste of herbs. Some people are more sensitive to the harmful effects of salt than others—but we could all benefit by avoiding the "salt mines"!

In the Scripture salt was an essential part of every Old Testament sacrifice, signifying that only the righteousness of Christ could make the offering acceptable to God. (See Lev. 2:13.) In the New Testament Christ challenges us, "You are the salt of the earth" (Matt. 5:13, NKJV).

In Palestine salt was used for flavoring and preserving. It was gathered from marshes along the seashore or from inland lakes. If left in contact with the ground, or exposed to rain or sun, the soluble salt itself would wash away, leaving only insipid impurities. In other words, it lost its flavor! As Christians we won't do others much good if we don't mingle with them and let our flavor (Christ's righteousness) rub off, or if we lose the characteristics that make us Christian. As Christ says in Mark 9:50, to get along with each other we need His "salt"!

Ask Christ for an extra scoop and see what a difference it can make in your life today. KAY KUZMA

True Olympians

Do you not know that in a race all the runners run, but only one gets the prize? Run in such a way as to get the prize. 1 Cor. 9:24, NIV.

MILO OF CROTON, the greatest of the ancient Greek athletes, earned his legendary fame as a mighty, fearless wrestler. In a bout, three falls to the knees constituted defeat, but Milo was never once brought to his knees. He began intensive training in 536 B.C. Each day, so the story goes, Milo would lift his baby bull to his shoulders and walk as far as he could. This continued week after week, with Milo increasing in strength and size as his bull increased in weight. After four years of this regimen, Milo went, with his bull, to his first Olympics. To impress the crowd, he sacrificed his faithful bull and then carried the massive carcass 400 meters around the stadium on his shoulders. In his first bout Milo was victorious, starting his illustrious athletic career.

The Greek Olympic Games began in 776 B.C.. They were held every fourth year until A.D. 393, when the Christian emperor Theodosius I ordered that all pagan centers be closed.

The apostle Paul used the games to illustrate various Christian concepts. He noted the single-hearted purpose, perseverance, and endurance displayed by the athletes, but he strongly reasoned that our goal should be something far greater than fame or an olive wreath crown "that will not last" (1 Cor. 9:25, NKJV). The goal should be eternal life (1 Tim. 6:12; Phil. 3:14). In striving for this goal, we depend totally on God as the source of energy and strength, giving Him the praise for success; we work with others and for others, not against them.

Aesop, a sixth-century B.C. philosopher on the island of Samos, once met a boastful victor in one of the contact sports. Aesop asked him if his opponent was the stronger man of the two.

"Don't say that," replied the athlete. "My strength proved to be much greater."

"Well, then, you simpleton," said Aesop, "what honor have you earned if, being the stronger, you prevailed over a weaker man? You might be tolerated if you were telling us that by skill you overcame a man who was superior to you in bodily strength."

Thus Aesop illustrated the irrationality of human competition. The apostle Paul lifts us above such behavior, leading us to depend on the everlasting arms of strength, which empower us to lift others higher—the true spirit of real Olympians.

What are you doing to lift others higher?　　　　　DAVID C. NIEMAN

Don't Turn Off Your Conscience!

For he is cast into a net by his own feet, and he walks into a snare. Job 18:8, NKJV.

WHEN I WENT TO the Amazon with students from Loma Linda University, I was terrified of all the bats. They flew around us every night—zooming close and then abruptly darting away. One night I was preaching in the church, and a bat came straight toward me. Instinctively I tried to defend myself with the Bible in my hand.

Then came the night we had to sleep in an open-air shelter—a kind of thatched-roof hut without windows. When darkness approached I began to worry about the bats flying around. I asked the local people, "Are the bats vegetarian or blood suckers?"

They told me that the bats could bite, but we should not worry about that. They assured me they were not dangerous. But that didn't help much.

Still scared, I remembered a friend in south Brazil who used to hang bottles in the open windows of a barn to prevent the bats from biting the horses. I decided to do that. I collected what I could find—bottles, shoes, stones, and sticks—and hung them around the palm shelter.

The bats came and surrounded the place all night long but did not fly inside. Their sound "radar" told them that there were obstacles in the window and they avoided the opening.

Later I learned how biologists catch bats to study. They go to their cave and put a net in the cave's opening. The bats fly into the net because they do not know the obstacle is there. The bat specialists found out that the bats are so used to entering and exiting by that opening without meeting any obstacles that they turn off their radar equipment. And thus the researchers can easily catch them.

That is the same thing that happens to many humans. We think we know our way well. We trust too much in ourselves, and we do not recognize danger. No problem with questionable friends, no problem with a little alcohol, no problem with a little vice—just for fun—and we fall into the trap. This trap can take our happiness, our health, and many times, our lives. Watch out for Satan's nets; don't turn off your spiritual radar.

Is your conscience strong enough to avoid sin? What could you do to be more perceptive to Satan's snares?　　　　　　　　HILDEMAR DOS SANTOS

Enough to Make a Saint Swear

So then, my beloved brethren, let every man be swift to hear, slow to speak, slow to wrath. James 1:19, NKJV.

IF EVER THE SAYING "enough to make a saint swear" could be applied to a man, it was today. Everything went wrong for my dad. He had hit his thumb with the hammer and had bumped his head on the rafters. He had fallen off the ladder, smashed his toes, and pinched his fingers in the garage door. About a week earlier, he had torn a ligament in his knee and could hardly walk. All morning Dad had patiently put up with us kids fighting. And as if this wasn't enough to test a man's patience, in a moment of carelessness I had left the parrot's cage door open and our beautiful parrot, worth more than $1,500, had escaped.

I expected a barrage of "How could you! Why did you? When will you ever learn?" and other bits and phrases meant to chastise and instruct. But instead, he quietly and painfully began hobbling around the neighborhood, chasing the parrot that his careless son had let out of the house.

Any normal man under these circumstances would have been raving mad, but Dad was not angry. Because of the awful pain, he fought to keep back the tears, but he didn't show anger toward me or criticize what I'd done.

The hours passed; Dad's limp got worse as he ran first one place and then another, trying to keep the parrot in view. Every so often he would say a short prayer and then press persistently on. After avoiding Dad for more than two hours, the bird landed on a neighbor's roof. My dad's hopes soared as he got a ladder and slowly climbed onto the roof. He prayed a silent prayer and walked over to the panting bird. The nearly exhausted man spoke softly to the parrot. Slowly, ever so slowly and cautiously, he reached out his hand for the bird—and waited—and prayed again. After what seemed like hours, the bird stepped onto his hand. Quickly Dad tucked the bird inside his coat and headed home.

With the parrot safely in its cage, Dad sat down on the couch, exhausted, his knee throbbing with pain. Then with tears in his eyes he looked at me. "I love you, son," he said.

"I'm sorry, Dad. I'm so sorry," I sobbed.

"I know," he said, "I know."

Thank You, heavenly Father, for being so patient with me when I make foolish mistakes.   JON SANDBERG

JUNE 13

I'm Thankful for My Body

*Dear friend, I pray that you may enjoy good health and that all may
go well with you, even as your soul is getting along well. 3 John 2, NIV.*

WHEN I WAS A young boy my grandfather told me I could do whatever
I set my heart on doing. I had been born a dwarf, and had to accept that I
was never going to grow to a normal stature. But in spite of being small, I
had big ambitions to be successful and independent in this big world. And
God has allowed my dreams to come true.

Some people may think it strange that I thank God for the body He
gave me. I can walk, talk, and drive. But most of all, I'm thankful that my
body is healthy, and I'm thankful I have had an opportunity to learn how
to keep it healthy.

I wasn't always health conscious. I used to eat animal products.
However, when I married, my wife, Tena, would not allow me to eat any
of the unclean flesh foods that are mentioned in Leviticus 11. Then after
several years we decided to gradually give up animal products and reduce
salt intake. We have found that by reducing the size of portions we eat and
eating only two substantial meals a day, we sleep better. Now we have
given up all dairy products, and both of us feel better, think better, and
have lost weight. I've learned that my body is very important to God—it
is the temple of God (1 Cor. 6:19). And I am what I eat!

Because we're so small (Tena is 3'9" and I'm 4'), Tena and I have
found that we have many opportunities to tell others about God and the
importance of living a healthy lifestyle. For example, when children see us
out shopping and ask, "Why are you so little?" we explain this is the way
God created us. He loves us, and we like ourselves because we love Jesus.
And sometimes, with a twinkle in my eye, I tell them to eat all their vegetables so that they can grow big and strong!

People sometimes comment, "You look so happy and radiant." When
we tell them our age, they can't believe it, so we share with them our
healthy lifestyle. We're disproving the research on dwarfism that says little
people don't live beyond 60 years of age! We are in our mid-60s and are
in great health, speaking and singing duets in church, and traveling around
the world helping to build mission schools, churches, and orphanages.

*Thank You, God, for the body You created for me. Help me to treat it the way
You designed it should be treated!*   GEORGE A. BAEHM III

174

IOU's Can Keep Love Alive

[Love] . . . keeps no record of wrongs. 1 Cor. 13:5, NIV.

DEBT IS USUALLY not a good thing—at least, not when we consider what is personally owed to us. UOMe's (You Owe Me) can destroy a marriage. If your mind dwells on UOMe's you'll constantly be thinking of the wrongs, the slights, or the injustices you have suffered, instead of talking it out and canceling the debt by forgiving and forgetting. UOMe's get stuffed into dark closets of your mind and tend to be pulled out in times of stress in order to hurt the other or cause the other feelings of guilt. So ban UOMe's in your marriage.

Instead, concentrate on the IOUs. "IOU for taking on the responsibility of a family; IOU for loving me enough to overlook my moods; IOU for letting me pursue my hobbies without question; IOU for absorbing financial burdens; IOU for being kind enough to leave me alone when I need aloneness. IOU for believing in me and encouraging me to become everything God made me to be." Get the idea?

Here are 10 IOUs that are guaranteed to make your marriage more meaningful:

1. IOU respect, because you are God's chosen one for me; You are royalty—a child of the King.

2. IOU the courtesy of remembering only your good points.

3. IOU Christlike words and actions. (I can do this only if I have a daily relationship with Christ.)

4. IOU hugs and kisses, gentle touches, and caring caresses.

5. IOU at least three compliments a day.

6. IOU the benefit of the doubt; even if what you say is hard to believe. I'll trust—not argue.

7. IOU forgiveness, for God has already forgiven me.

8. IOU the words, "I'm sorry," when I've been selfish or wronged you in some way.

9. IOU thanks for the kind things you do, for loving me; and for just being you.

10. IOU my time—time to listen, to laugh, to play, to worship together, to love.

To keep relationships happy and healthy, remember that love keeps no record of wrongs—no UOMe's. Concentrate on giving away IOUs of love and see what a difference it makes.

Is there someone to whom you need to give an IOU? KAY KUZMA

175

Is Your Environment Killing You?

Then the Lord God planted a garden in Eden, in the east,
and there he placed the man he had created. Gen. 2:8, NLT.

YOU'VE HEARD OF Pavlov and his dogs? After allowing them to smell meat while listening to a bell, he discovered that the sound of the bell alone could induce salivation. The same thing can happen in your body. Just about anything in the environment can elicit an automatic response after an association has been established. Cancer patients, upon returning to the clinic where they received chemotherapy, will sometimes re-experience the side effects of the treatment even though they do not get any medication. Pictures in the room, the fragrance worn by a staff member, or even the background music are responsible. Research underscores why it is essential to pay attention to anything at home or work that may negatively impact your health.

We will all remember where we were when we heard of the attack on the World Trade Center in New York. Those who were there will do more than remember. The slightest reminder may trigger the same stress response they experienced during the attack. An extreme result is a condition called Post Traumatic Stress Disorder, or PTSD. The more emotions associated with an event, the more likely it will leave a permanent memory in our brain. We live among triggers of both unhealthy and healthy responses. That's why people remember weddings! For optimal health, create an environment that will remind you of the positive; remove those things that might trigger anxiety.

Take a moment to think about your personal space—both at home and in your workplace. Are your surroundings cheerful and healthy? Are they places that nurture your soul and recharge your spirit? Do you feel calm and happy when you're in them? Do they provide you with comfort, offer you an opportunity for growth, and give you a sense of peace?

Before his death, Henri Matisse, the great modern French painter, spent many months bedridden with colon cancer. His family moved his bed so that he could take in the view of the countryside from his bedroom window. More important, they kept changing what was on his window sill—so he could be continually inspired to paint. He did some of his most famous pieces from his bed. Why not take a cue from the Matisse family? Add a little visual spice to your space.

Think about it—the closer we come to making our personal environments like the original garden home, the more of its benefits we will experience! DES CUMMINGS, JR.

Using God-Designed Fuel for Our Bodies

God said, "See, I have given you every herb that yields
seed which is on the face of all the earth, and every tree whose
fruit yields seed; to you it shall be for food." Gen. 1:29, NKJV.

GOD DESIGNED THE human body and created the fuel on which it should operate, but man has pretty much eaten whatever tasted good. The result has been a shorter life span and an increase of disease. Take cancer for example.

Scientists reported in a 1991 issue of *American Journal of Epidemiology* that one particular group of foods, if eaten twice a day, would lower lung cancer by 74 percent. What is this group? Fruit. Another group of foods have been shown to decrease prostate cancer by 40 percent and pancreatic cancer by 50 percent. What are they? Beans, tomatoes, or dried fruit.

Here's an interesting discovery: Beta carotene as a supplement was discovered to increase the death rate of smokers by 18 percent, so smokers are advised to not take this supplement. But when beta carotene is eaten naturally in foods such as apricots or carrots, it's useful.

Meat is commonly associated with a greater risk for cancer. For example, the use of hamburgers had increased the risk of non–Hodgkin's Lymphoma by 2.35 times. (JAMA, 1996)

What are the consequences of having meat as a major part of one's diet? The person gets less fiber and more animal fat, hormones, viruses, and chemicals such as benzophrenes. Plus, there is a greater risk for early maturation and obesity. Contrast this to a plant-based diet that is high in phytochemicals, fiber, and vitamins A and C, among other things, without any harmful animal fat. Ovary cancer of women is also dose-response related to meat, as well as to eggs. (*American Journal of Epidemiology,* 1999)

In 1992 the evidence in favor of a plant-based diet had become so strong that *Nutrition and Cancer* journal stated that high consumers of fruits and vegetables have only half the risk of cancer as compared to low consumers. Vitamins A and C (which primarily come from plant foods) have long been associated with good health. The *American Journal of Clinical Nutrition* (1986) reported a study where those over 65 years of age who were high consumers of foods containing Vitamins A and C have 30 percent the overall death rate, as well as cancer death rate, as compared to those who were low consumers.

Thank You, God, for designing a plant-based, "high-octane" diet to fuel my body.   JOHN A. SCHARFFENBERG

The Healing Power of Fellowship

*How wonderful it is, how pleasant, for God's
people to live together in harmony! Ps. 133:1, TEV.*

IN HIS BOOK *Love and Survival* Dr. Dean Ornish, known for his work in reversing heart disease, writes about the power of love and intimacy in the healing process. "I am not aware of any other factor in medicine—not diet, not smoking, not exercise, not stress, not genetics, not drugs, not surgery—that has a greater impact on our quality of life, incidence of illness, and the premature death from all causes." He goes on to say that loneliness and isolation increase the likelihood that we may engage in harmful behaviors such as smoking and overeating; that we may get certain diseases or die prematurely; and that we will not fully experience the joy of everyday life. "In short," Ornish observes, "anything that promotes a sense of isolation often leads to illness and suffering. Anything that promotes a sense of love and intimacy, connection and community, is healing."

Research at University of California at Irvine reinforces this observation. It was found that loneliness and lack of emotional support can cause a three-fold increase in the odds of being diagnosed with a heart condition, while having just one person available for emotional support served to be enough to reduce the risk of heart disease!

It's amazing, isn't it, that just one person can make such a difference in a person's well-being. What are you doing to be this kind of a friend? Are you a part of a small group sharing together, studying God's Word together, serving together to help others, and suffering together?

The Bible commands this type of relationship, to enter into each other's pain and grief and carry each other's burdens. Paul says, "Share each other's troubles and problems, and in this way obey the law of Christ" (Gal. 6:2, NLT).

Job cried, "A despairing man should have the devotion of his friends, even though he forsakes the fear of the Almighty" (Job 6:14, NIV). Rick Warren, in his book *The Purpose Driven Life,* puts it this way, "It is in the times of deep crisis, grief, and doubt that we need each other most. When circumstances crush us to the point that our faith falters, that's when we need believing friends the most. We need a small group of friends to have faith in God for us and to pull us through. In a small group, the Body of Christ is real and tangible even when God seems distant."

If Job were suffering in your neighborhood or church today, would you be the friend that would give him the intimate fellowship needed to increase his chances of surviving—and thriving?   KAY KUZMA

Now Is the Time to Quit

And they were greatly astonished, saying among themselves, "Who then can be saved?" But Jesus looked at them and said, "With men it is impossible, but not with God; for with God all things are possible." Mark 10:26, 27, NKJV.

"FIVE DAYS AGO three jumbo jets crashed in California. More than a thousand people died. Four days ago, three more planes crashed outside of Miami, killing everyone. Three days ago planes crashed in Denver, Boston, and Atlanta, with no survivors. Yesterday another thousand died in airline tragedies. So far today two planes have gone down. In the past five days alone the average daily death count has been 1,000 people."

These air crashes didn't happen—but suppose they had? If 1,000 people died every day in air tragedies there would be a cry of panic from the public demanding an investigation. Warnings would spread: "Don't fly!" Congress would pass emergency regulations. Yet every day in the United States at least 1,000 people die from a preventable, self-inflicted cause—smoking, or the use of tobacco products! In fact, cigarettes kill more Americans annually than AIDS, cocaine, heroin, alcohol, automobiles, homicide, suicide, and fire combined.

C. Everett Koop, former U.S. surgeon general, once stated, "Smoking cessation represents the single most important step that smokers can take to enhance the length and quality of their lives." And here's the good news: Unless there is already onset of disease, regardless of how long you have smoked you can enjoy good health after quitting. Other benefits include: (1) You'll have fewer days of illness, fewer health complaints, better overall health status, and fewer lung problems. And you'll spend less money for cold remedies, health care, and life insurance. (2) If you quit smoking by age 50, you have half the risk of dying in the next 15 years than smokers. (3) Your chances of a stroke decline quickly after you quit, as does the risk of lung and other cancers, heart attack, and chronic lung disease. (4) You're 50 percent less likely to suffer from impotence than are smokers.

God's will for you is to prosper and have good health. But His blessing of health will never be yours if you keep putting tobacco into your body. It's a poison. Tobacco, a legal drug, can be even more addictive than illegal ones, but with God nothing is impossible. For those who smoke or chew, now is the time to quit.

Whatever you're trying to overcome, give it to God. Let His willpower become yours. JAN W. KUZMA and CECIL MURPHEY

Anger Control

"Be angry, and do not sin": do not let the sun go down on your wrath. . . .
Let no corrupt word proceed out of your mouth. . . . Let all bitterness, wrath, anger,
clamor, and evil speaking be put away from you, with all malice. Eph. 4:26-31, NKJV.

IF YOU'RE LIKE most people, hardly a day goes by that you don't encounter situations that make you angry—people who break line, hectic traffic, an employer who criticizes and blames unjustly, your best friend's betrayal, your spouse's infidelities, your child's deviant lifestyle, or sexual abuse.

You are angry and miserable. Your mind screams for revenge. You want to tell people off. You are ready to fight. But as a Christian, how should you handle such burning anger? The Bible isn't usually thought of as a textbook on anger control. But the Apostle Paul's treatment of the subject in Ephesians is effective modern-day psychology.

First, Paul says *it's all right to be angry*. There are a lot of injustices and actual crimes that should make a Christian angry. The qualifier is, "Don't sin." Don't do something that hurts you or others or breaks your relationship with God.

Second, *get rid of the anger as soon as possible*. "Don't let the sun go down on your wrath." Talk about it. Pray for the other person. Reconcile. If you keep the anger and bitterness inside it festers. If you sleep on your anger it gets processed and filed in your brain and makes a stronger mark on your psyche. The sooner it's settled the sooner you can get back on track with God.

Third, *don't let unwholesome talk come out of your mouth!* Expressing your anger verbally is damaging. Not only does it make reconciliation difficult, but the risk of heart attack more than doubles in the two hours following an episode of moderate or greater anger. Is it worth it?

Fourth, *be kind and tenderhearted*. It's a well-known fact that feelings follow behavior. Act in a kind way and your heart will soften. Do something nice for the person who has wronged you, and you'll be surprised how this prepares you for the final step in anger control.

Fifth. *Forgive*—not because the person has repented or feels sorry, but because God has forgiven you.

The next time you start to get hot under the collar, try handling your anger the biblical way. Impossible? Remember, Christ makes all things possible!

Forgiving Father, when I get angry, help me to do what Jesus would do.

GLADYS HOLLINGSEAD

Dead Fly Perfume

Dead flies will cause even a bottle of perfume to stink! Yes, an ounce of
foolishness can outweigh a pound of wisdom and honor. Eccl. 10:1, NLT.

"IS THAT ALL YOU got her?" my brother and I exclaimed in disgust as
Dad gave a small bottle to Mom for her birthday.

"Look, boys. It's lilac perfume," she said as she gave Dad a big hug and
an extra long kiss.

"And it smells *sooo* good!" We could tell that Mom thought it was special, but what in the world was per—per—per—whatever you call it?
Then she opened the delicate little jar and let the fragrance curl up around
our noses, and we began to realize the value of that little gift.

A few minutes later we nonchalantly asked Dad, "How do people
make perfume?"

"I don't know," he said as he scratched his chin and grinned.
"Probably with fly juice!"

The back door banged as we ran toward the barn where the lilac bush
grew. Soon we had a pie plate heaped with fresh lilac blossoms. Catching
flies was a little harder, but we managed to get quite a few and carefully
sprinkled them over the fragrant flowers.

"Now what?" we wondered. It still wasn't perfume! After much de-
liberation we decided to add water and cook the whole concoction in the
sun. When it was finished we would strain it into a nice bottle and present
it to Mom. As the sweet smell filled the room she would beam all over and
hug us close. We could hardly wait. We put the pan up on the chicken
coop roof and went off to play. Every few hours we carefully checked it,
but the aroma seemed to move farther and farther from the sweet fragrance
we had anticipated. Within a day or two our career as makers of fine lilac
perfume had ended.

Several years ago as I told Mom the story (she had never known) she
began to cry and gave me a great big hug as if I had done something special. To her, love wasn't shown by the magnificence of the gift but by the
feelings that had gone into it.

When later I found the proverb about the dead flies in the perfume, I
thought, How true! But how did Solomon know? I wonder if he ever gave
his mom dead-fly perfume!

Is a gift of love ever really a failure—even if it doesn't turn out the way we had
hoped? What could you do today to give a little love?   HOMER TRECARTIN

Destroying Madness

Then they spat on Him, and took the reed and struck Him on the head.
And when they had mocked Him, they took the robe off Him, put His own
clothes on Him, and led Him away to be crucified. Matt. 27:30, 31, NKJV.

MAD COW DISEASE, when contracted by humans, causes incurable brain deterioration (similar to Alzheimer's) and a horrible death. That's why authorities slaughtered millions of potentially infected cattle in the United Kingdom in 1996. But the disease is still alive and well, posing a threat to anyone eating beef or beef by-products. The disease-causing prions are passed easily to other animal species, and they can't be killed, even by pasteurization or freezing!

How is mad cow disease spread? By bovine cannibalism! The "rendering" process takes the inedible remains of slaughtered animals, including dead pets and road kill, grinds and cooks them up into an unidentifiable mess. This "food" is fed to beef and dairy cows as a protein supplement to increase production of beef and milk. Humans get CJD (the variant human form) by eating parts of infected cattle—the brain, spinal cord, gut, and bone marrow, or possibly by drinking infected milk.

The prion, a protein devoid of genetic material, does not trigger a specific antibody; therefore, the body's immune system does not recognize it as an enemy. Human food sources most likely to be contaminated include sausages, hot dogs, and ground beef or meats labeled "mechanically separated." The only cows that you can safely presume are not eating animal by-products are certified organic cattle, which must be fed a plant-based diet.

Beware: the disease can go undetected for years, and there is no test to detect infected animals before they die. That's why it's so scary!

I wonder how long the prion of sin and rebellion existed in Lucifer's mind before it revealed itself? God could have "nipped it in the bud." He could have destroyed Lucifer's "madness" before the deadly agent had mutated and entered the minds of one-third of the angels and then humanity. But He didn't. Sin had to be allowed to run its course. Not until evil was developed to such an extent that it killed God's Son would the created beings of the universe truly understand it's hideous nature and serve God out of love instead of force!

Reflect on Calvary. How do you feel about a God who values your freedom of choice so much that He allowed people to kill His Son rather than force them into submission?   RISÉ RAFFERTY

Moment of Truth

*The Lord God had planted a garden in the east, in Eden. . . . And the
Lord God made all kinds of trees grow out of the ground—trees that
were pleasing to the eye and good for food. Gen. 2:8, 9, NIV.*

I GUESS I ASKED for it. I'd been feeling a little stressed out, and I thought
it was time for a medical checkup. However, I wasn't prepared for the call
I received a few days later.

"Your cholesterol level of 258 mg/percent (6.6 mmol/l) is very high,"
said the nurse. "The doctor wants you to begin medication immediately to
get it down to more ideal levels of 150 to 170 (3.9 to 4.4 mmol/l)."

I *walked* to the pharmacy to pick up my medicine. (I thought exercise
was necessary to keep cholesterol moving! I later learned my reasoning was
wrong, but exercise is good for the heart.) And I started taking those little
pills every day, without fail.

The moment of truth came, however, when I picked up a pharmaceutical
company's brochure. On the back I found a food chart giving cholesterol and
fat contents for a wide range of basic foodstuffs and prepared meals. It wasn't
the first time I had seen such a chart, but this time I looked at it more closely.
That's when something struck me with the force of a revelation. Clearly, some
foods are higher in cholesterol and fat than others. But the bottom-line reality
is that fruits, grains, and vegetables have no cholesterol, are very low in fat, and
are high in certain fibers that help lower the blood cholesterol.

Thousands of years ago this kind of diet was spelled out by our
Creator. God told Adam and Eve, "I have given you every plant yielding
seed which is upon the face of all the earth, and every tree with seed in its
fruit; you shall have them for food" (Gen. 1:29, RSV).

It's been only four weeks since that moment of truth and lifestyle
change. Yesterday I had another blood test. The result was terrific: my
cholesterol was down to 124 mg/percent (3.2 mmol/l)! My doctor took
me off the cholesterol-lowering drug, saying, "You don't need this anymore. Your diet change certainly made a difference. Stay with it, and you
won't have to worry about drug side effects, seeing the pharmacist, or seeing me!" Great news!

More good news: I've lost weight, gained energy, regained an incredible taste appreciation for simpler foods, and—very important, I'm feeling
much better. What a way to be!

*Thank You, God, for reawakening me to the knowledge You gave us in the
Garden of Eden.* LINCOLN STEED

God Will Guard Your Heart

*And the peace of God, which transcends all understanding, will
guard your hearts and your minds in Christ Jesus. Phil. 4:7, NIV.*

IT WAS 6:30 THAT morning of June 23, 1997, and I was doing my daily
exercise. Suddenly my arms went numb, and I felt a terrible explosion and
pressure in my chest and upper body. I felt paralyzed and realized I was
having a heart attack. I was only 51 years old. I was shocked!

My husband called 911 and within three minutes the paramedics were
trying to get me stabilized. I was rushed to the closest hospital by ambulance and administered morphine and other drugs. It was too much for my
heart, and I felt that I was slipping away. My husband quickly told the doctors my history of drug reactions, and they immediately changed the medication. After three and one-half hours, the attack ended and I was stable.

The next day it was determined that my left anterior descending artery
had an 80 percent blockage with an L-shaped bend. During the attack, a
blood clot had formed, resulting in complete blockage. Two days later,
medication had dissolved the clot significantly and the doctors successfully
completed an angioplasty.

My cardiologists told me I would not have survived if I had not been
in such overall good health and had a strong immune system. Most women
who have a myocardial infarction like mine usually die. Heart attacks are
the biggest killers of women—247,000 per year; it takes more lives of
women and men than any other disease. Three of my grandparents and
two uncles died of heart failure, so my congenital defect demonstrates that
genes played a significant role. It's like having to paddle a canoe upstream.

But the best part of this story is that I discovered God's peace throughout this experience. While in the ambulance, faced with death, I told God
that if I were to die right then it would be OK. But if He wanted me to
live, I would know that He had more purpose for my life. Peace came as
I trusted God for the outcome. I'm thankful that I have a personal God
who guards my heart, and for the wonderful doctors and nurses who are
His instruments.

Now, with my cholesterol at 163, walking one or two miles every day,
taking the best nutritional supplements I can get, and keeping God's peace
in my life, I'm feeling great!

Peace is a gift. Why not ask God to guard your heart and give you peace today?

KATHY CORWIN

God's Sound System

*The Lord came and stood and called as at other times, "Samuel! Samuel!"
And Samuel answered, "Speak, for Your servant hears." Then the Lord
said to Samuel: "Behold, I will do something in Israel at which both
ears of everyone who hears it will tingle." 1 Sam. 3:10, 11, NKJV.*

DID YOU KNOW we don't really hear with our ears? Our ears are just elaborate canals that transmit sound waves to the part of our brain that interprets them as sounds. Any interference along the way distorts what is ultimately "heard."

How does God's specially-designed sound system work? There's the external ear, where the vibrations enter the canal. Then comes the eardrum, a thin piece of skin stretched over the canal; it separates the outer ear from the middle ear. The middle ear contains the "ear bones" (hammer, anvil, and stirrup). Sound strikes the eardrum and starts the three bones vibrating like a tuning fork—but more accurately! These in turn set up a series of vibrations in the fluid of the shell-shaped inner ear, or cochlea. The cochlea is in the form of a spiral. The central, closed end of the canal registers low tones and the outer extension registers high tones. Within the inner ear is the organ of Corti, which is made up of tiny cells that transfer the sound waves to the auditory nerves that carry them to the brain's hearing center.

One problem: How could this sound system handle the differences in air pressure on the two sides of the eardrum? That's why God created the Eustachian tube; it goes from the inner side of the eardrum to the throat. Enough air enters this tube by way of the throat to keep the air pressure equal, making it easier for the eardrum to move with the sound waves that enter the ear.

Satan would like nothing better than to mess up this marvelously designed sound system so we can't hear accurately what is said to us (for relationships are built on words), or enjoy the beautiful strains of inspirational music, or perceive the sounds of God's nature—the wind, the waterfall, the chirping cicadas, the crackling campfire. Satan does this most effectively with infections and loud sustained noises (such as rock music) and by encouraging a sedentary lifestyle. Yes, research has found that healthy people retain more hearing capacity than others. One explanation might be that regular exercise improves the flow of oxygen-rich blood through the tiny blood vessels in the ear.

Lord, help me keep my ears healthy, so I can hear You talking to me as Samuel did, and be able to respond, "Speak, Lord, for your servant hears."

KAY KUZMA

The Greatest Joy

*Bear with each other and forgive whatever grievances you may have
against one another. Forgive as the Lord forgave you. And over all these virtues
put on love, which binds them all together in perfect unity. Col. 3:13, 14, NIV.*

IT IS WONDERFUL and affirming to have a kitten rub against our leg,
but it's infinitely better to hear kind words or feel an encouraging hug
from a friend. Our greatest joy is found in sharing ideas, hurts, looks, hugs,
squeezes, and hopes with others.

When Jesus taught service, He sent disciples out two by two. When
Paul was called to minister in Macedonia, he asked Silas and Dr. Luke to
come along. When Saul was lonely, he asked David to fill the quiet with
music. When Dorcas awoke each morning, she helped her neighbors.

People are at their best when living for others. Yet those same relationships bring our greatest challenges. People are wonderful and people
are awful! That's where the Creator comes in, carrying a supply of "relationship tools," ready with an apprenticeship on love:

How to trade grudges for appreciation. "Do not be overcome by evil,
but overcome evil with good" (Rom. 12:21, NIV).

How to think of others first. "Love your neighbor as yourself" (Lev.
19:18, NIV).

How to say hard things softly. "Let your conversation be always full of
grace, seasoned with salt, so that you may know how to answer everyone"
(Col. 4:6, NIV).

How to be patient with the impatient. "Everyone should be quick to
listen, slow to speak and slow to become angry" (James 1:19, NIV).

Want a little more joy in your life? You can go down to the animal
shelter and pick up a little kitten—or you can choose to develop your
human relationships by affirming friendships through e-mail, on the
phone, or face-to-face. Share a story. Talk about kids, jokes, work, shopping, cars. Be funny and hopeful. Make eye contact and say "hello" when
you meet someone in the hallway or at the market. Comment on what
they are wearing or on the "good, bad, or ugly" of today's weather. Talk
with someone you love. Turn off the computer, stereo, and TV. Eliminate
all the distractions and focus on the other person. Ask honest questions.
Listen. Encourage. Love.

*Here is how George Eliot prayed: "May every soul that touches mine, be it by
the slightest contact, get therefore some good, some little grace, one kindly thought,
to make this life worthwhile."* DICK DUERKSEN

Why Mozart Died so Young

And the swine, though it divides the hoof, having cloven hooves, yet does not chew the cud, is unclean to you. Their flesh you shall not eat, and their carcasses you shall not touch. They are unclean to you." Lev. 11:7, 8, NKJV.

WHAT REALLY KILLED Wolfgang Amadeus Mozart? According to a 2001 article published in the *Journal of the American Medical Association,* the culprit was likely trichinosis, the worm infestation caused by eating undercooked pork. This could explain all of Mozart's symptoms, which included fever, rash, limb pain, and swelling.

Mozart died at the age of 35. Years later, in 1846, Dr. Joseph Leidy of Philadelphia was eating a slice of ham for lunch when he noticed some funny-looking spots in it. He thought, *Those spots look familiar. I saw those very same spots in the muscle tissue of a corpse I was dissecting the other day!* He put his ham under a microscope. What he discovered was truly horrifying: it was full of tiny little worms we now call Trichina. The worms work their way into the muscles and can eventually kill the host. In human beings they come almost exclusively from eating pork products.

Mozart wrote a letter to his wife 44 days before his mysterious illness began: "What do I smell? . . . Pork cutlets! Che Gusto [What a delicious taste]; I eat to your health." He died 15 days after he became ill. Trichinosis has an incubation period of around 50 days. Mozart's symptoms were similar to those of others who eat parasite-infested pork.

Dr. Don Colbert, in his book *What Would Jesus Eat?* states, "Many people declare today that pork is a safe meat to eat in modern times. I disagree. Pigs eat enormous amounts of food, and this dilutes the hydrochloric acid in a pig's stomach. This in turn allows toxins, viruses, parasites, and bacteria to be absorbed into the animals' flesh. Besides being gluttons, swine are also extremely filthy animals. They will eat garbage, feces, and even decaying flesh. Pigs readily harbor parasites including Trichinella, the pork tapeworm, and toxoplasmosis."

Yes, cooking pork at temperatures of 160° F or greater will kill the parasites, but what about the center of the chops or steaks that are so often served rare? It's safer to eat what God tells us to eat (see Leviticus 11), and avoid the possibility of being eaten by worms!

Is there anything in your diet that God calls unclean? Maybe it's time to clean up your eating habits! SHAWN BOONSTRA

Finding the Fountain of Youth

*For our citizenship is in heaven, from which we also eagerly wait for the
Savior, the Lord Jesus Christ, who will transform our lowly body
that it may be conformed to His glorious body. Phil. 3:20, 21, NKJV.*

IN 1509 SPANISH explorer Juan Ponce de Leon heard stories from the
Indians in Puerto Rico of an island called Bimini where there was a fountain that could keep a person young forever. To find it became his passion.
He sailed north, but instead of the "fountain" he discovered Florida. For
12 more years he continued searching; alas, in 1521, he died of an Indian
arrow at 61 years of age.

Centuries later, people are still searching for the legendary spring of
youthful vitality, but unfortunately most are still looking in the wrong
places—at special diets and therapies or in their medicine cabinets. Christ's
gift of eternal life, with His promise that we'll be given new bodies, is the
ultimate answer to the search. But short of heaven, the best source is simply activity. Yes, that's right, if you want to find the fountain of youth you
can't sit there in your easy chair and dream about it. You've got to get up
and start walking!

As a person ages there's a loss in the ability to see, hear, smell, and taste;
there's loss in teeth and bone mass in the jaw area, decreased ability to digest and absorb food, and reduction in muscle and bone mass throughout
the body. Memory, judgment, reaction time, and balance may be affected.
And there's diminished liver and kidney function and a decrease in heart
and lung fitness. Almost all the deterioration attributed to aging can be explained by the fact that people tend to exercise less as they age. All cells,
tissues, and organs start to age when their particular activity is impaired!

The ancient Greek physician Hippocrates observed, "All parts of the
body that have a function, if used in moderation and exercised in labors in
which each is accustomed, become thereby healthy and well-developed,
and age more slowly, but if unused and left idle, they become liable to disease, defective in growth, and age quickly."

Sadly, although most would love to find the Fountain of Youth, 70 percent of Americans are not physically active. Inactivity is one of the greatest
public health challenges of this century! The incidence of stroke and type 2
diabetes could be lowered, high blood pressure could be prevented or reduced, and bone fractures would occur less often if people just moved more!

*So get going. Move those muscles and praise the Lord for His promise of eter-
nal life!*   KAY KUZMA

A Life That Knows No Limitations

I can do all things through Christ who strengthens me. Phil 4:13, NKJV.

IT WAS A BEAUTIFUL May day in 1995 during a cross-country riding event when Christopher Reeve's thoroughbred, Eastern Express, balked at a rail jump, pitching his rider forward. Reeve's hands were tangled in the horse's bridle, and he landed head first, fracturing the uppermost vertebrae in his spine. He was instantly paralyzed from the neck down and unable to breathe. Prompt medical attention saved his life. Delicate surgery stabilized the shattered C1-C2 vertebrae and literally reattached Reeve's head to his spine.

Reeve, best known for his role as Superman, learned to "fly" outside his body in a way few people have the strength or courage to do. Instead of giving up and becoming a prisoner of paralysis, he pushed himself to keep up a grueling regimen of four or more hours of physical therapy each day in hope that, against all odds, some movement and sensation would be regained.

In 2002 he could breathe on his own for up to two hours, move his fingers on his left hand, and move his right wrist. He could straighten his arms and legs and, in a swimming pool, initiate a step and push off against the wall. Most satisfying, Chris regained physical sensation in at least 70 percent of his body. He could feel the hand of his wife, Dana, on his. His progress had medical scientists rethinking their position that spinal tissue can never regrow.

Christopher Reeve is featured on the Web site "rolemodel.net" with this comment, "All of us are, in some way, prisoners in life—some by limited thinking, others by physical limitation. But rarely has a man demonstrated such a wonderful ability to face limitation, to cry for all that it has robbed him of, and then step beyond it into a life that knows no limitation. Each morning, being human, Christopher sheds a few tears. But then he brushes them away, stops feeling sorry for himself, and goes on to be an example to others."

He continued his acting and directing careers. He maintained an impressive speaking schedule, wrote books, and was a political activist for spinal cord injuries. He created his own freedom to be truly alive. What can we Christians learn from this man who believed that nothing was impossible?

Regardless of your limitations, continue to say, "I can do all things through Christ who strengthens me!" KAY KUZMA

Note: Christopher Reeve died on October 11, 2004, at the age of 52.

Don't Drink Your Way to Depression

For God has not given us the spirit of fear, but of power
and of love and of a sound mind. 2 Tim. 1:7, NKJV.

A WOMAN IN her 50s told me the following story:

"When I was in my late teens, living a secular lifestyle, I had my first anxious and blue period. For about five days I had a vague sense of dread and moped around lifeless. I found pleasure in almost nothing, and wondered why I had been born. As the years went by, the blue periods increased. I expected some day to require hospitalization and medications. I was never entirely peaceful.

"When I was 33 years old I became a Seventh-day Adventist Christian and learned healthful living was important. I began to exercise, to eat only at mealtimes, and stopped drinking the eight to 10 cups of coffee, tea, or colas I had consumed daily since my early teens. Almost immediately, I noticed I was steadier on my feet. Within a month the chronic anxiety from my stressful job diminished, but it was almost 18 months before I realized I had gone a year without any depression. It's now been more than 20 years."

More than 150 years ago God impressed Ellen G. White that coffee and tea artificially stimulated the system and then caused depression. (See *Counsels on Health,* p. 124.) Now we know the real culprit is caffeine. What does medical literature have to say about the dangers of caffeine in coffee, tea, colas, and chocolate? Not only do these caffeinated beverages cause depression, but they also increase the risk of headaches, infertility, chronic anxiety, allergies, muscular tremors, osteoporosis, and a host of other problems. The more caffeine, the higher the risk (*Internal Medicine News,* May 15, 1981, p. 6). Not until we did this research did we realize that substances with caffeine are on the list of the top 10 food groups causing food sensitivities, surpassed only by milk. If people only realized the dangers, they could enjoy the many healthful substitutes that are currently available.

God promises that we will avoid the diseases of the "Egyptians" (Ex. 15:26) if we follow His health principles. Most of us won't know until eternity just how blessed we have been by following a healthy lifestyle and how many diseases we have avoided because we "diligently" listened to the Lord.

Thank You, Creator God, for giving Your children knowledge about how to have peace and a sound mind—and help me to say no to beverages that might cause depression.   AGATHA THRASH

God's Grief Recovery Plan

*And God will wipe away every tear from their eyes; there shall be
no more death, nor sorrow, nor crying. There shall be no more pain,
for the former things have passed away. Rev. 21:4, NKJV.*

IN THE MANY YEARS since I was widowed, I have observed how others faced grief and compensated for their loss. In my case, I was so involved in the rearing of my daughters and my work as a dean of girls and teacher that, although there was a time of grieving, I was too busy to linger long at the ashes of a dead flame.

Those of my friends who have coped best were those who set about to plan and implement change. Mary nursed her husband through a long illness. After he closed his eyes in death, she reviewed her assets: relatively good health, a comfortable home, a small retirement pension. As the days passed, changes appeared in her home: new paint to lighten the dark walls, new carpet in the living area, rearranged furniture, a rose garden. Today, at 92, she still drives her own car, is active in her church, and is surrounded by friends who cherish her for her cheerful outlook.

When Margaret was left alone her health deteriorated, and she lost interest in life. Because she doesn't drive, she spent her days in solitude with only her dog, a cat, and the telephone. One day I called her. "Margaret, would you be interested in having a Bible study group at your home?" She responded with eagerness. Now every Tuesday morning I pick up the women who no longer drive and we meet at Margaret's home. This has developed into a support group as we add newly-widowed members. We study the Bible, have a prayer session, and share our joys and sorrows. We are blessed and our faith is strengthened by sharing answers to prayers.

The poet Emily Dickinson wrote:

> The bustle in the house the morning after death
> Is solemnest of industries enacted upon earth—
> The sweeping up the heart and putting love away
> We shall not want to use again until eternity.

Death, loss, and grief are all part of life on this earth, but we have the assurance of a better future when God wipes away our tears and for eternity we can use again our heart's love.

Thank You, heavenly Father, for Your grief recovery plan—and until You come and wipe away all our tears, help us to reach out and wipe each other's tears.

VELDA NELSON

Smog Alert

Do not be deceived, God is not mocked; for whatever
a man sows that he will also reap. Gal. 6:7, NKJV.

WHEN WAS THE LAST time you thanked the Lord for the air you breathe? It's a wonderful, free gift that is absolutely essential to life, yet we inhale and exhale 17,000 times a day without giving it so much as a thought. Maybe we should, because the clean air that God made for us on the second day of Creation has become dangerously contaminated by man's inventions. It's called smog.

Smog is a slow but deadly killer. It hangs around cities and industrialized valleys all over the world, slowly poisoning people. Smog is air that is contaminated by waste products from industries, factories, automobiles, trucks, airplanes, burning, and anything that puts noxious fumes, dust particles, and other poisons into the air. Smog is dirty, toxic air—and we breathe it!

When smog attacks, the entire respiratory system is damaged. First, the delicate lining of the nose gets inflamed, leaving it much more sensitive to germ or allergy attacks. Second, the action of the cilia, or hairlike, processes that normally beat many times a second, pushing foreign particles and irritants up out of the air passages, are slowed down or halted, leaving the lungs vulnerable to smog poisons. Smog irritates the lining of the air tubes and causes them to produce thickened mucus, which interferes with breathing, causes coughing, and triggers asthma attacks and emphysema. When smog makes breathing difficult, foreign matter such as dirt, bacteria, and viruses may accumulate in the lungs. Then of course there's the ultimate dreaded disease—cancer—that attacks weakened lungs!

Smog irritates the eyes. Even our brains are affected, because smog destroys the finest part of our oxygen supply—the electrified oxygen. Even though the oxygen percentage in the ambient air may be very close to normal, when the electrified oxygen is destroyed, vitality, creativity, and productivity of the mind, either intellectually or spiritually, can be markedly compromised. That's why, in a subtle way, smog may compromise the finest quality of our lives.

The smog of air pollution that poisons the body reminds me that there is smog of the mind and soul as well. We basically reap what we sow. Sow smog—reap ill health, decreased mental effectiveness and spiritual dullness.

Lord, forgive us for what we have done to the good air You created for us to breathe.

BERNELL E. BALDWIN

A Comforter in Shoes

Share the happiness of those who are happy,
and the sorrow of those who are sad. Rom. 12:15, Phillips.

I DISCOVERED HIM a bit apart from the rest of the picnickers. His head was bent over his dimpled hands, which were covered with at least a half dozen butterflies clinging to his fingers. Eagerly we rejoined the rest so he could show his mother this marvel! A few months later those same small hands were no longer dimpled, but scarred with needle pricks in search of good veins. His luxuriant hair was thin and strawlike, and in a short time he was gone—a victim of leukemia.

Meg, his mother and my dear friend, was devastated. What could be said or done for her that would assuage her grief? Flowers? A careful note in a card? Nothing seemed adequate. We all tried to keep her busy so she wouldn't cry.

Meg stopped by my house unexpectedly one afternoon while my mother was visiting me. I had a quick errand to run and left the two together until I could get back. Upon my return, somewhat later than I had hoped, I found my friend in my mother's arms, both their faces streaked with tears. They hadn't needed me. Meg picked up her bag, smiled through her tears, and said, "I've got to go." She left the room with a more buoyant step than when she came.

A few years later Meg asked me, "Remember when I was with your mother that afternoon after Randy's death? That was the first time anyone had let me talk about him—about how precious and special he was, about his illness, his death, the giving up, the letting go. She let me unload all my grief and heartbreak. Your mother cared enough about me to listen! I'll never forget it!"

Why could I not have been so sensitive to her needs? Perhaps I feared personal suffering too much to let myself be vulnerable to her woe.

The comforting work that my mother performed that day was similar to that of the Holy Spirit—who is often referred to as the Comforter. God's Spirit isn't busy doing comforting things for us or giving comforting information. He's just there—and the healing comes as we share what's on our heart, like Meg shared with my mother. In a way, my mother was like God's Spirit in shoes. I want to be like that, too.

Thank You, Holy Spirit, for being there for me. Help me to be there for others.

ROSE NELL BRANDT

Grandma, Get With It!

Even a child is known by his deeds, whether
what he does is pure and right. Prov. 20:11, NKJV.

BRYAN'S GRANDMOTHER made the best Toll House cookies in the world. Like the widow's flask of oil, her cookie jar was never empty. Kids, grandkids, and friends alike anticipated munching those crispy rich delicacies filled with gooey globs of chocolate. Five-year-old Bryan especially loved visiting Grandma. One night after supper and storytime, Grandma felt like rewarding Bryan for being such a good boy all day. She offered him a cookie.

"But Grandma," the little boy said earnestly, "I've already brushed my teeth!"

The next morning a somewhat chastened Grandma tried another treat. At breakfast she produced a box of Fruit Loops—a surefire hit with any kid. This time Bryan's voice dripped reproach. "Grandma!" he exclaimed. "Do you want me to get holes in my teeth?"

Suddenly Grandma remembered Proverbs 22:6, about training a child right. "I guess 5 years old is not too early to start," she reflected. "It's this grandma that needs to 'get with it'!"

The good news is that children can be taught—and the younger they get started, the better. Here are some tips for building good health habits early in life.

Three meals a day at regular times, with lots of whole grains, fruits, and vegetables. Discourage snacks for a better appetite for nutritious food at mealtimes. If a snack is needed, offer a piece of fresh fruit. And give plenty of water. Save sodas for special occasions.

Daily exercise—preferably outdoors—for at least an hour.

Adequate rest. Teenagers do best on nine hours of sleep a night, and younger ones need more. Put the kids to bed early enough so they awaken naturally in time for a healthy breakfast.

Control TV. The hours a child watches TV relate directly to weight gain and elevated blood cholesterol levels.

Cultivate a wide range of interests. Schedule library visits, music lessons, arts and crafts, hobbies, and family outings. Children who spend time with their parents and develop deep spiritual roots experience less stress and improved mental health.

Set a good example. The life choices you are modeling day by day are the strongest determinants of your children's future behavior.

Lord, help me realize that living "Your way" helps open up spiritual channels as well.   AILEEN LUDINGTON

Sign on to Sabbath Freedom

Each week, work for six days only. The seventh day is a day of total rest, a holy day that belongs to the Lord. Anyone who works on that day will die. Ex. 35:2, NLT.

THE FOURTH DAY of July is a grand date in United States history, for it commemorates the adoption in 1776 of the Declaration of Independence. By opting for self-governance rather than rulership by a distant nation, the founders of this country signed a document that relinquished all guarantees of a predictable, routine life in favor of freedom. It is difficult to imagine the psychological burdens that were shed by people just from the knowledge that all potential oppressions could be eliminated by this formal announcement of independence.

In a way, God did the same with His "Declaration of Sabbath." Though few people in the world have the luxury of democratic freedom, everyone has been given the freedom to have an individual relationship with God by making use of His gift of Sabbath time. Without compelling or prodding, God introduces us to an experience so lofty that many fight its benefits and blessings because they are unfamiliar with them. The Sabbath, established in perpetuity on the seventh day of Creation week, was designated by God as a day of rest. Sabbath is better than an idea—it is a reality!

Signing on to this day provides an opportunity for us to capture the essence of independence. The Sabbath is a space when the whole world gives way to our personal quiet time, uninterrupted, and ungoverned by any entity or being but God! Within the Sabbath we have freedom from worry, bills, work, deadlines, and pressure to produce and perform.

God gave humanity one common Declaration of Independence—the Sabbath, to be commemorated every seventh day. This 24-hour oasis in the midst of a barren and desolate, unfeeling world, refreshes the thirsty soul. Rather than a burden, the Sabbath has at its core an emotionally cleansing effect that allows for quiet reflection and contemplation. Without its incorporation into the weekly life, we would rush to our ultimate end uninterrupted, lacking due notice that our arrival at life's conclusion is no longer a future event but a present reality!

Sabbath offers freedom from an oppressive and destructive world. Sabbath—enter into its obligations! Relish its quiet! Bask in its solitude! Submerge into the most soul-refreshing time that you will ever achieve in a 168-hour week.

Sign onto Sabbath and find true freedom!   SAMUEL THOMAS, JR.

Consider the Lilies

Therefore I say to you, do not worry about your life. . . . Consider the lilies of the field, how they grow: they neither toil or spin; and yet, I say to you that even Solomon in all his glory was not arrayed like one of these. Matt. 6:25-29, NKJV.

IF YOU'RE AN anxious person, you likely feel jittery when routine is broken. Your sensation of being on edge and suffering muscle tension results in more fatigue, so you go to bed early. But after a few hours, you awaken and can't get back to sleep. Then you start worrying about not getting enough sleep and having to get up at 6:00 a.m. You drag yourself out of bed and, since you're still tired, you fumble, breaking something expensive, and you burst into tears. Then you begin hunting for your shopping list that someone has moved—and you can't find your keys. In 30 minutes you're due at your part-time job, where your supervisor recently complained, "If you can't move faster and quit obsessing over these stock labels, I'll have to put you back in." (He may as well have said Siberia in January.) Why can't you calm down? You're so anxious there is a good possibility you'll lose your job, the respect of your coworkers, and your savings. You go to bed worrying about that.

What can you do to stop the downward spiral of depression? How can you get through daily tasks and relationships when you are constantly tense, anxious, having panic attacks, or experiencing obsessive and compulsive symptoms?

It's best to realize that these conditions may not be controllable by will power, organization, Scripture, and prayer alone. It could be a tendency you've inherited. You may not be able to beat the blues by yourself—you may need professional intervention. If a physician suggests you take some medication, be sure to ask what your diagnosis is, how long it's anticipated you'll need the antidepressant—and then do your own research. It may be something you'll need all your life.

In addition, I'd suggest this prescription (it's totally safe—and it's free!): Read Matthew 6:25-34. Reflect on yourself as a lily. Imagine yourself in God's hands, with a gentle rain softly touching your face. Recall that you, as God said, are worth so much more than a lily. Take a deep, slow breath; release it slowly, close your eyes, and softly say, "I am worth far more than a lily; God will be with me." Meditate on a similar Bible promise every day, and believe that, regardless of your human hereditary weaknesses, God loves you without reservation.

Jesus, the next time I start to worry I will remember what You said about my value.
THAIS THRASHER

We're All Born Choosers

And whatever you do, do it heartily, as to the Lord and not to men,
knowing that from the Lord you will receive the reward of
the inheritance; for you serve the Lord Christ. Col. 3:23, 24, NKJV.

AS A CHILD, Ljiljana Ljubisic had a tough time enrolling in the public school system in Yugoslavia. In the 1960s and 1970s blind children were usually institutionalized. Lilo remembers school—both in Yugoslavia and later in Canada—as being hard on her. Kids made fun of this five-foot-eleven blind girl wearing big sunglasses. To read a book she had to press her nose against the page and at the end of the day would have a big black ink mark on her nose from the print. There was physical pain, too. Even a limited amount of light hurt Lilo's eyes, and many times tears would stream down her face.

Life began to change for Lilo when her physical education teacher insisted she try sports. To that point she had always spent the recess and physical education periods studying alone in the library. After all, she was blind. But her teacher would not take no for an answer and gave her a crash course in volleyball serving. Lilo determined to perfect her newly acquired skill, and began practicing alone in a dark gym. Two weeks later her teacher suggested she play a real game. The idea seemed preposterous. The teacher modified the rules. Lilo would serve all the time—and would do nothing but serve. Two captains were selected to pick their teams. Lilo was chosen last.

Lilo prepared to serve. Taking a deep breath, she brought her hand back and swung. The ball whizzed over the net and landed with a thud on the court. Fourteen more serves and the game was over. Each serve hit its mark and not one was returned!

Hard, grueling hours, days, and years of practicing followed. Competitions and travel have taken Lilo to all five continents. In the 1988 Paralympic games in Seoul she won a bronze medal in the shot put. In the 1992 Barcelona games she won gold medals in the discus and shot put. In the 1996 games in Atlanta she broke two world records for the totally blind (shot put, 10.99 meters; discus, 40.40 meters), earning her two bronze medals.

"No one is born a winner," Lilo says. "No one is born a loser. We're all born choosers. The Bible says we have the power of choice. I choose to be positive. I choose to have goals. I choose to do the best with what I have."

What are you choosing today?   ALEX BRYAN

The Boomerang Effect

I am the vine, you are the branches. He who abides in Me, and I in him, bears much fruit; for without Me you can do nothing. John 15:5, NKJV.

EVER SINCE DR. ROBERT ADER defined the psychoneuroimmunology field, studies have shown the positive impact of loving others. Take for example, the study by Nancy Collins at the University of California at Los Angeles on economically disadvantaged pregnant women. Would social support and loving care improve their physical and mental outcomes in pregnancy? Yes! Those who received quality loving prenatal care experienced fewer difficulties in labor. They delivered babies with higher birth weight, the babies were healthier, and these mothers experienced less postnatal depression.

Giving love and support has a boomerang effect—the giver as well as the receiver gets health benefits from doing good.

An amazing study supporting the benefits of doing good was done at Cornell University by three researchers, Moon, McClain, and Williams, and was published in the *American Journal of Sociology*. Starting in 1956, the study followed 427 married women with children for a period of 30 years. The researchers were surprised to find that 52 percent of the women who did not belong to volunteer organizations at the beginning of the study had experienced a major illness 30 years later, compared with only 36 percent of the women who had belonged to a volunteer organization. Other factors, such as the number of children, whether or not a woman worked in an office or as a housewife, education, social class and so on, did not affect their longevity. To summarize: the women who volunteered to help others had better immune systems, which resulted in longer life. As Ellen White once said: "The pleasure of doing good animates the mind and vibrates through the whole body" (*Testimonies for the Church*, vol. 2, p. 534).

What does it take to consistently follow God's "love one another" commandment? (See John 15:17.) When we truly love God and have a strong and healthy vertical relationship with Him, we will automatically produce a strong and healthy horizontal relationship with one another. If, as branches, we are firmly connected to the True Vine, we will automatically bear such fruits as accepting others, forgiving others, supporting others, praying for others, and encouraging, helping, and loving others. And as a result, we can enjoy the boomerang effect. Helping others helps you!

Ask God to impress you with what you could do for others. Write down each idea and then choose one; do it, and enjoy the boomerang effect!

KATHLEEN H. LIWIDJAJA-KUNTARAF

The Real Culprit

*Though He slay me, yet will I trust Him. Even so, I will defend my
own ways before Him. He also shall be my salvation. Job 13:15, 16, NKJV.*

IF THERE'S ANYONE who knew a thing or two about suffering, it was
Job. As I've revisited his story, it's opened windows of understanding for
me in my quest for an answer to the great Why.

The book of Job recounts a time when Satan challenged God about
Job—a saintly and prosperous man who walked closely with God. "Do You
think Job worships You for nothing?" Satan asked God. "You never let anything bad happen to him—and just look at all You've given him." Now notice carefully what Satan says next: "But stretch out your hand and strike
everything he has, and he will surely curse you to *your* face" (Job 1:11, NIV).

And then notice God's reply: "Very well, then, everything he has is in
your hands, but on the man himself do not lay a finger" (verse 12).

So Satan slaughters Job's family—all but his wife. He destroys his flocks
and herds and crops. But to Satan's great consternation, Job doesn't turn
against God. So the devil returns to God, intent on carrying things a step
further. "A man will give all he has for his own life," Satan argues. "But
stretch out *your* hand and strike his flesh and bones, and he will surely curse
you to your face" (Job 2:4).

And again God makes clear who the real villain is: "Very well, then, he
is in *your* hands; but you must spare his life" (verse 6). Then, just so none
of us could miss it, the writer next says that "Satan went out from the presence of the Lord and afflicted Job with painful sores" (verse 7, NIV).

Who afflicted Job? It was Satan, not God!

Satan's grand strategy in the war of evil against good is to make it seem
that God is against us, because he knows that children don't rebel against
parents when they are convinced their parents love them. But they do
rebel against parents whom they feel don't care.

Sometimes when bad things happen we may see evidences as to why
God permitted it; other times we remain in the dark. In such cases such as
the latter, we must fall back on our trust in the God we have come to
know, and say as Job did, "I will trust Him even if I die!"

*In the past few weeks have you felt you've been caught in the middle of the
fight between good and evil? Now is the time to fall a little deeper in love with
God—and trust Him completely.* KEN MCFARLAND

An Olympic Lesson

And Elisha prayed, and said, "Lord, I pray, open his eyes that he may see." Then the Lord opened the eyes of the young man, and he saw. And behold, the mountain was full of horses and chariots of fire all around Elisha. 2 Kings 6:17, NKJV.

ATLANTA, JULY 23, 1996: Never before in 100 years of Olympic games had the U.S. women's gymnastic team been so close to Olympic gold. They trailed Russia by only a few tenths of a point. Tension mounted. The pressure was on 17-year-old Kerri Strugs, the last gymnast to vault. She had two tries—her higher score would count. If high enough the U.S. would win; if not, Russia would take the coveted prize.

Kerri's first attempt was a dismal failure. She didn't complete the final revolution and fell backward on the mat. But the strike against her was worse than merely the psychological pain of failure in front of millions. When she fell, she badly sprained her ankle. Close-up camera shots caught the wince of pain on her face as she limped off the mat. She had one more try, but it was obvious to everyone watching that the U.S. was doomed. How could Kerri compete with a sprained ankle? Russia would win by default.

But the competition was not yet over. Limping into position, Kerri readied herself for what she knew she had to do. She had one more chance to win, and she was going to take it.

In disbelief I watched the telecast as Kerri sprinted down the mat, vaulted into the air, and executed a perfect landing on one foot! Then falling on the mat she gripped her ankle as sharp pains riveted through her body. But her courage, determination, and skill had secured the 1996 gold medal for the United States team.

I wonder if Kerri hadn't thought she'd make it if she would have gone through the pain. If she didn't have the driving dream to hope for the gold, would she have tried that second vault?

I've thought a lot about what it takes to succeed in life when you have a strike or two against you, as Kerri had, and I've concluded that it's your perception that makes the difference.

If you believe that everything is against you, like Elisha's servant did when he saw the enemy surrounding the city, then you'll give up. But if you see life through the eyes of positive expectation, you'll have the courage to fight on! Kerri believed she could do it. And that made all the difference.

Open my eyes that I may see life from Your perspective, where nothing is impossible. KAY KUZMA

Looking to the Light

The Lord is my light and my salvation; whom shall I fear? The Lord is the strength of my life; of whom shall I be afraid? Ps. 27:1, NKJV.

ONE MORNING A SMALL boy living on a North Dakota farm awoke in great pain. Recognizing their son was deathly ill, his parents were greatly alarmed. They rushed him to the nearest hospital, 75 miles away, where they were told that his appendix had ruptured. Peritonitis had set in, and poison was spreading rapidly through his body. Doctors quickly inserted a tube into his side and siphoned away the deadly toxin. Feverish days turned into frightening weeks.

Miraculously, the boy survived. Through the long months of isolation and recuperation in the family's farmhouse, a conviction grew within the youth that God had spared him. "It seemed to me that God had given me a second chance at life, and I prayed for guidance to use my life in ways that would please Him most," he would later write.

To pass the time, the boy began to play sounds on his father's old accordion. The more he played, the more he enjoyed it. Had it not been for the terrible ordeal of a ruptured appendix, the boy probably would never have developed an interest in music. But he emerged from that experience with a deep faith in God and confidence in himself. Following his interest in the accordion, Lawrence Welk left his North Dakota farm and became a gifted musician and host of one of American television's most popular programs.

Key to Welk's success was the fact that he chose to face the light rather than curse the darkness. Scripture constantly reminds us not to adopt the "victim" posture in life. We are urged, when in the midst of adversity and difficulty, to maintain confidence that the clouds will lift, that the darkness will give way to the dawn, that the power of God is not limited. Notice these compelling biblical passages (all from the New International Version):

Isaiah 41:10: "Do not fear, for I am with you; do not be dismayed, for I am your God."

Psalm 30:5: "Weeping may remain for a night, but rejoicing comes in the morning."

Psalm 118:6: "The Lord is with me; I will not be afraid."

Facing the light opens the windows of the soul, permitting the majestic grace of God to flow freely and creatively through our lives.

When darkness threatens to engulf you, partner with God and let His light shine.

VICTOR M. PARACHIN

Are You a Sheep or a Goat?

*When the Son of Man comes as King and all the angels with him, he will sit
on his royal throne. . . . Then he will divide [the people] into two groups,
just as a shepherd separates the sheep from the goats. He will put the
righteous people at his right and the others at his left. Matt. 25:31-33, TEV.*

GOD DOES NOT ultimately separate the righteous and wicked on the
basis of the evangelistic sermons we have preached, the diseases we have
cured, or even the miracles we received. Instead, He looks at whether people were better off for having met us. Did you give food to the hungry,
water to the thirsty, clothes to those who needed them, comfort to the suffering, friendship to those in prison? In the final judgment, titles, diplomas,
and baptismal statistics do not matter. God seems to care about tiny ges-
tures of kindness to people around us. Is this righteousness by small works?

Jesus adds an important detail to the parable that greatly appeals to me.
After He commends the sheep for their kind acts, the sheep ask, "What are
you talking about?" They are surprised that anyone would commend them
for their actions! How could this be?

The sheep are kind by their nature. They are kind people. Sheep do
not give a glass of water because they have been told to do so. They do
not visit a sick person because Jesus is king. They simply see a person in
need and help. It surprises them that anyone would notice these acts, much
less reward them. They are not seeking righteousness by small works!

By contrast, the goats would gladly do all of these acts if only someone would tell them they were required. When modern-day goats read
Matthew 25, they generate a list: "Food cupboard on Monday,
Community Services on Tuesday, Sunshine Band on Wednesday, and
prison ministry on Thursday." These are all worthy projects. Sheep do
them too. The acts are the same, but the attitudes behind them differ.

Throughout Matthew's gospel runs a theme—God is interested in attitudes. Jesus begins teaching by commending those who are poor in spirit,
sorrowful, gentle, merciful, and pure. He says that anger is as bad as murder and lust is as bad as adultery. He quotes Hosea: "I desire mercy, not
sacrifice" (Matt. 9:13, NIV). He tells His disciples that they must be like
little children.

What matters most in our lives on this earth? Jesus says that we should
be kind people who brighten our surroundings. God has this attribute. By
beholding His character, we become like Him.

*Are you a sheep or a goat? Do you need an attitude change before you meet
the King?*   DAN GIANG

Fearfully and Wonderfully Made

I praise you because I am fearfully and wonderfully made; your works are wonderful, I know that full well. Ps. 139:14, NIV.

I REMEMBER HOW amazed I was when I took a class in anatomy and physiology in college. I was awed at the complexities of the human body and its system of checks and balances. God designed everything to work so well together. Even though we eat different types of foods, our bodies try hard to make everything run smoothly. If there is too much sugar in the bloodstream, the pancreas excretes more insulin. If there is too little sugar, our stomach tells the brain to remind us to eat, or our body borrows from stored reserves.

We can even repair ourselves. The skin repairs a cut and broken bones can knit together again. If parts of the liver are removed, it can regenerate itself. After strokes or brain damage, nerves grow and alternate connections are made with repeated exercise. When a person exercises, the heart makes many more blood vessels to feed the heart. Then if there is a heart attack, these extra vessels, called "collateral circulation," can prevent much of the damage to the heart. It's kind of like congestion on the freeway. When one highway is clogged by an accident, we look for another route to get to our destination.

I had almost forgotten about my study of the human body until my daughter decided to follow in my footsteps and study nursing. She is now taking anatomy and has the same reactions that I had, as she sees how fearfully (awe-inspiring) and wonderfully we are made. I cannot wait until she sees for the first time a baby being born. I know she will get tears in her eyes as I did, and she will come home and tell me what a miracle it is.

Surely it is difficult to study science without admitting that there is a Master Designer. The world and our bodies are far too complex to have evolved by chance. Yes, since sin entered the world, there are some flaws in nature. And we know that if we don't treat our bodies the way they were designed to be treated—if we do not eat well and exercise—we may have poor health. However, when one considers how many people there are in the world who live a normal life span in the midst of so much sin and disease, it is amazing.

God, thank You for designing me in such a wonderful way; help me to take care of my body.   BONNIE SZUMSKI

I'm a Recovering Ego-holic

But these things I plan won't happen right away. Slowly, steadily,
surely, the time approaches when the vision will be fulfilled. If it
seems slow, do not despair, for these things will surely come to pass.
Just be patient! They will not be overdue a single day! Hab. 2:3, TLB.

LIKE THE PRODIGAL son, I loathed my rigorous church and home life;
I wanted to break free.

"Give me my space," this teenager screamed; so my parents gave me
SPACE and began my downfall. *S*—Smarts: the benefits of a strict home
and private schooling. *P*—Physically correct: vegetarian, athletic, tall, dark,
and, by some estimates, easy on the eyes! *A*—Articulate: well versed,
quick-witted. *C*—Charming/charismatic: an engaging, unabashed net-
worker. *E*—Ethical: honest; never smoked, drank, gambled, drugged,
overate, or had other addictions. But I became a well-educated, highly articulate, and charismatic "SPACE Cadet"—using God's gifts, without ac-
knowledging His gift-giving role. I was an *ego-holic!*

Ego-holism: "the compulsion to act and/or react excessively because of
feelings of inadequacy." It can be expressed in "big ego" ways—arrogance,
racism, sexism, selfishness, non-listening, or superficiality. It also can be expressed in "little ego" ways—procrastination, profanity, poor time management, flirtation, or mere spinelessness. Enough is never enough—whether
money, attention, clothes, beatings, degrees, sex, or even church attendance.

By January 1987 I was living lavishly and spending foolishly while
working for the world's largest public relations firm in Chicago. Then
everything crashed, and I crawled back to God through a gift: The *Life
Recovery Bible,* which addresses the addictive behaviors of Bible characters.
I learned that without God the Bible's "spirituality buffs" were originally
"puffs"! At age 40 I finally settled down and married. My "sandpaper"
wife, Elaine, began painfully smoothing my rough edges. As a new entrepreneur in 2001, I immediately gained and lost a major contract and was
told, "Talent is not your problem." Again my self-propelled ego had de-
railed me. This wake-up call finally forced me to acknowledge my addiction and begin deflating my ego through Christ.

My recovery model starts at the TOP: Target your problem; take full
Ownership of it; and Proceed immediately to turn your "lemons into
lemonade." I'm still struggling with selfishness, procrastination, arrogance,
disorganization, poor eye contact. But I'm in recovery—and it feels good!

Lord, help me acknowledge my ego-holic nature and walk humbly each day
with You.   TIM ALLSTON

Let's Spread the Good News

I will lead the blind by ways they have not known, along unfamiliar
paths I will guide them; I will turn the darkness into light
before them and make the rough places smooth. Isa. 42:16, NIV.

In my work for Christian Record Services I coordinate blind camp and visit the blind in their own homes, helping them make lifestyle changes to solve various health problems.

Alice wanted to go to camp, but she had rheumatoid arthritis and could not walk far. When I went to visit Alice my heart broke. She was a beautiful woman in her late 30s, born blind. Although she had been treated by her family as handicapped and retarded, she was highly intelligent, had a lovely speaking voice, and was skilled in reading Braille. She walked with pain, one foot was twisted, and she was overweight. Day after day she sat in her chair, listening to tapes.

I prayed for wisdom and suggested that she change her diet, take hot and cold showers for circulation, and use the stairs for exercise. All these changes would help her pain to be less, and then she could walk more and go to camp with us after six months.

She stopped drinking sodas and eating sugar. She began eating lots of vegetables and fruit, along with whole-grain cereals and bread. After four months of following the complete program, her pain was gone, and she could walk much further than ever before. She began to attend Braille Institute and learned to walk with a cane. Now she is very active and involved in training courses.

Later she told me that the reason she was so willing to make drastic lifestyle changes was because her doctors had just told her that the only solution to her pain was to amputate both feet! Now she praises God for His miracle of healing!

Bill had out-of-control diabetes; his blood sugar levels were between 180 and 300, and he was miserable to be around. Fearing kidney failure, he began coming to our weekly support group. In only six months his mood swings, frustration, anger, and anxiety attacks were gone, and his blood sugar level was 100 or less. Bill is leading a productive life now, filled with gratitude and open to the gospel.

My heart is heavy when I think of the thousands who need help. Many blind people are angry, frustrated, and unpleasant people simply because their blood sugar is out of balance. But this can be reversed. God is still performing miracles. We must spread the good news!

God of miracles, work in my life today and give me courage to spread the good news.   MOLLY LESICK

Forgiveness in Room 283

[He] forgives all your sins and heals all your diseases. Ps. 103:3, NIV.

THE NURSE CAME TO the room where I was visiting a patient. "Chaplain," she said, "the woman in room 283 wants to talk with you."

I found my way to room 283. As I seated myself in a chair near the bed the woman asked, "Chaplain, will you forgive me?"

Somewhat stunned, I replied, "I have visited with you several times, and you have never offended me in any way. What do you mean, will I forgive you?"

Then she told her story. "When I was a young woman I began to sell my body for money. This went on for some time until I discovered I had a venereal disease. It was necessary for me to have surgery to remove the diseased organs of my body. Later I married, but I never told my husband about my past life. Chaplain, I have carried the burden of my sin all of my life, and I cannot bear it any longer. You are the only person to whom I have told this story. Please, forgive me."

I told her that she had not sinned against me, but she had violated her body and sinned against God. Then I said, "Let me share some good news with you." Turning to 1 John 1:9, I read, "'If we confess our sins, he is faithful and just and will forgive us our sins and purify us from all unrighteousness'" (NIV).

"How do I confess?" she asked.

"We simply pray to God and ask for forgiveness."

She said, "Will you pray, asking God to forgive me? I don't know how to pray."

I explained that prayer is simply talking to God as we would talk to a friend. I pointed out that she had told me her story with ease. Then I told her to talk to God just as she had talked to me and ask Him to forgive her. She began to pray, asking for forgiveness. In the nearly 50 years of my ministry, I have never heard a prayer like hers. It was so touching that I wept.

God gave her forgiveness, and she had peace. She used to cry out in the night, but not after finding peace with herself and God.

Notice the order of God's benefits for us in Psalm 103:3. The Bible lists forgiveness for spiritual disease first and then healing from physical diseases!

Perhaps it is time to pray the prayer of forgiveness as did the woman in room 283. Why wait?   KENNETH H. LIVESAY

JULY 15

The Great Physical
Therapist's Exercise Plan

Therefore, strengthen your feeble arms and weak knees. "Make level paths for your feet," so that the lame may not be disabled, but rather healed." Heb. 12:12, 13, NIV.

A FEW YEARS AGO my back failed me. I couldn't stand or sit or lie on my side for more than a few seconds without great pain. The only comfortable position was flat on my back, floating on narcotics. The doctor in the pain clinic injected cortisone into my spine. The chiropractor tweaked my vertebrae. The elders anointed me. There was no apparent effect.

I feared I would never stand or even sit again. When my wife took me to the doctor's office, she carried a foam pallet for me. I lay on the waiting room floor like the man at the Pool of Bethesda, waiting for an angel to stir the waters.

Finally, after six weeks, I went to a neurosurgeon. He said, "Stand on your left leg and rise up onto your toes." My brain said, "I will," but my body did not respond. "O wretched man that I am! who shall deliver me from this body of death?" (Rom. 7:24).

The surgeon said, "If you're willing, I'll operate tomorrow."

"I'm willing," I said. "The surgery scares me, but it can't be worse than the way I am now."

When I awoke, the sciatic nerve pain was gone. The next morning I sat up to eat breakfast, then slowly walked the hospital halls, praising God. But I didn't run and jump. That took time. First came several months of exercising numb muscles, waiting for nerves to recover.

In our spiritual life it's not enough to submit to the knife of the Great Surgeon. We also need the guiding hand of the Great Physical Therapist. He gives us exercises that strengthen us. He asks us to come (Matt. 11:28). He tells us to go (Matt. 28:18-20). He gives us challenges (1 Cor. 10:13). He asks us to follow (Matt. 4:19). The exercises are progressive, building us without discouraging us (Phil. 4:13). (See also Hebrews 12:1-13.)

My late grandmother had both arthritic knees replaced. She was soon walking a mile a day—more than she'd been able to walk for years. But she didn't continue with her bending and stretching exercises, because they hurt. Scar tissue formed in her joints. Soon she could not walk more than a few yards, and the pain returned.

Spiritually, a lot of us are in a similar condition!

Lord, what spiritual exercises do You want me to do today?

ED CHRISTIAN

The Man in White

The Son of man came not to be ministered unto, but to minister. Matt. 20:28.

"HELLO, DOCTOR; come quickly. The patient in room 15 is not well."
I breathe deeply and close my eyes. All I need is a sound, undisturbed sleep
after having been on duty for two days and two nights. I've seen more than
200 patients in the past 48 hours, and tomorrow I'll be on duty again. My
head is empty. My body is numb from fatigue. The telephone falls from
my hand before the caller finishes. Sleep . . . sleep . . . sleep is the only
thing I can concentrate on.

Still, the demands are relentless: "Hello, Doctor; come quickly . . .
Hello, Doctor . . . Hello." Like a robot I put on my white coat. In my
head there is one sentence playing again and again like a broken record:
"You are the man in white in this place of soiled linen . . ."

Yes, death, here we are again, I think as I attend to another patient. *You
want to win. I've fought you many times. But God will have the last word, not you.*

Last night it was a young mother. At 3:00 a.m. it was a little boy. Their
eyes looked to me with confidence. I wanted to scream. The word AIDS
pierced my brain. I don't wear God's mantle. I'm less than the little finger
on His mighty hand. Still, I fight sin, darkness, and the devil.

I seem to have forgotten the ones who walked out through the hospital door wrapped in joy, their bodies restored to health. I did wonder about
their souls, but only for a moment. I had to run to attend to others. I still
wish I knew the answers. But how do I heal the unhealable?

I learn to be humble, to work instead of sleep, to pray instead of cry.
And on I run down the corridor to Room 15. "Here I am, my friend." I
understand the question in your eyes: *Why me? My children are still young;
my task is far from finished.* I hold your hand. I give you an injection to
soothe your pain. But I want to cry. *O Lord, I'm losing a friend.* Yet the man
in white is not supposed to cry. They don't want my tears or my feelings.
Only my skill, my brain, my sleep, my life.

O Lord, how do *You* bear the misery of this world? How do *You* heal?
The fragment "We have to pray to comfort God" rings in my ear. Is that
true, Lord? Does my prayer console You as it comforts me? So hear my
prayer then: *Here am I, Lord. Help me make it through another day. My task is
with the ones who live.*

Lord, be with all the medical personnel who are giving their lives to save others. Amen.

VERENA JAGGI—Written as a tribute to her husband,
a physician at Malamulo Hospital in Malawi, Africa.

And God Made the Butterfly

Through him all things were made; without him nothing was made that has been made. In him was life, and that life was the light of men. John 1:3, 4, NIV.

ON SUNDAY, JULY 18, 1999, Ron Bottomly had taken his wife and daughters to the Portland airport for a trip to California. After seeing them off, he walked toward the closest exit out of the airport mall area to the parking lot. There was a surprisingly large number of people passing back and forth, so he decided he could just as easily walk down the mall, past the shops, and take the next exit.

As he walked he noticed a beautiful glass butterfly in the window of the Made in Oregon store. He decided to check the price because his wife, Kathy, collected butterflies. Finding it a little more than his budget would allow, he turned to leave the store. As he stepped out he saw a gentleman had collapsed directly in front of him. Ron, a skilled ICU nurse, knelt beside the man, proceeded to do an assessment, and started cardiac pulmonary resuscitation (CPR). When the paramedics arrived he helped them start the intravenous and other emergency procedures. The gentleman was "shocked" and after about the fifth try, a palpable pulse was felt. Forty-five minutes after his collapse, the man was loaded into the ambulance and taken to the hospital with his heart beating.

A couple weeks later Ron received a package from Irene, the daughter of the man whose life he had saved. Inside was an exquisite glass ornament hanging from a metal stand and a letter that explained why she believed Ron unknowingly played a part in a divine intervention.

First, the fact that Ron was there at the right time and in the right place and was a trained medical ICU nurse, was a miracle. The large number of people at the exit was unusual for Sunday morning, but more strange was the glass butterfly. If Ron hadn't gone in to check the price, he would have already walked past the place when her father collapsed. Thinking the butterfly would be an appropriate thank-you gift for Ron, Irene and her sister went back to the shop, but there were no butterflies—and the shopkeeper said there never had been. They checked all the stores nearby. Nothing. "Unless both of us misunderstood what you said about the butterflies," Irene wrote, "my 13-year-old son, Brad, came up with the best explanation. God created an illusion to keep you nearby."

What an awesome God we serve—Creator of all, even butterflies in the mall.

DONNA BECHTHOLD

Scars

He will wipe away every tear from their eyes. There will be no more death or mourning or crying or pain, for the old order of things has passed away. Rev. 21:4, NIV.

DO YOU HAVE any scars from accidents in the past? I have a few, and there is a story behind each of them. There is a faint scar on the back of my right hand that I have grown fond of through the years, where the family dog bit me the day she died.

She had wandered out into the street against my orders and had been hit by a truck right before my eyes. As she lay dying in the middle of the road, I realized that I had to get her out of the way of traffic, so I grabbed her collar to drag her off to the side of the road. The pain must have been excruciating, because she suddenly chomped down on my hand to get me to stop. She sunk her teeth into my flesh, leaving a deep puncture wound. A minute later she took her last breath. Today the small scar is a reminder to me of a German shepherd I loved dearly as a boy.

It is interesting that God made our bodies to heal from injury, but also to scar. It may simply be the result of sin that we do not regenerate new tissue perfectly, but I do not resent those little bumps and creases. They remind me of mistakes, awaken memories of past events, and provide visual learning tools for my children. When they ask "How did you do that?" it affords me an opportunity to share experiences that may save them from future pain.

There are other kinds of scars—emotional ones, the kind you can't see—that we carry with us as well. Many emotional scars do not heal perfectly either, but leave a faint trace as a sad reminder of past mistakes. They may be caused by strangers, friends, or even family members.

You may wonder how these scars can ever be removed. God heals all scars, and transforms a heart of stone into a heart of flesh (Eze. 11:19). At the Second Coming we will not only be given perfect new bodies, but the pain and sorrow of this life will be purged as well, for as our text for today assures us, "He will wipe away every tear from their eyes."

What lessons have you learned from the scars in your life that have made you a better person?
LARRY RICHARDSON

Throw Away Your Coat!

Then Jesus said to him, "Go your way; your faith has made you well." And immediately he received his sight and followed Jesus on the road. Mark 10:52, NKJV.

BART WAS BLIND, and so had become a professional beggar at the gates of Jericho. He made more noise than a dozen normal beggars, and many wished that he had been cursed with silence rather than darkness. Bart survived through the generosity of passing merchants, all of whom were being robbed by the tax collectors. "Don't give it all to the robbers from Rome," he would shout. "Give some to one who really needs it! Help out old Bart. Come on, every dinero adds up toward a meal for a blind man."

Every day was the same. Until Jesus came to town. The stories preceded him. "Jesus," they said, "can restore the sight of the blind." It was a tale beyond belief, yet worth believing. So Bart began shouting for Jesus to notice him and "have mercy." Louder, louder, and louder! Until everyone shouted for him to be silent. Everyone except Jesus.

Instead of joining the crowd's put-downs, Jesus called for Bart to join Him down toward the river Jordan. Throwing his coat aside, Bart jumped to his feet and came to Jesus (Mark 10:50). His coat? That's like a street person giving up her shopping cart. Like a deaf man closing his eyes. Like an artist giving up his brushes, a computer programmer throwing away her laptop, or a fisherman leaving his line. Bart's coat was all he had. It was where he kept his money, and his dried mutton. Without it he would be bankrupt and starving. And, being blind, if he dropped it he would never be able to find it again.

Throwing his coat aside, he came to Jesus. The Healer had called, His voice promising new life—*eyes*—for Blind Bart. Nothing would slow the beggar down, hold him back or compromise his sprint. Not even his most treasured possession. There could be nothing between Bart and his Savior.

That's the requirement for all of us, the true cost of accepting God's gift of complete healing, of sprinting to His promise of new life. We must turn totally to the Savior and allow Him to restructure our values. He promises to replace our deafness with hearing, our weakness with energy, our anger with love, our blindness with sight! He is calling. Throw away your coat. Sprint to the voice of new hope.

Is there anything holding you back from sprinting to Christ?

DICK DUERKSEN

Reinforcing the Guard

*Do you not know that you are the temple of God and
that the Spirit of God dwells in you? 1 Cor. 3:16, NKJV.*

PICTURE YOURSELF AS a sacred temple. Every day, enemies attempt
to destroy you. The battles are waging around you and inside you. You
can win each skirmish, but only if your temple guard (natural killer cells)
stay vigilant.

Anything that weakens your energy, circulation, health, alertness, outlook, and perception gives the invaders an advantage. Pollutants, chemicals, sugar, and stress continually barrage your body's defense team. Your
enemies—bacteria, viruses, cancer cells, fungi—assault your body through
any opening—your mouth, eyes, nose, an open sore, or even skin pores.
How will you handle the next onslaught? Will you lose the battle to a flu
bug, cold, or bronchial infection? Or will you take charge and fight? It all
depends on how healthy your immune system is. Here are some boosters:

Keep your immune system guard in top-notch shape with a healthy lifestyle
and outlook. Embrace laughter, optimism, faith, and good relationships.

At the first sign of a cold (within 10 to 20 minutes), take a healthy dose
of a number of natural immune boosters: echinacia (usually with gold-
enseal), quercitin, vitamin C, garlic (raw garlic is best), and zinc are the
most common.

Oxygen and sunshine kills germs. Spend a few minutes deeply breathing warm air and feel the sun on your face or exposed skin. Or, if you can't
go outside, at least open the window for a few minutes to freshen stale indoor air; pull the blinds and let the sun shine in.

Drink lots and lots of water—but limit sweet fruit juices because sugar
suppresses the immune system. Instead, peel a grapefruit, leaving ample
white pulp, blend it in a little water, and drink it! (You can do it!) Eat sparingly. Your defense system works best when body energy isn't diverted to
your digestive system. Take a few charcoal tablets between meals.

And don't forget the benefits of hydrotherapy. Try a hot shower and
a short, but stimulating, cold rinse. Repeat it a few times and you will feel
what it does to your circulation!

*God has given you incredible power over the organisms and environmental poi-
sons that invade His "temple." Use it!*   KAY and JAN W. KUZMA

Only a Prayer Away

Your righteousness reaches to the skies, O God, you who
have done great things. Who, O God, is like you? Ps. 71:19, NIV.

"OH, WHAT ARE WE going to do?" muttered Pam. As she continued to express her concern, I shared with her how I used to let worry and anxiety control me until I learned what it did to my body.

"I know you're right," she responded. "I'm damaging my body and only hurting myself. But how can I change?"

For me, the first step was to recognize and admit that I had a problem. Watching a film on what stress does—lowering the immune system paving the way to all types of diseases—helped me determine that worry did not fit into my life plan—and it certainly wasn't God's plan for me!

Instead of sitting around worrying, I learned to take action on my feelings. When I sense a negative worry creeping into my thoughts, I walk. If I'm at work, I take a break to walk out those feelings. If I'm home, I walk outside. Previously I had a treadmill that I used for my "negative thought" workouts.

"But," I said to Pam, "I've found something even better than walking. The best way to reduce my negative feelings is to pray." When I mentioned prayer to Pam her comment was, "But God's so far away, how can He help me down here?"

I could relate to what Pam was saying. He is far away physically, but experience had taught me that He's only a prayer away.

The next morning I prayed that as I read my usual three of four chapters from God's Word, I would recognize an answer to Pam's question. I found the first part of the answer in Psalm 71:3: "Be my rock of refuge, to which I can always go" (NIV). Reaching up to Him shortens the distance between. The chasm is bridged, however, when He reaches down to us with His angel host. Psalm 103:19-22 says, "The Lord has established his throne in heaven, and his kingdom rules over all. Praise the Lord, you his angels, you mighty ones who do his bidding, who obey his word. Praise the Lord, all his heavenly hosts, you his servants who do his will. . . . Praise the Lord, O my soul" (NIV).

Why should we worry when God has promised us refuge when we ask—and sends His servant angels to meet our needs? He is only a prayer away. "Who, O God, is like you?"

God will do His part to reach down to you—are you reaching up to Him
in prayer? RITA STEVENS

Soul Truth

*For the Lord himself shall descend from heaven with a shout,
with the voice of the archangel, and with the trump of God:
and the dead in Christ shall rise first. 1 Thess. 4:16.*

AS SCIENTISTS PROBE ever deeper into the biochemical reactions within our brain, the notion of the soul as a separate entity becomes increasingly suspect. And those people, Christians or other, who believe in the soul as the guarantee of immortal life find their hope threatened.

Francis Crick, who with James Watson discovered the double helix of DNA 50 years ago, has spent many years researching consciousness, partly with the goal of disproving the soul. Crick, now 86, claims that he and other researchers have found the group of cells from the back of the cortex to parts of the frontal cortex that are responsible for generating consciousness and one's sense of the self. He believes that "one day all humanity will come to accept that the concept of souls and the promise of eternal life were a deception—just as they now accept that the earth is not flat." This statement is part right and part wrong.

Right: that the concept of souls is a deception. It has no biblical basis. The Scriptures teach that we are whole beings, with body, mind, and breath inseparably linked. The Creation account establishes the reality: "The Lord God formed man of the dust of the ground, and breathed into his nostrils the breath of life; and man became a living soul" (Gen. 2:7). Adam does not receive a soul; he becomes a soul as he receives life-breath from God. And when that life-breath ceases—when he dies—his existence ceases.

Wrong: that the promise of eternal life is a deception. If the promise were dependent on an immortal soul—an idea that comes from ancient Greek philosophy—it would be a cruel lie. But it isn't. It springs from Jesus Christ, the conqueror of sin and the grave, He who died on Calvary but who is alive forevermore and who assures us: "Because I live, you also will live" (John 14:19, NIV).

Resurrection itself is a notion beyond human reasoning. Nothing—nothing!—continues beyond the grave. But in God's memory nothing is lost: we "sleep," safe in Him. And at our Lord's return we rise from the dead as new beings, with new bodies but with the old "us" keyed in by the fingers of a loving Father. The idea stretches our minds. It would stretch our faith also except for one fact: Jesus did it! He died and rose again! And so shall we.

Thank You, Lord, for Your promise of the resurrection and whole-person life forever with You.
WILLIAM G. JOHNSSON

Too Much Isn't Better

Then the Lord God took the man and put him in the garden of Eden to tend and keep it. Gen. 2:15, NKJV.

I LOVE GARDENING, but it's hard work. I think that's why God placed Adam and Eve in a garden and told them to take care of it. He knew humans need exercise. The evidence is mounting: Exercise reduces the risk of cancer. In 11 studies relating exercise to breast cancer approximately half showed a protective effect of exercise. One study even showed that 12-year-old girls who exercised had less breast cancer later in life than those who didn't.

In a longitudinal study of more than 17,000 Harvard alumni, researchers found that those who were overweight in young adulthood and middle-age had a higher risk of colon cancer—unless they were physically active. They also found that those who were most active had considerably less lung cancer after smoking. Researchers concluded that exercise boosts the immune system.

In the Nurses' Health Study of approximately 86,000 nurses, exercise reduced the risk of colon cancer by almost half. The more time spent sitting, the higher the risk for colo/rectal cancer.

Why is it that exercise helps reduce cancer risk? It usually prevents overweight—and being overweight is associated with cancer. It improves the body's response to insulin. Those who exercise tend to eat more fruits and vegetables. It helps in moving the food through the intestines more quickly, giving carcinogens less time to act. And exercise reduces estrogen production, which is related to breast cancer.

But just like most good things, too much is not necessarily better. David Nieman, while at Loma Linda University, showed that brisk walking for 45 minutes five times a week for 15 weeks boosted the activity of natural killer cells that help to knock out viruses and malignancies in the body's cells. The walkers had as many colds and flu episodes but these didn't last as long.

However, the natural killer cell activity was lessened 25 to 46 percent by running for three hours, and this effect lasted for 21 hours. In the 1987 Los Angeles Marathon, 13 percent of the runners came down with colds or the flu within a week after the race, compared to only 2 percent who trained for the race but didn't run.

Thank You, God, for letting me learn what's good for me. Now give me the willpower to get up and get the exercise I need to keep healthy. Amen.

JOHN A. SCHARFFENBERG

My Spiritual Resurrection

*I have been crucified with Christ; it is no longer
I who live, but Christ lives in me. Gal. 2:20, NKJV.*

MY MOM'S SUICIDE rocked my life. My first reaction was shock. Then denial. Then anger. *(How could she do this to me? To my kids?)* Then guilt. *(Why didn't I do something more?)*

As I tried to put the pieces of my life together, I questioned God's role in Mom's suffering (she was manic-depressive) and her subsequent choice to end her life. Blindly, I saw only two options: (1) God didn't fulfill His promise to not allow any temptation beyond what Mom could bear; or (2) Mom just blew it! Either way, it was a losing situation. Either God or Mom screwed up, and that conclusion almost destroyed my relationship with God.

Over the next year or two I really struggled with my spiritual life. In retrospect, I think it was a combination of my relatively sterile spiritual life before Mom's death, her suicide itself, and the subsequent questions it raised in my mind about God's role in our lives. Also, I attended a large, impersonal church where I had no support group to listen, encourage, and reinforce to me the truth that God loves and Satan destroys.

I'm embarrassed to say that I almost gave up on God. I kept going to church, but mainly for the kids' sake. Even though I was struggling, I still believed in a God to whom I wanted my kids to relate. I didn't want them to grow up not going to church because of me.

Before making a final choice to bail out on God, I committed to do some more reading and investigating. I read a book by Philip Yancey, *Where Is God When It Hurts?* That really helped me to "wake up and smell the roses!" My family also began attending a smaller church where I became involved and made friends who loved me, regardless—and I began therapy.

Over the past five years I've really come alive spiritually! I've benefited from four small groups (one secular recovery group and three spiritually based groups). I've had a much more meaningful devotional and prayer life, and I've been much more active in my church. It's been wonderful— like my own spiritual resurrection! I wonder why it took me so long (30 years) to get connected with God.

God, You are so good! You have big, strong shoulders to lean on when I feel weak. You patiently listen to me when I question You and Your ways—and You love me, regardless. Thank You! ROB THOMAS

Avoiding Posttraumatic Sin

The next day John saw Jesus coming toward him, and said, "Behold!
The Lamb of God who takes away the sin of the world!" John 1:29, NKJV.

POST-TRAUMATIC STRESS DISORDER is the clinical name given to the syndrome we see when those who live through crisis suffer from permanently altered nervous systems that continue to destroy them long after the bullets of abuse stop flying.

Jack was a typical Vietnam veteran of the 80s: shoulder-length hair; combat fatigues and boots; a wide, hyper-vigilant stare; increased startle reaction at loud noises; unable to sit still; a social isolate. He'd been through an alcohol treatment program and remained sober for three years. Then, on the anniversary of Tet 1968, when his compound had been overrun by Viet Cong and his buddies killed, he relapsed by drinking to almost unconsciousness, hoping it would kill him—and the memory. Now, two weeks later, he continued to feel suicidal, and so he came to see me.

He discussed in detail the loss of his best friend who died in his arms; the devastation they had wreaked on a village known to harbor North Vietnamese military, and his shooting of a little girl wearing a backpack full of ammunition who was running toward a group of enemy soldiers. He sobbed uncontrollably at times, sharing his intense guilt, anxiety, anger, and pain. Being taught to hate and destroy human beings, and experiencing horrifying combat scenes, had scarred him for life.

He avoided contact with most of society, lived in a remote shack near the mountains, and had not been able to work for the past seven years. He could barely make ends meet on the small check he received. I insisted he begin attending Alcoholics Anonymous again and prescribed medication to lift the weight of his depression and help him sleep without being awakened by vivid nightmares.

Like the combat-beleaguered veteran, our nervous systems become permanently altered by our encounters with sin. When we participate in sin there is no going back to erase the imprint on our brain neurons. Jack had no choice at the time of his combat experience, but in our daily lives we *can* choose to reject temptation. With God's strength we can move closer to Him each day and shut the doors a little tighter against evil.

Have you called on Jesus today and asked Him to take away your sins—and to keep you from temptation? Jesus is the only way to avoid the posttraumatic sin syndrome.   THAIS THRASHER

Our Marvelous Designer

I will praise You, for I am fearfully and wonderfully made; marvelous are Your works, and that my soul knows very well. Ps. 139:14, NKJV.

MARVELOUS DESIGN IS demonstrated in the eye. Light travels through the pupil to the retina in the back of the eye. There it is registered chemically in the rod and cone cells, which transmit sight through nerves to the back of the skull where we "see" in the posterior lobe of the brain. The ability to see is tremendously complex.

The chemical basis for sight is as important as the nerves. If an image is held stationary on the retina, the participating photoreceptors (rods and cones) would soon be chemically fatigued, and the image would fade. Microscopically small and rapid eye movements guarantee that an image registers on one set of cells until it is chemically exhausted and then moves to another while the first cells are restored. Cellular level movement constantly sweeps across the retina, enabling sight to be chemically processed by fresh photoreceptors. The exterior eye muscles make these movements possible.

Each eye is equipped with three pairs of taut, elastic muscles. As with other skeletal muscles of the body, almost all of which work in pairs, each eye muscle vies with its counterpart to pull the eye in different directions. Among them, these six muscles allow eye movement in every direction. Each eye muscle originates on bone within the eye socket and attaches to the eyeball itself, just behind the pupil. Constant tension helps make these eye muscles among the fastest and most accurate in the body. Capable of seven coordinated movements, they give humans one of nature's most advanced tracking systems. In addition to the invisible microscopic movement from cell to cell, these muscles enable us to maintain binocular vision—the ability to visualize depth and distance.

An important eye muscle is the superior oblique, which can function only by virtue of the muscle having a tendon that passes through a pulley-like growth of bone. This allows the muscle to be active at an almost 90 degree angle. The eye and its chemical and neuromuscular control is probably the body's best example of design by a Creator God. It could not have evolved by random evolutionary changes.

Although, according to 1 Corinthians 13:12, we see only "dimly" now, what wonderful glories we can anticipate in the new earth when our marvelous Designer will give us "full vision"!

In God's design for your eye, doesn't it make you want to shout, "Praise the Lord"!   P. WILLIAM DYSINGER

Changing Dietary Habits

I will give you a new heart and put a new spirit in you. Eze. 36:26, NIV.

MOM WAS A SUPERB cook and made the best white-flour tortillas. One noon we came from working in the field and sat down to a delicious meal. When we reached for the tortillas and uncovered them, we were disgusted. They were brown and stiff. Horrors! We were hungry. Who would dare feed anyone shoe leather like these lousy tortillas?

Incensed deprecations were hurled at Mom, who had lovingly offered us the best she knew. She had read that whole wheat was better than white flour, though the entrenched custom is to use white tortillas.

Poor Mom, she had to bear with a family who should have been thanking her for her love. She undoubtedly wept alone in her closet. What brutality on our part. I hate to think of it!

But Mom was much bigger than to succumb to our stupid nonsense. She happily returned to making white-flour tortillas. But then one day she put just a little whole wheat in the dough. When we saw little brown specks in our favorite white tortillas, a howl of protest went up immediately. But we were hungry and, because the tortillas were not much different than usual, we began to eat them. For some time after that we had the same tortillas with a few brown specks, even though we grumbled some about them.

Then one day we saw more brown spots than previously, though not greatly different than before. Again a howl of protest went up. But again we were hungry enough to eat them, with grumbling. A few days later the tortillas were again darker than before. This continued for a long time until Mom had us eating the best tortillas in town, with the best nutrition. And they were delicious to us. All credit is due to God, who selected a loving mother who was willing to withstand the assaults of an ungracious, unthankful family.

Now a white tortilla is insipid and rubbery to me. It takes time to change dietary habits, but when there is love it can be done, even with the most culturally ingrained taste habits. Dietary habits are difficult to change, but you can choose new ones.

Take heart! A change in a health habit is but a glimpse of the transforming changes God desires to make in our lives, if we allow Him.

Are you willing to make the changes God wants to make in your life?

ALBERT SANCHEZ

It's Not How You Walk

He has shown you, O man, what is good; and what does the Lord require of you but to do justly, to love mercy, and to walk humbly with your God? Micah 6:8, NKJV.

IN 1978 CAROL SCHULLER lost her leg in a motorcycle accident. Her body may have been broken but her courageous spirit carried her through seven months of hospitalization, intravenous feedings, collapsed veins, and a raging infection that threatened her life; then as a "handicapped" person, the struggle to feel normal and whole again.

Carol loved to play softball, so the summer after her accident she signed up for the team. At the time, Carol's artificial leg was attached just below the knee, which was so stiff she could hardly bend it. Running was out of the question. When she was asked how she expected to play softball when she couldn't run, she answered, "When you hit home runs, you don't have to run!" That season she hit enough home runs to justify her position on the team.

Six surgeries later, Carol took up skiing and won a gold medal in the qualifying races that admitted her to the elite corps of skiers participating in the 1983 National Ski Championships.

When Carol was 17, the Schuller family took a Hawaiian cruise. The weather was beautiful and Carol was not ashamed to be seen in shorts or swimming attire, even though people looked at her and wondered what had happened.

There was a talent show the last night of the cruise. Carol came on stage in a beautiful full-length dress and said, "I really don't know what talent is, but I thought this would be a good chance for me to give what I think I owe you all—an explanation. I was in a motorcycle accident. I almost died. They amputated my leg below the knee, and later, they amputated through the knee. I spent seven months in the hospital, with intravenous antibiotics to fight infection. If I've one talent, it's this: during that time, my faith became very real to me. I look at you girls who walk without a limp, and wish I could walk that way. I can't, but this is what I've learned: It's not how you walk that counts, but who walks with you and with whom you walk."

She paused, and then said, "I'd like to sing a song about my friend, my Lord." She sang, "And He walks with me, and He talks with me . . ." There was not a dry eye in the audience.

Regardless of what has happened to you, like Carol, you can hold on and make the most of it. As Carol's dad, Robert H. Schuller, often says, "Tough times never last, but tough people do."   KAY KUZMA

None of These Diseases!

If you diligently heed the voice of the Lord your God and do what is right in His sight, give ear to His commandments and keep all His statutes, I will put none of the diseases on you which I have brought on the Egyptians. For I am the Lord who heals you. Ex. 15:26, NKJV.

MY EXPERIENCE WITH AIDS patients can be summarized by three cases. The first was a man with peptic ulcers. He was a highly stressed person; several times he came to me because of pain in his stomach. Shortly before he became my patient he had hemorrhaged and was given a blood transfusion. At that time there was no concern about HIV infection, so the blood was not tested. Ten years later he developed AIDS and in six months he was dead.

The second one was a drug addict. He shot heroin for many years. When he came to my office he was really motivated to start a new life, but it was too late. A lab test found he was HIV positive. He left my office and after two or three months came back with a major infection in his bluish arm, a sign that he had gone back to drugs. That was the last time I saw him.

The third patient was a good Christian who came to me for a physical examination. Just one thing concerned me—some nodules in the left side of his neck. I checked them and asked for lab tests. The finding? He was HIV positive. Checking back with the patient I discovered he had been involved in homosexuality, but five years earlier had accepted Christ and given up that lifestyle. Short of a miracle, he is probably dead by now.

These three cases represent the three main ways AIDS is spread: blood, drugs, and sex. But the point is that all three men could be alive and healthy today if they had developed attitudes and behaviors that were based on God's commandments. If we live as God says we should, there would be no need for burning anger and bitter resentment that so often causes ulcers, nor would people be involved with drugs or self-gratifying sexual behavior.

Exodus 15:26 sums it up well. If you follow God's commandments, "none of these diseases will fall upon you." What God promised to do for His people was not so complex, miraculous, or supernatural as it might appear. Quite simply, God was saying, "I made you and know what's good for you. Follow My prescription for health, because how you choose to live your life today will affect your life tomorrow."

Are you living today for what you would like to be tomorrow?

HILDEMAR DOS SANTOS

He Still Cares

Therefore humble yourselves under the mighty hand of God, that He may exalt you in due time, casting all your care upon Him, for He cares for you. 1 Peter 5:6, 7, NKJV.

IT WAS JULY, 1995. My 10-year-old daughter was lying in the hospital bed with 19 wires and tubes attached to her highly fevered body. The doctors had induced a coma because of a severe head injury, the result of a fall from a horse.

Doctors were very worried because she had a concussion the size of a big grapefruit on the left side of her brain. Their concern was that Nicky's ICP (inner cranial pressure) was high and climbing. The doctors and nurses were trying desperately to bring the ICP down by increasing the dosage of mannitol, but it was all in vain; the ICP kept rising. They all had very troubled looks on their faces.

Meanwhile I prayed, "Lord, please save my little girl and please protect her mind from confusion." Then the words of Psalm 71:1 came to mind: "In Thee, O Lord, do I put my trust: let me never be put to confusion."

Suddenly I felt a tap on my shoulder. It was my friend Cindy Keenan. She saw the despair on my face and noticed that Nicky's ICP was very high. She looked at me and said, "Nicole, let's sing Nicky's favorite song, 'I Cast All My Cares Upon You.'"

Cindy and I were on opposite sides of the bed, and we began to sing softly. As we finished I lifted my head, and I couldn't believe my eyes. The ICP was dropping, dropping. It dropped lower than it ever had been. When medicines failed, the Creator stepped in.

Nicky has done exceptionally well in her studies. She cares for others and has lots of friends. Her principal affectionately calls her the social butterfly. I have told her over and over that God has a special plan for her, and I thank Him that her mind is healthy. A few years ago she even became a paid author for sharing her story in the December 1998 issue of *Children's Mission.*

I don't know what the future holds, but I do know that God works miracles when we cast all our cares upon Him.

If you have problems and worries today, give them to the Lord—for He does care for you.   NICOLE SYDENHAM

Accepting Truth

*Be diligent to present yourself approved to God, a worker who does not
need to be ashamed, rightly dividing the word of truth. 2 Tim. 2:15, NKJV.*

AFTER BEGINNING HIS ministry in Capernaum, Jesus returned to
Nazareth to preach in His home synagogue. His neighbors took offense.
How could this poor carpenter's son, this self-taught preacher, stand before
them and impart new information? They were so angered at His presump-
tion that they were ready to throw Him over a cliff. This rejection led Jesus
to utter sadly the now-famous phrase, "No prophet is accepted in his own
country." (See Luke 4:16-24.)

It is tempting to emphasize new scientific research and neglect to
credit the pioneering efforts of those who laid the foundation. Dr. Winea
Simpson was a foundation-builder who received little recognition. In the
1950s she began to gather data about maternal smoking habits and premature births. Her results established, for the first time in history, an epidemi-
ological link between the two. Her findings were published in reputable
journals, yet few took notice.

"Who is this woman?" medical researchers asked. "She's a graduate of a
small religious medical school (now known world-wide as Loma Linda
University). What are her qualifications? How does she presume to enter the
rarefied atmosphere of the world of research? Who is she to challenge smoking—America's favorite habit?" By the 1950s smoking had gained great popularity. Tobacco companies were lining up celebrities, including doctors, to
give testimonials; the general public viewed smoking as stylish, acceptable.
The associations that we now take for granted between smoking and lung
cancer, coronary disease, and chronic lung disease, had yet to be established.

Years passed. Dr. Simpson pursued other research interests. Twenty years
later scientists dusted off her report, repeated and elaborated on her experi-
ments, and confirmed her findings. Dr. Todd Fraser, a renowned research
professor at Harvard University, visited Loma Linda and took time to visit
Winea at her home. He said that meeting her was the highlight of his trip.

Could it be we are in danger of rejecting Bible truth because the
Christian community at large is following tradition, rather than accepting
light discovered by those without prestigious academic degrees or the
right connections?

*Are there Bible doctrines you've accepted because your parents or your church
have said they are true? Isn't it time you begin your own research to see what the
Bible really says?* JAN W. KUZMA

Preventing Emotional Anemia

*And be kind to one another, tenderhearted, forgiving one
another, even as God in Christ also forgave you. Eph. 4:32, NKJV.*

LOVE CANNOT EXIST without expression. That's why so many marriages are running on empty, or suffering from what family counselor Dr. A. Horowitz calls emotional anemia. Emotional anemia is when a person does not give or accept feelings of appreciation, affection, or closeness. If this condition is not caught early and corrected the relationship can die.

The following prescription will protect your marriage from suffering from emotional anemia. Here is what husband and wife must give to each other every day:

One daily comment of appreciation for something the other says or does. *Two* compliments every day. More is even better! *Three* significant hugs daily, not just a quick embrace when heading off to work. *Four* kisses. Here, variety is the spice of life. Vary your style! *Five:* Share a moment of beauty—an extravagant sunset, a flower breaking into bloom, a tree in blossom. *Six:* Recall a special memory from any part of your marriage: a wedding memory, the thrill of holding a newly-born child, a birthday celebration, a special vacation or family reunion.

Seven: Participate in a devotional time together. Let this become a daily ritual to which you both look forward. Read something special, sing praises and pray as you walk hand-in-hand in your own "garden of Eden." Discuss what a Bible passage is saying to each of you personally and how it might affect your marriage and life plan. Nothing is as significantly bonding as a wife and husband praying out loud together, mentioning one another by name in the prayer, sometimes while holding each other close.

You have just read seven powerful steps to nurture a marriage. They can take only a few minutes out of the day's activities—perhaps at different times and on different occasions. But they will never be insignificant! When these seven preventative measures happen in your relationship, your marriage will never be threatened with emotional anemia.

And here's a promise: What may start out as a daily prescription will likely turn out to be an eagerly anticipated delight!

Does your marriage show signs of becoming emotionally anemic? Is there anything on this list you haven't been doing? If so, begin today to follow these prescriptions.

ALBERTA MAZAT

Take It Easy!

Let your moderation be known unto all men. The Lord is at hand. Phil. 4:5.

WHAT REALLY HAPPENED to Jim Fixx, the legendary runner of the 1980s? He completed 20 marathons; he ran an average of 60 miles a week, racking up a total of 37,000 miles. Then he dropped dead of a heart attack at 52 years of age. An autopsy revealed that his coronary arteries were almost blocked, and he had scar tissue from two previous heart attacks. Why?

The reason can be summed up in one word: moderation, or rather, lack of it. Thinking his intense running schedule would keep him fit, he paid no attention to his diet. Ultra-marathon runner Stan Cottrell once said he saw Fixx stuff himself with four donuts before speaking at a conference, giving the excuse, "I didn't have time for breakfast."

God gave us bodies that can tolerate almost anything—in small amounts. But even good things can be bad if overdone. Health demands that we avoid extremes! Long-lived people observe the principle of moderation in their lives. They generally eat smaller, simpler meals. Many exercise extensively, but they walk rather than run. They live at a slightly slower pace, yet they feel they accomplish what they need to do. They are flexible people who accept the joys and disappointments in life as expressions of the will of God.

Dr. Robert Samp at the University of Wisconsin confirmed that almost all long-lived people have a conservative, middle-of-the-road outlook and personality. They take prudent risks but no unnecessary or hazardous ones.

Dr. Dean Ornish has stated that most degenerative diseases are diseases of excess, caused by eating an overabundance of food or dietary fat; indulging in alcohol, caffeine, or cigarettes; exercising excessively; or developing an extremely stressful response to life events.

You can go to extremes even in health reform. You can be absolutely correct and rigidly adhere to diet and exercise—and still be miserable. It's been found that those who hate exercise do not gain as much of the benefit!

Moderation preserves your health, helps you maintain your energy level, gives you a sense of having control over your desires, postpones the occurrence of disease, provides a "safety" mechanism when you erroneously adopt bad health practices, and introduces balance into your life.

Lord, help me to live a balanced life—spiritually, physically, emotionally, and socially. JAN W. KUZMA and CECIL MURPHEY

A Cheerful Heart

A cheerful heart is good medicine, but a crushed spirit dries up the bones. Prov. 17:22, NIV.

THREE OR FOUR TIMES a week I walk around my country neighborhood. I pass horse farms, a goat farm, and a llama farm. I take exercising seriously, so to get my quota of movement I usually am rushing to make sure I cover four-plus miles. After my walk-run, many times I still feel tense as I rush to my next activity or appointment.

One day I decided to slow down and enjoy my walk. As I passed the goat farm, three goats were standing like statues on an old broken-down table left in the yard. I giggled at the odd sight. The horses were frisky at the next farm, chasing each other in glee. I smiled. The expression on the llamas' faces made me laugh as they stared dolefully at me. By this time I was in a great, relaxed mood.

The chipmunks were scampering all around me in the trees as I walked down our long, wooded driveway, and they made me chuckle. I reflected on the difference of how I felt after this walk—relaxed and ready to slow down and share some joy with others. Had I actually gotten more out of my exercising by enjoying myself than by pushing to reach my four-mile goal?

The part of the brain that enables us to exercise, the motor cortex, lies only a few millimeters from the part of the brain that deals with thought and feeling. Could there be a crossover effect? I know exercising helps with depression, but if you're happy and laughing, do you get more out of your exercise, as well? In a study at Loma Linda University, 50 students were put on a high-cholesterol diet and then asked to choose an exercise program they enjoyed—volleyball, tennis, swimming, or running. Within three days the cholesterol level of every student had dropped. But when the students were asked to exercise on treadmills, no reduction in cholesterol was found. No enjoyment—no cholesterol benefit. Interesting!

I think that's what God meant in Proverbs 17:22—when you laugh and are cheerful, you feel better, you get more out of your exercise, and your joy is contagious. It ends up being good medicine for yourself—and for those around you.

Start a joyful fad today—slow down and start laughing. You'll be surprised at how many smiles you'll get and how much better you'll feel.   SANDY CLAY

Getting Rid of the Plaque of Sin

Here is a trustworthy saying that deserves full acceptance: Christ Jesus came into the world to save sinners—of whom I am the worst. 1 Tim. 1:15, NIV.

MANY TIMES, WHEN I examine someone's teeth and tell them they have cavities and gum disease, they're shocked. "I don't understand," they say. "I brush my teeth!"

To me this shows the influence of advertising. The subtle message is that if you use our mouthwash, toothpaste, or tooth brush, you won't need the dentist. But that's not true! Here's why:

The main cause of tooth decay and periodontal (gum) disease is the bacterial plaque that forms on your teeth. It is fed by improper diet. One of the best ways to ensure that you can have clean, healthy, disease-free teeth and gums is to make sure that the bacterial plaque is properly removed.

How do you know you have properly removed the plaque from your teeth and gums? Have you ever washed your car and thought you did an excellent job until, when it dried, you see the dirt left behind? Have you ever done the same when you are washing windows, only to leave telltale streaks after it dries?

That same thing happens when you brush your teeth. Even though you think you're doing a good job, the chances are great that you're leaving behind some bacterial plaque.

One way you can see if you have left behind any plaque is to stain the bacterial plaque with a dye solution. The remaining plaque can be seen like the dirt left behind on the car or the windows. Then you can brush off and floss away the remaining plaque and get your teeth clean. But since few take the time to use a dye solution after each brushing, it is a good idea to visit your dentist or dental hygienist at least every six months, so the bacterial plaque you left behind can be removed.

Jesus is the dye solution that discloses the condition of our heart. We need Jesus' help daily to get rid of the "plaque" of sin in our lives, just like we need to brush and floss daily. Satan is falsely advertising that we do not need Jesus. We are led to believe that we can take care of our own problems. Satan offers false substitutes for our joy and happiness. All the time, we are leaving the plaque of sin to eat away at our hearts, and only Jesus can remove it and make us spiritually clean.

Lord, examine the condition of my heart today and remove the "plaque of sin" that causes decay in my life.   EDDIE C. TOWLES

Reaping What You Sow

Be not deceived; God is not mocked: for whatsoever
a man soweth, that shall he also reap. Gal. 6:7.

I'VE LEARNED THAT faithful attention to little things is what eventually leads to health, happiness, and success. Here's a story that I remember when I'm tempted to cheat on small stuff.

A young builder was asked by a retired couple to construct a retirement home for them. The elderly couple carefully instructed the builder in regard to their desired floor plan, and emphasized that they wanted only the highest quality materials to be used.

The builder, however, decided to use low-quality materials and charge a high price, figuring that the elderly couple would never know the difference. In this way he could earn a bigger profit.

During the time period that the home was under construction, the builder married, and the newlyweds often visited with the elderly couple. Shortly before the owners were to move into their new house, they asked the builder and his bride to come see them. The elderly gentleman explained that because the newlyweds had become like children to them, and because they were struggling to get established, the elderly couple wanted to give them the newly constructed house as a wedding gift.

As the unselfish gentleman handed the builder the keys, the builder's heart sank, and he almost cried. All during the construction he had used the cheapest materials. And now the inferior house was his. If only he had followed the old man's instructions. If only he had been honest. If only . . . But alas, it was too late! For as long as he lived in that house he was painfully reminded of the small decisions he had made that ultimately determined his destiny.

Here's the formula to remember: Decisions shape behavior, behavior forms habits, habits mold bodies and character, and that determines destiny. It's the faithful attention you give the little things that will determine the end result.

Take your body, for example. It may not immediately show on the outside what you're putting inside, but it's the little things that will ultimately make a difference—such as drinking enough water; breathing deeply; getting adequate sleep; avoiding harmful substances such as alcohol, caffeine drinks, and tobacco; and eating green leafy vegetables rather than pasta and pastries! What you sow you'll ultimately reap!

Think about it—are you sowing today what you ultimately want to reap?

JUDITH GETCHELL

Breathe In—Deeply

*Let us therefore come boldly to the throne of grace, that we may
obtain mercy and find grace to help in time of need. Heb. 4:16, NKJV.*

PART OF THE QUALITY of your life depends on how well you inhale and exhale. If you're typical, you use less than half your lung capacity when breathing. Shallow, improper breathing reduces vitality and causes your metabolic rate to slow down, bringing on fatigue and exhaustion. It affects memory, creativity, and concentration, as well as judgment and willpower. In extreme cases, it can lead to anemia and depression.

Breathing also affects your emotions—and strong emotions affect your breathing. When you're afraid, extremely nervous, or angry, you take rapid, shallow breaths. When contented, more relaxed breathing. Basically, strong emotions and shallow breathing go together. Suppression of emotion results in muscle tension that limits respiration. Just watch a child, when angry, pull in the shoulders and constrict chest and throat muscles to prevent screaming! But breathing deeply and slowly has a calming, relaxing effect.

Carry your head up, back straight, chest out, shoulders back. Do this exercise 10 times a day: Breathe slowly, mouth closed, expand the lower ribs while breathing in; then take one more whiff. With open mouth, let the air out until every bit is gone. Make deep breathing a habit!

Prayer is the breath of our souls. Rapid, shallow praying is unhealthy—it compromises the quality of our spiritual lives. Yet most of us use only half our "lung" capacity when praying! We rattle off a few clichés and think we've fulfilled our religious obligations. But prayer isn't an obligation or a sacrifice we make to God. It's an absolute necessity for spiritual life, a privilege that our Creator God granted us so that we could have instant access to the Intellect of the universe; a communication system that requires no dial tone or chat room in order to talk to God.

Prayer is so powerful. Through it we become charged with energy, powered with motivation, and fueled with courage. Through it we have access to whatever we need, for God said, "Ask and you will receive." Through this connection to the God of Creation and Life, we can have an immune atmosphere around us to protect us from the germs and disease of the "god" of death and destruction.

Is your quality of life being compromised by shallow breathing? Why not take some deep breaths right now—both of air and of prayer!

KAY and JAN W. KUZMA

Pesticide Poisoning

I am the vine, you are the branches. He who abides in Me, and I in him, bears much fruit; for without Me you can do nothing. John 15:5, NKJV.

PESTICIDES ARE POISONOUS compounds designed to kill insects, weeds, and fungal pests that damage crops. The question is: Do the thousands of pesticides in use today, harm more than agricultural pests? While certain pesticides are "approved" for use, the potential long-term dangers of overuse have been difficult to document. John Wargo, a Yale University researcher, says, "No one really knows what a lifetime of consuming the tiny quantities of pesticides found on foods might do to a person."

Many pesticides approved by the Environmental Protection Agency (EPA) were registered long before extensive research linked these chemicals to cancer and other diseases. Now the EPA considers 60 percent of all herbicides, 90 percent of all fungicides, and 30 percent of all insecticides as potentially cancer-causing. Many are so toxic that human contact is prohibited.

Farmers and their families are another at-risk population. High exposure to certain pesticides places farmers at increased risk for cancer, including leukemia, non-Hodgkin's lymphoma, and cancers of the brain, prostate, and stomach.

When seeking to decrease pesticide residue, buying organic produce is an important option. Organic farmers are allowed to use only natural pesticides such as soaps, insecticidal compounds extracted from plants, bacteria, and a few types of metals and minerals. If you don't eat organic produce, you can reduce pesticide residues by peeling and washing fruits and vegetables with soap.

The battle against insects, weeds, and fungal pests is like our sin problem. Sin destroys, eating away our very life. Our human way of dealing with sin, our attempts to change and reform, are like the pesticides. In appearance, our "fruit" looks healthy. Our lives seem different. But our cure has only added to the damage. Our "good fruits" are still motivated by the old principles of self-interest and our desire to earn heaven or to look good to others.

God's remedy goes down deep—to the root level. His life-giving Spirit nourishes the soil of the soul, feeding the roots and causing the branches to flourish with the fruits of the Spirit. God's way is Jesus. He is the organic way. He's the answer to the blight of sin.

Ask yourself, In my fight against sin, have I gone "organic," or am I trying to kill sin myself? RISË RAFFERTY

First I Gave Him My Heart

But God shows his great love for us in this way:
Christ died for us while we were still sinners. Rom. 5:8, NCV.

BOB PRYOR HAD been feeling unusually tired, so he came to Florida Hospital. Sadly, the news wasn't good. After more than 37 years of diabetes disease, his kidneys were shutting down. Not much time remained.

He needed a kidney transplant to save his life. As doctors talked with Bob and his wife, Sandy, they explained the best donor would likely be one of Bob's siblings. Sandy refused. She wanted to be the donor herself. She wanted to be tested first. The doctors explained that the chances of a good kidney match were far greater with a blood relative. But Sandy insisted on being tested anyway. So the doctors agreed.

The results were remarkable. Sandy and Bob's blood makeup turned out to be very similar. The chance of a successful transplant was high. So the surgery was approved and Sandy was elated. Though the sacrifices would be many, Sandy was ready. Surgery would last more than three hours. Recovery would take more than two months. Time away from work would be financially tough. Their three children would have to be cared for by others. But none of these concerns frightened Sandy. She was willing to accept any and all risks to save the one she loved. When asked why, she replied, "I gave him my heart 19 years ago," she said. "What's a kidney?"

When I open the Scriptures I find a similar story of a God willing to accept any and all risks to save the one He loves. And the one He loves is you. God was ready to make the ultimate sacrifice rather than be without you. He willingly went to the cross to defeat the disease of death. There is nothing God won't do to win your love. There is nothing He won't give to secure your devotion.

Sandy gave Bob her heart long ago. Giving her kidney was simply more evidence of her love. God gave you His heart long ago. Giving His life for you was simply more evidence of His love. But just as Bob had to accept Sandy's sacrifice for him, you must accept God's sacrifice too. Perhaps the decision is easier when you discover all God has done to win you. Before asking for your trust, He gave you His devotion. Before asking for your faith, He gave you His life. Before asking for obedience, He gave you His heart.

God's love is vast. His commitment is deep. His loyalty is eternal. How can you be absolutely sure? First, He gave you His heart. Praise Him for His gift of life.

TODD CHOBOTAR

Dying the Way We Live

For none of us lives to himself alone and none of us dies to himself alone. . . .
So, whether we live or die, we belong to the Lord. Rom. 14:7, 8, NIV.

"I HATE THAT COLOR!" Estelle wadded up the nightgown and threw it onto the floor. Deliberately, she turned her wheelchair and ran over the pink gown. I watched tears trickle down her daughter's face. "You don't do anything right. You never did!" Estelle wheeled out of the room.

I had come to the nursing home to visit Rosemary, an elderly relative who was dying of cancer. In a small room with two beds, it was impossible to pretend I hadn't heard. I looked at the daughter, trying to think of a comforting comment. I suggested that her mother had gotten cranky in her old age. The daughter shook her head. "She's always been difficult. But she's worse now."

A few minutes later, Estelle rolled her wheelchair back into the room. She paused and scrutinized the top of her dresser. "You moved my letters! They belong on the left side! People can't leave anything alone in this awful place." I tried to concentrate on talking with Rosemary, but Estelle's voice grew louder with her complaints about the food, the temperature, and the incompetent staff at the nursing home.

A few minutes later, Estelle's daughter and I walked together to the elevator. "You know, I've figured out something," she said. "People die the way they live, don't they? I keep thinking she's going to soften, to change, but she isn't. Look at Rosemary. I've never seen her cross, even when she's hurting. She's always considerate. When they're late bringing her medication, I can see the pain on her face, but she never complains." As we stepped into the elevator she said, "I'll bet she's always been sweet like that." I agreed, remembering what a kind, gentle woman she had always been.

Estelle died a few weeks later, after ranting most of the afternoon about the way her doctor ignored her. When Rosemary died, two of the nurses cried. I asked if they took the death of each patient that much to heart. "Oh, no," one of them said. "Rosemary was special. We used to find reasons to go in and see her. She was always thoughtful and encouraging."

Since then I've realized that people don't get harsh or mean just because they're old. Their behavior reflects the way they've lived.

God of loving grace, enable me to live each day in such a way that my life is a constant testimony of Your grace, so that when I die people will say that I died the way I lived.   CECIL MURPHEY

The Healing Effect of Imaging

The Lord is my shepherd; I shall not want. He makes me to lie down
in green pastures; He leads me beside the still waters. Ps. 23:1, 2, NKJV.

IMAGING (PICTURING something in our minds) can dramatically change our emotional state. It can arouse new determination to renounce self-defeating behaviors and negativism, and promote psychological growth. We can image scenes such as a walk through the woods, along a riverbank, or by the seashore—any peaceful, quiet experience. This is one way to induce restful feelings when we are anxious or apprehensive. People who image under these circumstances can recapture the peaceful emotions they have experienced at some previous time in their life. The associations made of such literal walks, with the accompanying feelings of restfulness and peace, are reawakened in the imaging experience.

The Psalms and the parables of Jesus provide a rich collection of descriptive life experiences for imaging. Jesus used imagery abundantly in His earthly ministry. An intimate relationship with Jesus generates a host of powerful experiences that become a part of the fabric of our mind. Resurrecting these experiences will vaporize any threatening cloud. As someone once said, "We have nothing to fear for the future except as we forget the way the Lord has led us."

Imaging can help addicts overcome their addictions. People who are vulnerable to the tactics of certain others, can often find help by visualizing themselves in the presence of these people and rehearsing how to handle the situation *before* their next encounter. Associations will be formed in the brain, and when the situation arises the associations will easily form again; the individual will experience the same strength and decisiveness they experienced in their imaging session.

Reliving your courting days through imaging can help you regenerate the positive experiences of those days. The images awakened arouse the same romantic emotions you experienced then, and current bonding is strengthened. The formation of mental images of fondest dreams and hopes yet to be fulfilled adds another dimension to the benefits to be gained from imaging. This exercise awakens hope, assurance, and the will to make a marriage work.

To recall and relive the positive experiences of the past does much to counteract discouragement and depression.

Picture the pastoral scene of Psalm 23 and see if it has a calming effect on you.

ELDEN M. CHALMERS

The Six Facets of Intimacy

The man and his wife were both naked, and they felt no shame. Gen. 2:25, NIV.

THE CONDITION OF Adam and Eve being naked and not ashamed goes beyond mere physical nakedness to total honesty and openness. *Intimacy!* That's what every married couple wants, but few experience. In fact, the bride and groom walking down the aisle after saying "I do" are heading for isolation and alienation *unless* they intentionally love and energetically nurture each other daily.

Marriages are under assault. The state of detachment is common, resulting in the tragedy of affairs and divorce. Other couples endure the tedium of a relationship that is an institution and not an alliance. Competing commitments of family, work, church, community, parents, friends, neighbors, and things leave couples exhausted. Before they know it, they are like passing couriers who can only wave and wish the other well. They may notice the growing distance, but endure it because they're too busy, tired, or selfish to exert the effort it takes to achieve true intimacy.

True intimacy is like a six-faceted diamond. To experience the closeness and openness God wants you to have in marriage, couples must share all the dimensions of intimacy.

1. Emotional intimacy: The result of sharing private feelings and listening to each other's emotional highs and lows makes couples feel supported and cared for.

2. Intellectual intimacy: Sharing ideas, opinions, and information without fear or embarrassment is deeply satisfying and stimulating.

3. Recreational intimacy: Having a recreational companion is high on a man's list of what he wants in a wife. But wives, too, glow when their husbands are willing to share activities, sports events, and fun times with them.

4. Sexual intimacy: Couples must demonstrate a mutual genuine interest in satisfying the needs of each other and being able to openly dialog their desires and insecurities.

5. Social intimacy: It's good to share and enjoy friends in common.

6. Spiritual intimacy: Being able to share similar beliefs about God and honestly discussing one's personal spiritual journey transforms individuals into soul mates!

Only in the context of this six-faceted kind of nakedness can husbands and wives truly experience the joy that God means for them to experience.

How is your Marital Intimacy Quotient? What could you do today to increase your "MIQ"?
ELAINE and WILLIE OLIVER

Forever Changed

As he [Saul] neared Damascus on his journey, suddenly a light from heaven flashed around him. He fell to the ground and heard a voice say to him, "Saul, Saul, why do you persecute me?" Acts 9:3, 4, NIV.

I WAS BROUGHT up with good moral values, but by the time I was stationed at Fort Riley, Kansas, I was living merely for the pleasures and excitement of the world. I was a tough guy who boxed and wrestled for the Army. I drank, played drums for dance bands, and frequented night clubs. I knew better, but I thought this was the way to enjoy life.

Every night, however, I loved to walk by myself and just think, enjoying the night air before going back to my room to sleep. One night as I was out walking around the base, I passed the base church. Suddenly I heard a voice. It said, "Why are you living like this, Gary?"

I turned around and was ready to hit whoever was playing this joke on me. But nobody was there. I was puzzled. I walked on for a while, and the voice came again, "Gary, why are you living like this? Your parents did not bring you up this way."

At that point I looked behind me, but all that was there was the church with its doors wide open. A very bright light was on inside and a beautiful light shown outside. I don't know what came over me, but I was irresistibly pulled toward that church. I went inside and walked to the front, knelt down, and gave my heart to the Lord.

I don't know how long I was there, but when I left the church and walked back to my room I was a very different man. I went to bed that night and knew I could never again live the kind of life I had lived before. My army buddies had called me "Parker the Drunk," but when I quit drinking and carousing, sent for the Voice of Prophecy Bible Correspondence Course and joined the church, I became known as "Preacher Parker."

When people tell me, "I can't quit drinking . . . or smoking . . . or . . ." I reply, "I know, I've been there. But God can. Give your life to Him and His power to resist temptation can be yours."

God spoke to Saul on the road to Damascus and to me on an army base. There is no place you can go that God cannot reach you with His life-changing love.

Are you struggling with some harmful habit or sin that you know you should give up? Why not give your life completely to the Lord and ask Him to give you His power to resist temptation? GARY PARKER

Meet My Family

Out of the mouth of babes and nursing infants You have ordained strength. Ps. 8:2, NKJV.

IT'S EASY TO FEEL sorry for yourself when you're wheelchair-bound as a quadriplegic. Feeling down and not worth much used to be a nearly normal state for me. Fortunately, it's now a rare exception. On the days when I feel the need for a pick-me-up, the mail carrier usually delivers an air mail letter from one of "my children" that puts things back into perspective. How or why I got started sponsoring children remains a mystery to me. Now I can't imagine not doing it.

Felipe was the first child I welcomed into "my family." He lives in the Philippines with his parents and seven siblings. His dad works on a sugar plantation while his mother, in addition to being a full-time mom, is a fish vendor. Felipe is a big help to his family by fetching water and tending the family's cow when he's not going to school.

I started to get to know Felipe seven years ago when he was seven. His mother and a sister wrote the first two letters to me. He started writing after that, first in Filipino and soon after in English. Now I can read his letters without the aid of a translator. His progress is exciting to see, and he's such a good and faithful letter writer.

Despite his poverty, Felipe has never complained. He and his family are so grateful to me for the little I do. They have an abundance of love for God, each other, and me, along with a faith that moves mountains. What touched me the most was when Felipe wrote, "I'm so glad you love me, even if I'm poor." How could I not?

This is such a good thing, I thought. *What could be better?* More children, of course!

Patryga, a 13-year-old from Poland, and Mohammed, a small boy from Sierra Leone, joined "my family" four years ago. Because of the war in his country, Mohammed is missing. It's not known if he's even alive. He'll never be forgotten.

Rose, a little Sioux Indian, looked like a princess doll when I first saw her picture. She moved before I got to really know her.

I live alone and I can't do all the things others do, but I can enjoy my children.

Thank You, God, for allowing me the honor and privilege of serving my little family. God, You are a lover of children. Put this same love in my heart to reach out to one of Your little ones. Amen. THERESE ALLEN

Only a Left-eye Blink

But do not forget to do good and to share, for with
such sacrifices God is well pleased. Heb. 13:16, NKJV.

DOMINIQUE BAUBY WAS the 43-year-old editor-in-chief of the French magazine *Elle* when he incurred a massive stroke that affected his brain stem. He describes "swimming up from the mists of coma" 20 days later and emerging to the maddening condition called locked-in syndrome, wherein the victim is paralyzed from head to toe, his mind fully intact, imprisoned inside his own body.

In Bauby's case, blinking his left eyelid was his only means of communication. He awoke from his coma to find a doctor sewing the right eyelid shut with a needle and thread "like he was darning a sock." His right ear was deaf; his left ear amplified and distorted any sounds farther than 10 feet away. He describes his condition: My head "weighs a ton, and something like an invisible diving bell holds my whole body prisoner." On many occasions, however, his mind "takes flight like a butterfly," which was the basis for the title of the book he authored, *The Diving Bell and the Butterfly,* by blinking out the letters one at a time. That's right; his transcriber recited the alphabet until Bauby blinked at the appropriate letter, building words one letter at a time.

He tells about reveling in simple pleasures and modest requests. "I would be the happiest of men," he announced, "if I could just swallow the overflow of saliva that endlessly floods my mouth." Ever fashion-conscious, he turned down a "hideous jogging suit" provided by the hospital for clothes he was accustomed to: "If I must drool, I may as well drool on cashmere."

He recalled how, on the final day before his former life was snuffed out, "I mechanically carried out all those simple acts that today seem miraculous to me: shaving, dressing, downing a hot chocolate." "How can I describe," he laments, "waking for the last time, heedless, perhaps a little grumpy, beside the lithe, warm body of a tall, dark-haired woman?"

Some of the hospital staff enraged him, particularly "those who wrenched my arm while putting me in my wheelchair, or left me all night long with the TV on, or let me lie in a painful position despite my protests." Yet he forgives them.

Dominique Bauby died two days after his book was published. As I now read his words I have to ask myself, "What am I doing with this enormous life of mine?"

Consider: What is God asking you to do with your life?   CHRIS BLAKE

AUGUST 16

My Friends Were My Dogs

*I will restore you to health and heal your wounds, . . . because you
are called an outcast, Zion for whom no one cares. Jer. 30:17, NIV.*

SIX MONTHS AFTER I'd presented my health seminar in his city, Arnold
told me this story:

"I mean it! My dogs were my closest friends because they did not insult me. I'm 42 years old, and a few months ago I weighed 290 pounds. I
avoided people because they either pitied me or preached at me. I guess I
was pitiable because I could not walk even half a block without severe leg
pain. My knees and feet hurt so badly that my physician wanted to put me
on a disability pension. But I wasn't ready to give up on life yet. Actually
I was raised a good Christian, but like so many of us boomers, I paid little
attention to my health. I ate what I pleased. It took a lot of suffering to finally wake me up.

"When I heard about a health lecture entitled, 'Eat More and Weigh
Less,' I thought, *Just what I need.* The week before, I had managed to go
without doughnuts for a whole week—then felt so deprived I ate a dozen
at one sitting. Yes, I definitely needed help.

"After Dr. Diehl's first lecture I kept going—attending the entire four-
week Coronary Health Improvement Project (CHIP). I bought a book
and some cassette tapes and followed the instructions carefully at home. It
felt good to start caring for my body in God's way.

"It's been six months now, and I'm sure you notice a big difference. I
have dropped 100 pounds. I am aiming to slowly lose another 30 pounds
to reach my normal weight. I have to tell you, you are right about eating
a lot of high-fiber plant food. With these changes in my diet I don't feel
hungry at all.

"I'm like a new person. My breathing is normal, I can see my feet, I
walk six miles a day without pain, my migraines have disappeared, I work
full time, and I'm back in church.

"But you made one mistake, Dr. Diehl. You said this way of eating
would save money. Have I got news for you—the program cost me a lot—
I've had to buy all new clothes! I'm not complaining, though. No, I'm not
complaining. Every way I look at it, I got a real bargain."

*Lord, thank You for reminding me that the basic principles You gave in Eden
are still amazingly effective in today's world.* HANS DIEHL

238

Replacing Shattered Dreams

For I know the plans I have for you, says the Lord. They are plans for good and not for evil, to give you a future and a hope. Jer. 29:11, TLB.

NINE MONTHS AFTER Donnie and I were married, he complained about weakness. I thought he wasn't eating right. Others mentioned he looked pale. I excused it as lack of sun. Then came the day when we had planned to rearrange our furniture, and Donnie complained he was too tired. I was upset. Donnie moved two things and was exhausted. I decided we had to find out what was wrong.

After hours of tests, the doctors finally announced, "We're shocked you're walking. Your hemoglobin count is only 5.8, and 14 is normal. We're hospitalizing you!"

A few days later we heard the dreaded word, leukemia. The next eight months were torturous. Three weeks of hospitalization for intensive chemotherapy and then a break at home, then more chemo. Then a remission, but he would go days without sleeping. He wouldn't stop eating, couldn't exercise, and looked bloated, so back to the hospital. Then two good months. Our hopes soared; we made plans. Then one day in October, Donnie held me close and hoarsely whispered, "The doctors say it's back." I think he knew he was dying.

I had put my faith in two things: God and nutrition. Not until family and physicians pleaded with me to turn off the respirator did I give up on both. I was angry. How could God do this to me? Mustard-seed faith was supposed to move mountains, but I had mountain-size faith and Donnie still died! All that juicing and herbs—nothing worked. At 24 years of age my future was gone! A *widow!*

I had always said nice things to God, but no longer. I told Him exactly how I felt. "I'm so mad at You right now I can't talk. Maybe later." I journaled and cried and held on to my pastor's words: "What God takes away He replaces threefold."

My daily drive to work became prayer time. "God, You promised me a future. How could You allow this?" Then occasionally I found myself thanking God for something, until the day I surprised myself by praising Him the whole way. God was working a miracle of healing for me!

He has now restored my passion for good nutrition and given me a wonderful new husband who absolutely adores me, a precious daughter, and a little one on the way.

Have you suffered a loss? Try thanking Him for little blessings and see if He doesn't have a miracle of healing in store for you, too. ANGELA KUZMA

Hospital for Sinners

If My people who are called by My name will humble themselves, and pray and seek My face, and turn from their wicked ways, then I will hear from heaven, and will forgive their sin and heal their land. 2 Chron. 7:14, NKJV.

I HAVE A FEAR and loathing of hospitals. I know them too intimately. As a severely asthmatic child in smoggy California, I visited the emergency room of St. Francis Hospital so regularly the nurses and I greeted each other by name. I even chose to give birth to my two children at home.

So when I recently admitted myself to the local medical center for out-patient surgery, it was with much sighing and trepidation. The anesthesiologist asked if I had any questions.

"Well, yes," I grimaced, as a nursing student wrestled an IV needle the size of crochet hook into my vein. "I don't smoke or drink or eat meat, and I weigh only 108 pounds, and I really don't like drugs, so probably the less medication I get, the better." She replied gravely, "I see," and before I could object she emptied the contents of a large-looking syringe into the needle. "What was that?" I asked with alarm. "Just a little anti-anxiety medication," she soothed.

As my head began to feel warm and mushy and the contours of the room went wiggly, all the conspiracy theories I had dismissed through the years took on sinister new possibilities. My last semirational thought was *They haven't put me under yet—I could still run for it!*

I've often heard it said that the church is not a country club for saints but a hospital for sinners. I've always appreciated that analogy. How true that each of us enters church fellowship morally and emotionally damaged, even diseased, in some fashion. How utterly not entitled we are to despise fellow patients because their deficiencies differ from (or disturbingly mirror) our own.

On the other hand, it also occurred to me that if the church is like a hospital, not everyone can be a patient—at least not all of the time. How grateful I was that there were people in that hospital who were well and capable. How comforting it was to see my nurse sitting faithfully by my side, clothed and in her right mind, with her sponge on a stick to quench my dry, thirsty lips.

I'm glad the church is becoming a safer haven for wounded souls. It's good to feel the chill of legalistic denial giving way to the warmth of spiritual and emotional honesty. I hope we don't stop short on our road to recovery!

Lord, help me to be a healer of wounded souls in my family, church, and community!
LESLIE KAY

Riding High, Feeling Low

I will give you a new heart and put a new spirit in you; I will remove from you your heart of stone and give you a heart of flesh. And I will put my Spirit in you and move you to follow my decrees and be careful to keep my laws. Eze. 36:26, 27, NIV.

I WAS RIDING HIGH in the business world. It was my twenty-fifth year in chamber of commerce management; I enjoyed hobnobbing with leaders in business, industry, and the professions, with movie and television stars, with leaders in local, state, and national politics. But I was not happy.

I had a beautiful, loving wife and four wonderful children. Some would say that I "had it made." But happiness was not part of my day. Oh, I had the pleasure of the success of many projects, but I was restless and depressed. The stress of it all was heavy—destructive. I was not a loving father, husband, or Christian. I was too busy for my family or for God.

Although people were praying for me, I didn't know it or care. I seemed to be caught in a whirlwind of success that was pulling my spirit down, and I didn't have the strength to resist.

Then in 1973 my wife and I attended a prayer seminar that revolutionized my life. I had read the Bible before. I carried it to church. I knew all the familiar stories. I had a pretty good handle on doctrine. And I prayed daily—short "please" and "thank you" type prayers. But I never put the Bible and prayer together. Never before had I read God's holy Book focusing on the promises and then actually taking God at His Word, accepting what He said as a personal message to me, believing it, and claiming it for myself.

I decided to experiment. As I began to search for promises that would meet the needs in my life, I came across Ezekiel 36:26, 27. From the depths of my unfulfilled spirit, I cried out to God, "Lord, give me a new heart and put a new spirit in me." And He did. Changes began happening in my life, and I began to feel hopeful for the first time in years.

No longer were my prayers like feathers flying in the wind. They became focused and specific. Miracles started happening, and I've never been the same since. I have discovered that God's Word contains the instructional package for peaceful, joyful living. All you have to do is accept it, believe it, and claim it.

Are you living a ho-hum life and can't seem to pull yourself out of the doldrums? Why not take God at His word, claim the promise for a new spirit, and see what a difference it makes. RUBEN NEUHARTH

Blessed Beyond Belief

I have seen his ways, and will heal him; I will also lead him,
and restore comforts to him and to his mourners. Isa. 57:18, NKJV.

"WHAT DOES A PERSON have to do to get some sleep around here?" I asked the nurses at 3 a.m.. I was frustrated and discouraged! I had been taken off morphine and released from ICU two days previously and hadn't had a wink of sleep since. The excruciating pain was unbearable. I couldn't find any restful position in the bed or chair. The nine ribs that had been broken 10 days earlier in an auto accident were causing me agony. The sleeping pills the nurse gave me brought four hours of sleep.

After 14 days of hospitalization I was released to go home and heal, but the doctors had concluded that I would never be able to do heavy physical labor again. Healing was a slow process. I couldn't stand for anything to touch the left side of my chest. The nerve damage was so severe that the left side of my body could break out in a sweat while the right side felt comfortable. I spent day and night in my rocker-recliner, but whenever I attempted to recline I had the horrible sensation of somebody crushing my chest. For three months I sat, ate, and slept in that chair.

Taking a shower by myself was scary. When I reached across my body to wash the right side with my left hand, the left shoulder blade got hung up on a broken rib. Oh! I thought I would die! If I didn't do the painful daily exercise of crawling up the wall with my fingers to stretch my left shoulder, it would freeze up, and I couldn't move it at all. There were many discouraging days when I felt helpless and hopeless, wondering when I would actually heal and to what extent.

When my wife and I celebrated the 10-year anniversary of my auto accident, we made it into a celebration of praise to God for what He has done for us. Though it was a year and a half before I could work again, God strengthened me even beyond my former abilities. I have returned to extremely heavy physical labor, and I know our God is an awesome God!

Consider this: "We all desire immediate and direct answers to our prayers, and are tempted to become discouraged when the answer is delayed or comes in an unlooked-for form. But God is too wise and good to answer our prayers always at just the time and in just the manner we desire. He will do more and better for us than to accomplish all our wishes" (Ellen White, *The Ministry of Healing*, pp. 230, 231).

If you are hurting, count your blessings and believe that God is in the process of healing you.   DAVID J. DILDINE

Hanging on to Your Seat, and Other Stress Reducers

Peace I leave with you, My peace I give to you; not as the world gives do I give to you. Let not your heart be troubled, neither let it be afraid. John 14:27, NKJV.

STRESS IS THE WAY the body reacts to change. Too much negative change makes an alarm go off. Your body gets ready to fight or flee. Blood pressure, heart rate, and blood flow to the muscles—all increase, while blood flow to the skin and kidneys decrease. You breathe faster, your hands get clammy, your mouth dries. Sound familiar?

Over the years our work has taken my husband and me to many countries. Living in some of the poorest and least politically stable countries of the world, and traveling by all sorts of transportation, we have encountered varied experiences, some definitely causing major stress!

Learning to put my complete trust in God has been a growth experience for me. Fear and anxiety were my natural, innate reaction in times of stress and uncertainty. However, God in His love has given me repeated opportunities to prove the validity of His words when He says, "Fear not" and "My peace I give to you." Believe me, I have claimed these promises hundreds of times!

For example, once while traveling by public bus along the Korakoram highway in Northern Pakistan toward the little kingdom of Hunza, fear struck relentlessly as the driver careened along mountain roads, around sharp corners on two wheels, and on the wrong side of the road! To one side of us the lofty Korakoram range (an extension of the Himalayas) rose to magnificent heights, while on the other side a precipitous drop of some 2,000 feet ended at the Indus River in the gorge below. Fear glued me to my seat. Claiming God's promises, "Peace I leave with you. . . . Let not your heart be troubled, neither let it be afraid," finally relaxed my tense body and brought peace to my mind, even to the point of knowing that whatever the outcome, God was in charge, and I could trust Him.

I have also found it helpful to conjure up a picture of Christ "at the helm" as the driver of the bus, plane, or whatever. I'll admit, it was hard imagining Him driving as close to the edge as some of our drivers did! Sometimes a song helps calm my fear. Life isn't as scary when you picture yourself "Safe in the arms of Jesus," or "Under His wings."

We don't always have control over the circumstances we find ourselves in, but how comforting to know the One who does.

Trusting our all in God's loving hands reduces negative stress and brings peace! Try it! YVONNE DYSINGER

Three Magic Words

Then the man said, "The woman whom You gave to be with me, she gave me of the tree, and I ate." And the Lord God said to the woman, "What is this you have done?" The woman said, "The serpent deceived me, and I ate." Gen. 3:12, 13, NKJV.

AFTER A PARTICULARLY grimy day in the backyard, my two brothers and I were ushered into the bathroom to shower before dinner. Mom told us to all get into the shower together. With mischief afoot, I hurried to finish first, then scampered out of the shower and leaned against the steamy glass door so no one else could get out. Push as they might, they could not overpower me.

Then Brad decided to use his bare bottom as a battering ram and began pounding on the glass door. I laughed hysterically at this hapless strategy until on his third butt-ram the glass door shattered, bringing Mom running to the bathroom. Fortunately, no one got cut, but there we stood with a mixture of shock, fear, and guilt all over our faces.

Mom surveyed the damage and demanded, "Who did this?" We all denied any responsibility. I didn't break the glass door—Brad's bottom did it. Brad claimed innocence, insisting that the door only broke because I held it shut. Little Tom said he was only a bystander.

I am convinced that there are three magic words that thrill the heart of every parent. And I don't mean "I love you." That endearing phrase comes in second place behind the seldom heard confession, "It's my fault." What a melody those words create in the home.

It reminds me of that sorry scene in the Garden of Eden when God asked His children what happened. Adam blamed Eve. Eve blamed the snake. And the snake blamed God. Blaming others could be considered a secondary sin—one that immediately follows the "original" one. A mistake is made—a sin is committed—and then without thinking, sin is stacked upon sin by falsely blaming someone else rather than admitting our error. The sad thing is that the secondary sin may be worse than the first because it causes alienation, hurt, distrust, and insecurity.

When people blame others instead of taking responsibility for their actions, a very unsafe environment is created. You never know when you'll be blamed for someone else's mistakes. If we would use the three magic words, "It's my fault," more often, instead of blaming others, we would create a magic world of love and forgiveness in the home.

Lord, when I'm tempted to blame others for my mistake, help me to admit, "It's my fault."   LARRY RICHARDSON

Accepting the Odd-shaped Pegs

But Jesus said, "Let the little children come to Me, and do not forbid them; for of such is the kingdom of heaven." Matt. 19:14, NKJV.

AS A CHILD I gave my teachers fits. I didn't mean to disrupt their classrooms, but no matter how hard I tried to be good, something always went wrong.

Now I'm a teacher. I remember that first day surrounded by 28 third graders. Even though I had promised to recognize and inspire the little misfits, I found myself praying for 28 left-brained children who would be excited about sitting still, listening carefully to me, and raising their hands to talk. It would make my life much easier—and I'd look a lot better as a teacher!

Just as I was beginning to think, *I can handle this,* Jenny showed up. She was defiant, rude, mean to the other students, and was dead set against doing anything I wanted her to do. I was so consumed with trying to deal with her unruliness that the uniqueness of the other students blurred. Just to manage, I toughened my stance, accepted less creativity, and life in Room 10 began to resemble a police state. Then her family moved. My heart ached for that little girl, for I knew she was merely trying to get the message across that she was hurting and angry because life had dealt her a bad hand.

Jenny's absence did give me the calm I needed to look more carefully at my other students. I discovered some less disruptive odd-shaped pegs who would be a challenge to me, if I were really going to be the kind of teacher I, as a kid, always wanted to have—one who would accept me for who I was, and adjust the curriculum to better meet my needs instead of criticizing me.

Why do I care so passionately about these children whom many consider to be trouble makers? Because I was one of them. I know how it feels to never get your name on the gold star list—even though you try very, very hard. I know how it hurts when a principal calls you a turkey. I know how my parents struggled to find ways to motivate me. But I was one of the lucky ones who, in spite of it all, felt loved.

Jesus wants the children to come to Him—just the way they are. He wants to meet their needs. Let's not turn the children away by forcing odd-shaped pegs into the pharisaical holes we've designed!

Lord, forgive me if I have hurt one of Your little children or kept them from coming to You. KEVIN KUZMA

Kissed by the Prince of the Universe

All the days of the oppressed are wretched, but the
cheerful heart has a continual feast. Prov. 15:15, NIV.

IT WAS THE SADDEST time of my life. My 17-year-old daughter was in a coma as a result of an accident, and our family could not communicate with her. It seemed like Becky was in a far away country with no ability to send messages. Would she wake up, and if she did, would she be OK? Yet we could find joy in our tragedy.

You might ask what we could find joyful about our circumstance. Well, she was still alive, and we had the love and support of family and friends. And we had God. Besides, God loved her more than we did. Jesus has promised that He will come soon and make all things new. If Becky never improved in this life, we knew that He would restore her at His second coming.

We could have been angry or bitter, but those feelings would have caused damage to our bodies. There are chemicals that are released when we smile or laugh. These endorphins bathe the brain and give us a feeling of well-being. If we are angry or depressed, we deplete the good chemicals. It is true that "a cheerful heart is good medicine, but a crushed spirit dries up the bones" (Prov. 17:22, NIV).

Do you remember the story in Acts 16 about Paul and Silas singing in prison? They had been flogged and thrown into a cell with chains on their feet. Yet they could sing praises to the Lord.

Therefore, my family chose to be joyful in our time of trouble. Oh, yes, I did shed tears, but I also looked for humorous things. Since our daughter had all of her hair shaved (because of brain surgery), we called her our G.I. Jane. I called her my sleeping beauty. I told her she needed a handsome prince to kiss her and wake her up.

The Prince of the universe did kiss her. Becky was fully restored to us many months later, and we are now singing songs of victory! There are many troubles in this world today, but it is possible to have joy in spite of any circumstance. Even if you have trouble and are not able to sing victory songs here on earth, remember that we will have eons of eternity to sing all those songs of praise and victory to the Prince, Jesus Christ.

If life seems a little dreary, remember that you too have been kissed by the Prince of the universe!   BONNIE SZUMSKI

Ministry Moments

But everything exposed by the light becomes visible, for it is light that makes everything visible. This is why it is said: "Wake up, O sleeper, rise from the dead, and Christ will shine on you." Eph. 5:13, 14, NIV.

THE HOLY SPIRIT rejoices in exposing God's children to His light. And if we are obedient to what God wants us to do we'll grow spiritually during these divine experiences.

Although I was born with and continue to foster a spirit of adventure, there are times when my Heavenly Father can both challenge and mystify me in my "going forth" on His behalf. I ask myself, "Why am I doing what I'm doing?"

Just such an incident occurred within a five-minute framework while the clerk checked out my grocery purchases in the supermarket line. I overhead a conversation between two other shoppers behind me in the next check-out lane.

Woman: "I haven't had a cigarette for two months. Now I'm buying a whole carton!"

Man: "If you've gone two months without, why are you giving into temptation now?"

With no preconceived plan, I asked the clerk to excuse me for a moment. I found myself climbing over the chromed banister between the check out lanes and going up to the lady shopper. I said, "You don't need a cigarette; you need a hug. God loves you so much I'm here to give it to you."

Without a second's hesitation she came directly toward me with arms outstretched to receive the promised hug and returned it with great enthusiasm and a beaming smile. She didn't say anything to me, but as she returned the cigarettes to the shelf behind her, she commented to her own checker, "Well, I don't really need a cigarette. I'll take a Twinkie instead."

I completed my purchase and walked out to the car asking God, "What was that all about?"

I've learned that God has many ministry moments planned for me where I can be used as a conduit for His light to shine through me—if I'm just awake to His nudging. And although He never explained to me the ministry moment at the checkout stand, I drove away with the peace of knowing that for that one single moment this woman had come to life and smiled in God's face as He reached out and hugged her with my arms.

What is the Holy Spirit nudging you to do today? Let Christ's light shine on you!

CATHERINE J. CARPENTER

Small, but Not Insignificant!

Thank you for making me so wonderfully complex! Your workmanship is marvelous—and how well I know it. Ps. 139:14, NLT.

RECENTLY THE HUBBLE telescope took a picture of a very tiny spot in the sky. In the picture, astonished astronomers counted 3,500 galaxies. To give you an idea of just how small a spot this was, if the moon were a pizza in the sky (about half the size of your thumb at arms length) and you made 15 cuts across and 15 cuts up and down, one of those little pizza squares would be about the size of the area photographed.

Each of those galaxies, like our own Milky Way, contains approximately 100 billion stars.

Many of the stars, perhaps most, have planets orbiting them. The Bible indicates that God has created other worlds, so there may be untold numbers of inhabited planets in these galaxies.

But that was one tiny spot—what about the rest of the sky? Astronomers once believed that the universe was not uniform. Now it appears that in any direction one would take this photograph, a similar number of galaxies would be seen, with their untold billions of stars and planets. In fact, it's conceivable there are more galaxies in the universe than grains of sand on the earth.

Now see yourself in this gigantic, unfathomable universe. It makes you feel pretty small and insignificant, doesn't it? But that's not the way God sees you. After all, if God knows the numbers of hairs on your head (Matt. 10:30), you must be pretty important to Him. And if He catches every one of your tears in His memory bottle (Ps. 56:8), obviously He cares.

Consider for a moment the condition of humans when they were first created. Adam and Eve were perfect, their bodies designed to last for eternity. Even after they sinned they lived almost a thousand years! And they had a mental capacity to store information forever! (They didn't need books or computers!) Incredible!

Obviously, sin has done a major number on these bodies and brains of ours. But in spite of our degenerated state, when we think about how our bodies and brains work it still boggles our minds—every bit as much as when we try to consider the vastness of the universe.

Teach me to treat my incredibly complex body today as the Master Creator designed it to be treated.   JIM BRACKETT

Four Hours to Live

*Behold, I will bring it health and healing; I will heal them
and reveal to them the abundance of peace and truth. Jer. 33:6, NKJV.*

I FELT A RAGE of terror and hurt spread through my body as the doctor told me, "You will want to call the relatives. Your mother has suffered a severe cerebral hemorrhage and has about four hours to live." Four hours to live? I looked at my watch and thought, "She will be dead by 4:00 p.m.!"

Just a few hours earlier my wife had called me at my office to tell me that my mother, 50 years old, had suffered a stroke and was being rushed to the hospital. Mother lived 130 miles away from us, and the hospital was 90 miles away. I rushed to the hospital to be with her.

Now, standing there in the hallway, a whole lifetime rushed through my mind. With tears coming almost uncontrollably, I walked to the pay phone and called my wife. I blurted out the story and asked her to call the head elder of the church where my wife and I had been taking Bible studies for a couple of months, and ask him to pray for Mother. I knew the pastor was out of town, but I had great confidence in the elder.

As my Aunt Helen and I sat together waiting for those four hours to pass, I prayed silently to the God whom I did not know very well. The four hours passed and two doctors, shaking their heads, came from my mother's room. My heart pounded as I rushed up to them and asked what was happening. With a great deal of excitement one doctor said, "She is breathing normally and has spoken to us. We now give her a chance."

Forty-two days later she walked out of the hospital. Within the next year my wife and I became converted Christians and were baptized into the Seventh-day Adventist Church. I entered college to study for the ministry. The following year Mother was baptized and then, over a period of years, my nephew and niece and their families have been baptized. When Mother was 71, she walked to the top of Stone Mountain in Stone Mountain, Georgia.

God says, "I will heal them and reveal to them the abundance of peace and truth." He is still doing just that! I praise Him for His continued working in my life and the lives of my family members. He will do the same for all who call on His name.

Lord, I call on Your name and ask You for health, for healing, for peace, and for truth. Amen. JIM COX

Wounding Words

With the tongue we praise our Lord and Father, and with it we curse men, who have been made in God's likeness. Out of the same mouth come praise and cursing. My brothers, this should not be. James 3:9, 10, NIV.

ONE RULE I HAVE endeavored to teach my children is that there are some things that are never spoken. No matter how aggravated, angry, or upset one may be, there is a line that must not be crossed. You may not say things that hurt other people. Words are like feathers in the wind: once spoken they may be repented of, apologized for, and forgiven, but they can never be erased from the hearer's psyche.

This is true for adults. Wounds caused by such words as "My mother was right; you'll never lose those extra pounds," or "I should have married John; he's made a success of himself," never heal. But it's our children who are especially vulnerable. Words that cause emotional reaction, especially if there is pain attached, become memories that haunt a person for a lifetime.

Sam was about 4 years old. A guest was helping in the kitchen and Sam, who was curious and needed to learn about everything going on around him, was on a small stool, lending a hand. Some mistake was made, and the guest said to Sam, "If you had a brain you'd be dangerous." Sam had never been spoken to like this before and left the kitchen in tears. The guest was shocked. This was just her way of relating to children; she hadn't meant to hurt Sam's feelings.

Twenty-two years later Sam and I were working in the kitchen when something slipped to the floor. Sam immediately responded, "Like ____ said, if I had a brain I'd be dangerous." The incident had not been alluded to in all that time, but the painful memory of those thoughtless words was still there.

How much more words must hurt when the stab is intentional. "I never wanted another child anyway"; "You're the dumbest kid on the face of the earth"; "She won't attract boys with that face." It's scary to realize that in a moment's thoughtlessness we can scar someone for life.

The world is cruel enough. Our families should be safe places with locks on the doors to safeguard our children from dangers that could harm their bodies—and locks on our tongues to safeguard them from words that could wound their sensitive souls.

Lord, help me to tame my tongue to never say anything I wouldn't want said to me. KATHY KUZMA

No Pity Party Allowed!

*"It is enough! Now, Lord, take my life, for I am
no better than my fathers!" 1 Kings 19:4, NKJV.*

FIRST KINGS 19 IS a favorite chapter of mine because it gives me a
glimpse of someone as human as I am. Here's the great Elijah sinking from
triumph to despair. He has just prayed and heavenly fire consumes his
water-logged sacrifice. Then he asks God for rain and after three years without a drop, there's a torrential downpour! But Elijah is just as subject to
human emotions as we are. We've all said at times, "I have had enough!"

But God doesn't answer Elijah's prayer to die; instead, He sends an
angel to feed him, not once but twice. When Elijah is strong again, he
travels on to Horeb, and what does he do? He hides in a cave!

God isn't going to let him get away with that, either. "What are you
doing *here*, Elijah, so far away from your duties? You, of all my people,
should have remained at your post! My past compassions to you should
have strengthened and served you *especially for a time such as this.*"

We need to know that God understands when we cry out in exhaustion, heartache, and despair. Just as He brought Elijah out of the cave, He
will bring us out of the darkness of whatever cave we are in now, into His
light once again (Ps. 18:28).

Elijah thought his labor was useless, that it had come to nothing.
Those with the highest and holiest purposes are the very ones who experience such intense dejection and rejection. Elijah's heart withered at the
thought that he had failed. So it is with all of us who feel we have failed
God, family, and church because of mistakes or our humanity.

This chapter tells us that God isn't going to let us get away with self-
pity. We are all subject to depression, but there is an angel to help us out
of our cave, if we believe.

God urges us, as He did Joshua, to "be strong and of a good courage"
(Joshua 1:6). An anonymous saint said, "So, in the Lord's ministry, the nucleus of the church was not found in the applauding multitudes on Olivet,
but in the few faithful ones in the garden of Gethsemane."

When you feel you have had enough, be the faithful one in
Gethsemane, kneeling with Jesus, who set His face toward Jerusalem, realizing what He was about to endure (Luke 9:51).

*Whatever you're facing today, set your face toward Jesus, and He'll give you
the strength to make it through.*   PAT NORDMAN

The Economics of God's Food Program

*Why do you spend money for what is not bread, and your wages for
what does not satisfy? Listen diligently to Me, and eat what is
good, and let your soul delight itself in abundance. Isa. 55:2, NKJV.*

THE UNITED STATES Department of Agriculture did a study to determine which foods provide the most nutrients for the dollar spent. For all the nutrients listed, potatoes and the cereal groups provide equally well the most nutrition for the money. Coming in next were legumes. And fourth, green and leafy vegetables. Notice that all of these foods were part of God's original diet.

The poorest buy for the dollar was sugar. Next to sugar—or the second worst buy for your money—was the meat and fish group. This is not to say there is not some good nutrition in meat or fish, but for the dollar spent, it was quite expensive.

In 1993 an analysis was made of the cost of food in India for the nutrients gained. In India beef is cheaper than chicken. Fish, however, is very expensive. The same number of rupees spent for lentils as for beef provided 3.5 times more calories, 3.5 times more protein, 19 times more calcium, 6.5 times more iron, 7 times more potassium, 12.5 times more vitamin B1, 3.6 times more riboflavin and 1.2 times more niacin than beef.

On the other hand, beef provided unhealthy saturated fat and was loaded with cholesterol, while the lentils had little fat and no cholesterol. The beef also had no carbohydrate and no fiber, which are essential to a healthy diet. A similar study was done in Latvia in 1993. Chicken was inexpensive. Yet grains and vegetables still had a great advantage over the chicken nutritionally for the money spent.

In summary, throughout the world the relative cost for nutrients purchased is high for meat and low for most plant foods. If getting the best buy for your money is important to you, God's original diet is by far the best. It is not only superior from the economic standpoint, but ideal for disease prevention. Why is it, then, that so many people spend wages for food that is nutritionally inferior when if they would eat what is good for them, the chances are that it would cost them less?

God asks you to be a faithful steward of what He has given you. The next time you go to the market, perhaps you should consider getting the most nutrition for your money and select a wide variety of plant-based foods.

JOHN A. SCHARFFENBERG

About Doubt

And Jesus said to him, "If you can! All things are possible to him who believes." Immediately the father of the child cried out and said, "I believe; help my unbelief!" Mark 9:23, 24, RSV.

FEW THINGS IN LIFE are as painful as doubting at a deep level. A man came to Jesus one day, cursed with such honesty that he was engaged in a titanic struggle with faith. He was desperate. His boy was possessed with demons trying to kill him. Somewhere he had heard that Jesus could heal the child but he did not really believe it. Yet more than anything else in the world he wanted his boy well again. And so he went to Christ.

Can you imagine the journey there? His friends walk with him and fill his ears with strong admonitions. "Say nothing of your unbelief. This is your only chance. It's for your kid. Don't reveal too much about your own convictions, and remember that a little pretending can go a long way."

Then he is face to face with Jesus, who confirms his worst fears by saying, "If you can believe, all things are possible." Oh, no. What now? Can he repress this cursed doubt and save his child? Can he just this once affirm what his mind denies? But he will not. He exercises his terrible honesty and cries out, "Lord, I believe; help my unbelief!"

The response of Jesus to such intellectual anguish is profoundly moving. All discussion about faith stops. Jesus is satisfied. The child is promptly healed. What does this demonstrate? It shows that double-mindedness does not shut us out of God's concern. It shows that God does not demand that we give up our intellectual honesty as the price of His love.

Nevertheless, we would miss half the story if we did not see that two people were healed that day—the boy and the father. As stated above, doubt is often an extremely painful condition. Mix insecurity, guilt, and confusion together and you have the emotional essence of doubt. Jesus did not leave him there.

What does this teach us about doubt? Live by what you believe and not by what you question. Unbelief is not home; nobody can live happily in it. What you accept, no matter how small, is a hundred times more important than what you reject. Chronic cynicism is a devastating disease. Refuse to cry, "Lord, I don't believe." For the benefit of your own soul, shout the honest, entire truth, "Lord, I believe; help my unbelief!"

Thank You, Lord, for not demanding perfect faith before working miracles in our lives. SMUTS VAN ROOYEN

Fighting Fibromyalgia

*Beloved, I pray that you may prosper in all things and be
in health, just as your soul prospers. 3 John 2, NKJV.*

IN 1993 I RODE the high road. I was awarded sales person of the year, got a raise, a car, and a promotion. I smiled a lot, looked good, and talked the talk. But inside, my life was a hollow black hole and every night I cried myself to sleep. I felt abandoned, unloved; no one really cared. God seemed to have gone on vacation a million miles from where I lived.

I worked hard and tried to play, but my heart wasn't in it; I was just too tired. Little by little my life ebbed away until at 103 pounds I couldn't get out of bed. That's when my mom started coming over and my children learned how to take care of themselves. I thought that I would never smile again.

To suffer from either depression or fibromyalgia would have been enough, but one perpetuates the other and who knows for sure which came first. Fibromyalgia is defined as a non-articular rheumatic condition affecting muscles, ligaments, and other fibrous tissues in the body. So when I said I felt like I had been hit by a Mack truck, I wasn't kidding.

Health professionals say that as many as 5 percent of the general public suffers with fibromyalgia, a condition caused by chronic stress. Overstress makes people irritable; they complain of being tired, unable to fall asleep, or obtain a restful night's sleep. They are plagued by aches and pains. They lack energy and enjoyment of life. They feel anxious, depressed, or unable to cope.

Finding healing when your emotional and physical health have been ripped away like two legs from a three-legged stool, is not easy. But if you keep breathing and God says, "Live," that seemingly fragile spiritual part of you will find the way.

My healing began when I attended Weimar Institute. The acronym that changed my life is NEWSTART®: Nutrition—eat right; Exercise—move, whether you feel like it or not; Water—drink lots; Sunshine—take time to let it into your life; Temperance—avoid artificial stress relievers such as coffee, alcohol, drugs, or sugar; Air—breathe fresh, clean air; Rest—take a Sabbath; Trust—find a personal relationship with God and nurture your own spiritual development.

If life has lost its meaning, let me recommend a new start!

Am I living by God's NEWSTART program for health and soul prosperity?

CATHY O'MALLEY

Drinking God's Stuff

Teach me Your way, O Lord, and lead me in a smooth path. Ps. 27:11, NKJV.

THE SEIZURES WEREN'T very frequent at first, so I passed them off as being stress-related. But I was wrong, almost dead wrong. They began to occur more frequently and more violently. The seizures became so severe that they would put me in bed for days at a time. I was concerned about driving and wouldn't even hold my new granddaughter, Savannah, for fear of dropping her. I even swallowed my male pride and asked for prayer during morning worship at Three Angels Broadcasting. But nothing seemed to calm this beast within.

I figured it was time for the hospital, the CAT scans, the EEGs, and the blood letting in order to find out what was causing the seizures. But all the tests were negative. So I thought, *Back to work and forget it.* But instead, it was back to bed, shaking violently and having several seizures a day. I was down for the count, and the count was almost to 10.

My wife, Mollie, has this saying: "God may not always be there when I want Him to be, but He's never late." His "never late" came in the form of a newsletter received by Mom Ford at 3ABN. The article was on aspartame, an ingredient found in diet sodas, the same diet sodas that I had been consuming more and more. (They were on sale; I couldn't pass that up!)

Mrs. Ford gave the article to Mollie. Mollie came home that evening with several gallons of water, propped me up in bed and said, "Here, drink this." I drank nothing but water for the next several days, every hour on the hour. We could see results in 24 hours. The seizures stopped immediately and the shaking began to dissipate. I was nearly killed by diet soda. I realize everyone isn't as sensitive to aspartame as I am. But if it happened to me I know it can happen to others.

As far as I'm concerned, aspartame is a killer, yet in 1999 it was in more than 7,000 products (maybe more today). I even found a Web site (www.dorway.com) declaring its harm. It's been months since I've had a seizure, and I'm now a certified water drinker—you know, the stuff God makes.

Just as acquiring a taste for a man-made thirst-quencher almost killed me, so can developing a taste for man-made philosophy and religious ritual. The only safe way is to drink the Living Water from His Word.

Lord, teach me Your ways.   HAL STEENSON

Crying Together

Rejoice with those who rejoice, and weep with those who weep. Rom. 12:15, NKJV.

MY DAUGHTER WASN'T expected home from her private Christian high school until 3 p.m. But in she marched at 11 a.m. with a firm declaration, "I'm never going back to that school again. Those kids aren't my type."

My husband had recently taken a pastoral call to this university town, and my daughter was new to this school. Approaching my 15-year old with what I thought was rational persuasion I reminded her that the law required her to be in school.

"Then you can call the local high school and enroll me there!" she declared. When I asked if something bad had happened she replied, "Yes, Dad spoke at chapel this morning and afterward some kids mocked me with words from his speech."

Perhaps it was just having fun on their part. Perhaps it was malicious. But whatever, it had inflicted pain. She wept. And I wept with her. It's not hard for a mother's heart to be touched by her child's pain. Once the tears were over, she checked her face in the mirror to be sure her eyes weren't swollen and red, ate some lunch, and announced she was ready to return to that "awful" school.

Three years later my daughter called from boarding school, where she had elected to spend her senior year. "I was up almost all night," she reported.

I asked if she had spent the time studying. Graduation was just around the corner. "No," she said, "I was up with Susan. Ben broke up with her yesterday. She was all shaken up over it!"

Some day Susan will laugh about it, I thought. Had my daughter tried to cheer her up? She's capable of witty repartee. Or perhaps she offered some advice?

"Susan needed lots of comfort. Lots of tears," my daughter continued.

"So what did you do?" I asked.

"I cried with her, Mom, like you did when I quit school!"

Young as my daughter is, she has learned when to eschew witty words and well-meaning advice, recognizing the inexpressible comfort of communal tears. She's not likely to question the truth of the biblical prescription "Weep with them that weep."

Offering advice or sharing cheer have their place, but it's not until you weep when another weeps that you're really connected.   EDNA MAYE LOVELESS

Learning to Lean

From the ends of the earth I call to you, I call as my heart grows
faint; lead me to the rock that is higher than I. Ps. 61:2, NIV.

ISN'T IT AMAZING how quickly life can change? Things we take for granted are suddenly gone or compromised. That's what happened to me recently. I was playing softball with our church group. We were losing badly. I had to think of some way to stop our losses, so I dove toward base and ended up breaking my leg, tearing my ACL (a ligament) and some cartilage, and falling right on my face. (Next time I'm going to try not to be quite so dramatic!)

Yes, sir. That game was over. We might have lost miserably, but the only thing people remember is the sight of me being carted off in the ambulance.

And I had to wonder, *Why? Why me? Why this? Why now? I certainly don't have time to be hobbling around on crutches.* With my leg in a cast, I can't drive. I've had to rely on the kindness of others to run errands for me, cook meals, and watch my children while I undergo hospital procedures and endure doctor's appointments.

It's hard to have to lean on others when you are as independent and self-sufficient as I am. And that may be why this happened. I've learned that it's OK to rely on others more. It's OK to need help. And it's OK if they let you down, or forget about you when your illness drags on. Now I know how it feels to be at the mercy of others for an extended period of time. People are busy with their own lives. Working me in isn't always easy. My friends have been great, but I know that after nearly three weeks of being an invalid, their lives have gone on. Mine is stuck.

I've also learned how my kids feel when they ask for something and I don't get it right away. It's hard to be dependent and patient at the same time. And when you are dependent you tend to demand a great deal. I've learned what it's like to ask for an ice pack or a glass of water and have to wait for it.

For right now, God's not only going to have to lead me to the Rock that is higher than I, He's going to have to give me a boost to get on top. But that's OK, because I'm learning to lean.

Lord, lead me in the way You want me to go, and if necessary give me a boost!

CÉLESTE PERRINO WALKER

Paying Grandma Back

God demonstrates his own love for us in this: While we were still sinners, Christ died for us. Rom. 5:8, NIV.

MY GRANDMOTHER WAS always doing something to help someone. She accomplished many good things even though she went nearly blind at a young age and spent her life in darkness.

In her village on the Canadian prairies nearly a century ago, she was known as the village "nurse" who treated the illnesses of any who needed her. Once she spent several days with a very sick young boy who was expected to die. She applied hot and cold water treatments and various remedies of the time, and persisted until the boy was on his way to recovery. The grateful family credited Grandma with saving their boy's life.

Thirty or 40 years later Grandma and Grandpa retired from the prairie farm and moved to White Rock, B.C., near Vancouver. An eye surgeon heard about Grandma and operated without charge, restoring much of her sight. I can remember, as a 12-year-old, the excitement at a family reunion over Grandma's ability to see again. She saw many of her 11 grown children for the first time, for they had been born after she was blind.

The eye surgeon was the little boy whose life she had saved so many years before.

But before we applaud Grandma's compassion for others I must tell the rest of the story. The reason Grandma had so much time for community service was because she kept her oldest daughter out of school most of the time; essentially she used her as an unpaid servant to keep the house and raise the 10 younger children.

Yet, isn't it true that most of us, at times, have two sides to our characters? I love Jesus, but I join the apostle Paul in wondering why I sometimes do the things I don't want to do (Rom. 7:15).

Grandma, in her human weakness, sometimes treated her loved ones badly. But at the same time her life revealed a compassion that wanted to serve God by reaching out to those in need.

When I recognize the reality of my own negative side, it is comforting to remember that our compassionate heavenly Father cared enough, even about my ornery grandmother, to bring relief to her in her old age through the boy she had helped so long before.

The true measure of character is not in how you treat strangers, but in how you treat the members of your family. Are there any changes you should be making in your life?   LEONARD BRAND

My Right Hand Versus God's

I have set the Lord always before me. Because He is at
my right hand, I shall not be moved. Ps. 16:8, NKJV.

KING DAVID NEVER knew when he composed this lovely psalm that he penned it just for me! But some day, I'll fill him in.

"Now why did you say that verse 8 of my sixteenth psalm held such significance for you, Cheryle?" the king may question with a curious twinkle in his eyes.

I'll turn toward him in all my new celestial beauty and explain, "Well, King, we find Satan busier than ever bringing heartaches and handicaps upon the human race. When I was born not much was known about the prognosis of oxygen-deprived babies. The doctor informed my parents that I had suffered a birth injury called cerebral palsy, which affected the motor portion of my brain. He said I probably wouldn't make it to my first year. But he underestimated a praying mother's determination to keep her infant daughter alive!

"As I grew, it became apparent that my right side was clearly affected. But in spite of the injury to the motor portion of my brain, I was able to do some things for myself. Most of my physical activities, however, were limited and had to be adjusted to wheelchair life.

"Now, here's where the blessing kicked in. Because of my many physical limitations, I learned that I must reach out for help. From childhood to adulthood I found that my most secure and comforting help came from the Lord. He was that someone *at my right hand.* Because I chose to make Him foremost in my heart and life, He's been there for me literally at my weakest point—my dysfunctional right hand. Sometimes He's been there through the willing hands of a college classmate. Sometimes in the helpful hands of one of my students. Always through the supporting arms of family and friends.

"I've rejoiced to see that no matter what I needed to accomplish—schooling, traveling, teaching, or just day-to-day activities—the Lord was there *at my right hand* to get the job done with *His right hand.* In fact, King David, your psalm ends with the best news of all: 'In our Lord's presence is complete joy. At His right hand are pleasures evermore' [verse 11, paraphrased]."

The Lord is at your right hand, too. Are you aware of His presence? Are you experiencing the joy that His presence brings? I hope so!

CHERYLE A. CHISHOLM

An Act of God?

There is a way that seems right to a man, but its
end is the way of death. Prov. 16:25, NKJV.

"I'M SORRY TO HAVE to tell you that you have a cancer." These words strike as a dagger to the heart of the patient sitting across from me. "Cancer? This isn't supposed to happen to me!"

As a cancer surgeon I have had to break this sad news to several thousand patients. Even though most had lifestyle practices known to cause cancer, the announcement almost always came as a shock. Nonsmokers were especially shocked!

There is now convincing evidence that as much as 80 percent of cancers are preventable or at least can be delayed. About one third of cancers are associated with smoking and drinking. Now it appears that another 50 percent may be related to diet and/or lack of exercise. More than 20 categories of cancer-inhibitory phytochemicals have been identified in practically all varieties of fruits, grains, nuts, and vegetables. Even smokers on a diet high in fruits and vegetables are reported as having a delayed onset of lung cancer.

What should you do to lower your risk of cancer? First, avoid tobacco and alcohol. Second, avoid meat, milk, eggs, cheese, and animal fats of all kinds; they have been identified as promoting increased risk for certain cancers. Increase your intake of fruits and vegetables, especially raw ones. Third, exercise. An active exercise program reduces the risk for certain malignancies.

I have been teaching community health education classes for many years. It is somewhat amazing and very gratifying to see the enthusiasm with which many, upon hearing these concepts for the first time, accept the principles of healthy living. It is also very disappointing to see so many of my church friends resist the special instructions God has given us, especially about diet.

More than a hundred years ago, before science discovered the same thing, God inspired Ellen White to write, "Grains, fruits, nuts, and vegetables constitute the diet chosen for us by our Creator. These foods, prepared in as simple and natural a manner as possible, are the most healthful and nourishing. They impart a strength, a power of endurance, and vigor of intellect, that are not afforded by a more complex and stimulating diet" (*Counsels on Diet and Foods,* p. 363).

Cancer is not an "act of God"; rather, God has acted to instruct His people in its prevention!

Lord, help me to follow the health principles You have given to Your people.

ARTHUR WEAVER

Faith or Fear?

The Lord is my light and my salvation—whom shall I fear? The Lord is the stronghold of my life—of whom shall I be afraid? Ps. 27:1, NIV.

MEN GENERALLY DO better than women on standardized math tests. But two psychologists, Diane Quinn and Steven Spencer, discovered that they could influence the outcome simply by changing the expectations. Half of the experimental group were told they were taking a standardized test designed to measure their math ability. The women scored 10 while the men typically scored 25. It would seem to indicate that men are smarter in math, right?

But wait. The other half of the experimental group was told they were being given a test that was "gender fair." In it, both sexes did equally well—both women and men scored 20! In other words, the women did better and the men, worse!

What made the difference? Their expectations! The same is true spiritually speaking: your faith determines your outcome. If you have hopes and dreams, they will probably come true. But if you live in fear, then it will probably be as Job said, "What I feared has come upon me; what I dreaded has happened to me" (Job 3:25, NIV).

Goliath, the Rambo and Terminator of the Philistines, challenged Israel to send over their best fighter to duel with him. "When the Israelites saw the man, they all ran from him in great fear" (1 Sam. 17:24, NIV). They were already defeated before they ever set foot on the field.

But David, even though smaller and less experienced, trusted in God. He killed the giant with a well-placed stone from his sheepherder's slingshot.

What is your Goliath? What do you fear? Is it an unsure job? Financial problems? Is your marriage falling apart? Are you worried about losing something you cherish? Is it a dreaded disease?

Regardless of the nature of your Goliath, God's message is, turn it over to God. Ask Him to help you to look at your problem through eyes of faith, seeing possibilities and positive outcomes.

Fear destroys and paralyzes. Faith empowers and frees. You can be more than a conqueror over your fears today by simply doing what Jesus said years ago to Jairus, the father of the little girl who had died: "Don't be afraid. Just believe."

Are you facing a Goliath? The outcome of your life will be determined by your faith or your fear! BILL TUCKER and TIM CROSBY

Learning Disabled but Leaning on God

But seek first his kingdom and his righteousness, and all
these things will be given to you as well. Matt. 6:33, NIV.

I HAVE A SEVERE learning disability—dyslexia-dysgraphia (a reading and writing disorder). My brain plays tricks on me. I see words backward. Even sentences get mixed up. I may write the last part of a sentence first, or start a word with the wrong letter and have to go back and fill in.

Learning to read was a nightmare. And spelling? Forget it! In school I was a failure. My way of coping was to just not care. I made recess a priority, but many times recess and field trips were denied me because my work wasn't done. I loved sports but my grades kept me from playing varsity. I felt frustrated because I knew I couldn't do any better.

When it came to testing, I didn't want anyone to know I was slower. I would start off trying to do the test correctly but when others were finishing up, I'd quickly guess or leave pages blank. I barely passed high school.

I've tried everything—different schools, tutors, various theories of instruction, color sheets over reading materials. But the only thing that helped was laborious practice. I got through college by going to study groups where students discussed reading assignments, or I had someone read them to me. I never took notes; I would just listen. When tested, I knew the information. By college, it didn't bother me to be the last one to finish a test, so I ended up with decent grades—a 2.98 GPA.

My year as a student missionary in Majuro changed my life. My fifth-grade students appreciated my efforts. An educational administrator told me I had a gift for teaching. I wondered if I could I be a teacher with my learning disabilities. "OK, God," I prayed, "if this is what You want me to do, I'll do my part and study hard."

There was just one problem—I had to pass the California Basic Educational Skills Test before student teaching. The first time I took it I failed all three sections. The next time I passed math. After a few more tries I passed reading. I took the test nine times before I passed the writing section!

All this has taught me patience—something that a lot of teachers don't have. I've also learned you don't have to worry about yourself. Wait on the Lord, and He'll come through.

Has life given you a challenge that you're working to overcome? Why not put God first and see how He works things out for you? TIMOTHY PIERCE

Who Am I?

I, when I am lifted up from the earth, will draw all men to myself. John 12:32, NIV.

THE SETTING IS Yankee Stadium. Runners are on first and third. The pitcher checks the runner on third base. Then, as he glances at the runner on first, his eyes focus on something happening in the stands. He sees a man in the throes of a heart attack. Immediately he is faced with a dilemma. Should he go on with the ball game or help the man who is having a heart attack?

What could a baseball pitcher do to save a heart attack victim? Usually nothing. But the pitcher on the mound at Yankee Stadium that day was Doc Medich. There was a reason his teammates called him "Doc." He was a senior medical student. Alerted to the crisis in the stands, Doc faced the question, *Who am I? Am I a baseball player trying to strike out my opponents, or am I a medical student trained to help people in a health crisis?*

Every day you face the same who-am-I question. How you answer it will determine your moves. The game that you are playing is not in a stadium; it is the game of life. Is your life objective that of having fun? Or is it gaining earthly possessions? Perhaps it's prosperity, the accumulation of wealth? Is your game to grab status and prestige? Do you desire influence and the power to control others? Or is it pleasure, travel, entertainment, or sports that you're after?

Each time you answer the who-am-I question you need to consider how Jesus Christ would have responded. You find His answer in Matthew 20:28, where He says, "The Son of Man did not come to be served, but to serve, and to give his life as a ransom for many" (NIV). Jesus came to this earth to minister. His goal was to serve others. He spent His entire life helping, healing, and caring for people.

That day in Yankee Stadium, Doc Medich threw one more pitch to the batter, and then answered the who-am-I question by jumping into the stands and helping to save the man's life. The game changed that afternoon because the pitcher took on the role of service.

Does your game of life need to change? Do you need to stop your current game and start another so that you can lift up Jesus and minister to His people?

Ask yourself the question "Who am I?" Is your answer consistent with the way you are playing your game of life?　　　　　　　　　　DAVID WHITE

Taming Children's Terror

God is our refuge and strength, a very present help in trouble. Therefore we
will not fear, even though the earth be removed, and though
the mountains be carried into the midst of the sea. Ps. 46:1, 2, NKJV.

SEPTEMBER 11, 2001: The day terrorists attacked the U.S. One week later here is what children were saying: "I worry about my mommy and daddy and the big buildings they work in exploding." "I saw the planes crashing. I'm afraid someone will get on with a bomb." "I feel so sorry for the people. I just can't stop thinking about it."

Children fear that which they don't understand. They fear dangerous things that they have no control over. They fear sudden tragic happenings that maim and kill, such as plane crashes, earthquakes, lightning, and explosions.

You can't prevent tragedy from striking your family. You can't prepare for every bad thing that could possibly happen to children. But you can provide a stable and secure environment where healing is possible and where their terrors can be listened to, talked out, and tamed.

Encourage your children to talk. Unresolved fear erupts in nightmares and behavior regressions. Talk about what's good in tragic situations rather than focusing on the pain, loss, and death. Tell them the truth. "Bad things may happen, but you can choose to smile, help others, and look for the good." Then hug your kids and tell them you love them and will protect them.

Turn off the TV. When children see a tragedy replayed on newscasts it's as if it's happening again and again. Instead, play soothing music or read to your children. Just hearing your voice is reassuring to them. Give the children something to do to help others.

Reassure them that God still holds the whole world in His hands. Read them Bible stories of God's deliverance, such as when Elisha's servant thought the enemy was going to attack, God helped him to see horses and chariots of fire protecting their city (2 Kings 6:17). Tell them about their guardian angel, who will never leave their side, even when bad things happen or Mommy and Daddy can't be there. Help them memorize Psalm 34:7: "The angel of the Lord encamps all around those who fear Him, and delivers them" (NKJV). Pray for courage. Pray that God will put a hedge of protection around your family and give you the faith needed to get through tough times.

Thank You, Father, for promising to help us in times of trouble.

KAY KUZMA

Volunteering Is Good for Your Health

And the King will tell them, "I assure you, when you did it to one of the least of these my brothers and sisters, you were doing it to me!" Matt. 25:40, NLT.

RON NEISH, AN Adventist chaplain, tells of spending seven days at ground zero right after that fateful day the World Trade Center towers were leveled. He saw firefighters and police officers work with zeal. He describes a long-retired New York firefighter, who must have been around 90, staggering along a cleared roadway. He wore his 1930s fire-fighter's outfit—an old-fashioned brim hat and a large coat that hung just above his ankles. Neish reports that the old gentleman became "a real and welcome part of the rescue program."

I can picture the elderly man waking up that Tuesday morning and watching the tragedy with the rest of us. His eyes fill with tears and compassion. And then he goes to the attic and takes out his 60-year-old uniform and answers the call of duty.

What is it that makes some people go out of their way to serve and to save? They may be old or young, rich or poor. They stand out from the crowd like a Mother Teresa or a Schindler. Not all are religious, but they willingly take risks for others. They exhibit a spirit of adventure and a love for people that keeps them service-oriented rather than merely thrill-seeking.

We find great reward in knowing we have helped someone, but science tells us that doing good also promotes health. In uncertain times like these, concern for others makes everyone better off, not only the victims but also those who help them.

Volunteering for community service may prolong your life. Researchers at the University of Michigan report that retired people who volunteer just 40 hours a year tend to live longer than those who don't. Volunteers are happier and experience more energy and control over their lives. In Canada almost one in four of those over 65 are volunteers. They enjoy an improved quality of life and increased physical activity. Maybe volunteerism should be part of the health message.

In this era of overt evil God wants us to do more than wring our hands. He wants us to offer people an alternative lifestyle of caring, of refusing to be sidetracked by nonessentials. It's time to avoid criticism and start encouraging; to forget our own low self-esteem and build up that of others; to prepare not just ourselves for Christ's second coming, but those around us.

Ask yourself, "Where could God use my gift of service?" and sign up as a volunteer today. ELLA M. RYDZEWSKI

Pardoned or Prevented?

Please forgive your servant's offense. . . . When the Lord has done for my master every good thing he promised concerning him and has appointed him leader over Israel, my master will not have on his conscience the staggering burden of needless bloodshed or of having avenged himself. 1 Sam. 25:28-31, NIV.

DAVID AND HIS MEN were in the desert and needed supplies, so David sent 10 men to ask Nabal, a rich sheep owner in the area, for help. After all, David's men had treated Nabal's shepherds kindly and had never taken anything from them, so David figured Nabal would certainly return the favor. Instead, Nabal insulted the men and sent them away empty-handed.

When David learned what happened, he was furious. He armed 200 men and was about to teach Nabal a "fatal" lesson when Abigail, Nabal's wife, intervened and talked some sense into David. "Why avenge yourself? You'll only end up having painful memories on your conscience. Let God, who has been so good to you, take care of the problem."

Abigail was a very wise woman. Not only did she save her husband's life, she also gave insightful counsel about what avenging does to the avenger! Had David committed the sin of getting even, he no doubt would have been pardoned, for "her husband . . . was surly and mean in his dealings." Abigail herself said, "He is such a wicked man that no one can talk to him." But the question arises: which is better, a pardoned or a prevented sin? In David's case, a prevented sin not only saved a family but it saved David's conscience and reputation as well.

There are times in our lives when a prevailing grace becomes a preventing grace, when a friend will remind us that it isn't our nature to say or do what we feel like at the time we're offended. The wisdom is in recognizing what our friend has done for us by stopping us before we foolishly act out our anger. David did; he realized what this perceptive wife of Nabal did for him and he exclaimed, "Praise be to the Lord, the God of Israel, who has sent you today to meet me. May you be blessed for your good judgment" (1 Sam. 25:32, 33 NIV).

The consequences of getting even can be immeasurable. When we are angry about unjust situations, the only course of safety is in following God's Word: "Blessed are the peacemakers" (Matt. 5:9) and "Be not be overcome by evil, but overcome evil with good" (Rom. 12:21).

Let God's Word be your "Abigail" to talk sense into you when you feel like getting even.   PAT NORDMAN

Thank You, Jesus, for the Pain

But to the degree that you share the sufferings of Christ, keep on rejoicing, so that also at the revelation of His glory you may rejoice with exultation. 1 Peter 4:13, NASB.

IT WAS SABBATH morning. I was walking back and forth in the shallow end of the pool in the Desert Springs Therapy Center. I had gone there to get some relief from the crippling arthritic pain I was experiencing. Because of the nerve compression and severe pain that occurred when there was weight on my spine, in the water was the only place I could exercise.

I longed for a peaceful time alone with God, but the quietness of the morning was destroyed by a patient named Linda who was berating the staff because doors had slammed during the night, keeping her awake. My first response was impatient irritation. How could she be so insensitive? It's almost impossible to keep doors from slamming when the desert wind is blowing hard, especially when patients such as I are on crutches. Then I realized that my door was one of those that had slammed. As I was leaving my room, I wasn't prepared for the blast of wind and before I knew what was happening, it banged shut. I couldn't help it! Nevertheless I felt impressed to go and apologize.

So I got out of the pool and hobbled over to Linda's door on my crutches. "Linda," I said, "Mine was one of the doors that slammed last night. I'm sorry." As I looked into her eyes I could see tears starting to form, and I knew I was talking to a woman who felt unloved. "You know, Linda," I said, "God loves you."

Linda left the center that day, but before leaving she accepted a Bible study lesson guide on God's love from the book of John. I had been able to get through to Linda, because I too was in pain.

The whole experience brought back to mind something that happened many years ago when the disease first threatened the active outdoor lifestyle I loved and at times made teaching my classes a nightmare of pain. One of my students once asked me if I had ever thanked the Lord for having ankylosing spondyltis. I wondered what was wrong with that student, and if she would pass my class!

I smiled. I had come a long way from that day. Now, because of experiences such as this one with Linda—experiences I wouldn't have if it weren't for the pain—I can honestly thank God.

Can you honestly say, "Thank You, God, for my pain"?

DAVID E. ABBEY

Reprogramming the Hard Drive

Remember, it is sin to know what you ought to do and then not do it. James 4:17, NLT.

A WOUND CAN BE cleaned, bound up, and in time it will usually heal. Many cancers can be cut out and, if they haven't spread, the prognosis can be fairly good. Chronic disease generally comes on slowly and one learns to cope. But a stroke hits like lightning and, depending on the location of the strike and its severity, can instantly change everything about you— your body functions, your energy level, your personality, your speech, and your ability to move, to analyze, to plan, and to execute actions. In one awful moment one can be tumbled from the height of functionality and productivity and rendered maimed, disabled, and in some cases paralyzed.

Having a stroke is like having your computer hard drive crash. Data is scrambled or inaccessible. Some information may be lost permanently. Certain functions no longer work. But unlike a computer, you can't just install a new hard drive! Destroyed brain cells can't be resurrected. But your brain does have the amazing power to reprogram itself—with the help of good nutrition, exercise, and a positive attitude.

If a lost function is performed over and over again, new pathways can be formed in the brain. Every time you focus your effort to perform a function that once was automatic—even though part of the brain's nerve system that performed that function may be destroyed or substantial amounts of wiring lost—your brain sprouts new connections to restore the function.

If part of the needed brain center is not destroyed, sometimes the brain instructs the remaining portion to carry the load. If the required parts are completely destroyed, the brain will, if possible, figure out new wiring to perform the function. In any case, the secret is persevering, focused effort. Do it enough, and eventually a new connection will be made.

The problem with most stroke patients is that they work hard for the first few months after the stroke and then become discouraged and quit exercising. If they could realize how close they are to making connections they would continue the hard work of rehabilitation.

Sin, like a stroke, also destroys connections. We need to cooperate with the Holy Spirit in restoring the connections.

Why not give God permission to immediately begin reprogramming your hard drive?   KAY KUZMA

Is Your Soul Thirsty?

As the hart panteth after the waterbrooks, so panteth my soul after thee,
O God. My soul thirsteth for God, for the living God. Ps. 42:1, 2.

WE MUST HAVE water to survive! Our bodies are more than 70 percent water; to keep them running smoothly we are told to drink eight glasses of water a day. You might survive for weeks without food by living on body reserves, but water is so integral to life—with every function depending on it—that most of us would die after three to four days. To skimp on water intake is to put your body in serious risk of malfunctioning.

To get the most out of your water intake, you should drink two cups before breakfast, two or three between breakfast and lunch, and two or three between lunch and supper. So that it doesn't interfere with digestion, wait an hour or two after eating and stop about 15 minutes before eating again. And don't depend on thirst—you need water way before you feel thirsty for it!

What a blessing to have running water in our homes, or go to the local store and buy a bottle! But imagine you're near Death Valley in the middle of summer. Your car broke down and you have no idea when help might arrive. You drank your last sip of water three hours ago. The desert is so hot that you see water shimmering in the distance, but it's only a mirage. Or imagine you've just hiked 10 strenuous miles, and your mouth is dry and your energy zapped. You reach for your canteen for a refreshing drink, but all the water has leaked out. It will be four more miles before you reach another source. As thirsty as you'd feel in these situations, that's how thirsty God wants you to be for Him!

David drew the corollary that our thirst for water is like our need for God. Pursued by King Saul, David cried, "O God, you are my God, earnestly I seek you; my soul thirsts for you, my body longs for you, in a dry and weary land where there is no water" (Ps. 63:1, NIV).

Our world is cut off from God by sin—a true desert in the midst of the universe. Are you aware of your critical need of spiritual water? The next time you take a refreshing drink of pure, cool water, consider also your soul thirst. How can you quench it? The answer is in Revelation 22:17: "Let him that is athirst come. And whosoever will, let him take the water of life freely!" Drink in spiritual water throughout the day—don't wait until you're thirsty.

Have you gotten your drink of living water yet? Come to Jesus, the source of the water of life, and let Him fill you to overflowing! JIM HINRICHS

Sunlight—One of God's Greatest Blessings

Then God said, "Let there be lights in the firmament of the heavens to
divide the day from the night; and let them be for signs and seasons,
and for days and years; and let them be for lights in the firmament of the
heavens to give light on the earth"; and it was so. Gen. 1:14, 15, NKJV.

THE SUN SHONE 24 HOURS a day on December 24, 1928, when Richard Byrd and a crew of 41 arrived in Antarctica, where they would spend the next 14 months. But when the days began to shorten there was a significant deterioration in the morale of the men. By April they lost the sun altogether and it did not appear for five months. Many became morose and depressed. Norman Vaughan wrote, "How can I explain the joyousness of the first few days of sunlight? We felt like prisoners who had received commutation of our sentences. A brightness appeared on our faces. We walked faster and moved with an energy we had long forgotten." Admiral Byrd's men suffered from what we now call SAD, "seasonal affective disorder." They were deprived of the endorphins that sunlight causes the brain to produce and that give a sense of well-being.

The sun is one of life's greatest blessings, yet we often take it for granted. We're basically unaware that the sun kills germs, prevents infections, and helps heal certain diseases by increasing the oxygen-carrying capacity of the red blood cells, thus boosting the immune system. Acne, psoriasis, pityriasis, rosacea, and ulceration of the skin, such as that caused by varicose veins, injury, and insect bites, all respond well to graded doses of sunlight. Tanned skin is three times more powerful in killing germs than untanned. However, too much sunlight damages skin, putting it at high risk for cancer. And repeated sunburn dehydrates and wrinkles skin. Moderation is important.

Without us even realizing it, every time we're out in the sun an incredible chemical reaction takes place, providing us with Vitamin D. We need 400 units each day, and we get all we need by exposing our faces to sunlight for just five minutes a day.

Sunlight strengthens your heart and improves circulation. Like exercise, it lowers the resting pulse rate, tunes up the heart muscle, and increases cardio-output by improving the heart's efficiency. It also tends to normalize blood pressure, whether it's high or low!

And finally, sunlight stimulates the thyroid gland to increase hormone production, which in turn increases your rate of metabolism and helps you burn calories!

Have you had your time in the sun today? Go for a good walk and let the sun revitalize you!   JAN W. KUZMA and CECIL MURPHEY

Restorative Dentistry

At that very time Jesus cured many who had diseases, sicknesses and evil spirits, and gave sight to many who were blind. Luke 7:21, NIV.

TOOTHACHES COME IN all shapes and sizes; they can range from a tiny nagging twinge to an excruciating, throbbing pain! From the moment patients suffering from toothaches arrive in my office their overwhelming desire is to be relieved of their pain. Often they don't care what I do to "fix it." They just want the pain to go away!

Giving them temporary relief is easy, but restoring the tooth so that it functions well for them is often a more complicated process. If a patient simply chooses to leave my office after I've relieved the pain but without "restoration," they are doomed to return again and again with the same problem. If they choose to have the tooth fully restored, they reap the long-term benefits of improved health!

While here on this earth Jesus showed us the ultimate in restorative medicine! He restored sight to the blind; working legs to the lame; noses, fingers, and toes to the lepers; healthy blood to the hemorrhaging; movement to the paralyzed; rational brains to the demented; and life to the dead. I have a feeling He even restored good teeth for rotten, aching ones! In a small way I like to compare His restorative mission to the world with the dentistry I practice every day!

But before the restoration, Jesus (as a good dentist would), first took care of the pain, the pain of a guilty conscience, by saying, "Your sins are forgiven." Jesus speaks to me today in the same way, promising me forgiveness—pain relief—so that I can see more clearly what I need to do to experience restoration! In my life, restoration can happen only when I am willing to admit that I have a problem and I need help.

Sometimes when patients no longer feel pain, they refuse to admit that the problem that caused the pain is still there. They may have a large cavity caused by poor dietary habits, smoking, poor oral hygiene, or just plain neglect. If they don't change their destructive habits, the pain will return.

The same is true in our spiritual lives. If we refuse to be restored by Jesus, the great Healer, our pain will grow until it becomes unbearable. By coming to Jesus—spending time communicating with Him each day—we can be forgiven and restored to His image.

Lord, sharpen my senses so that I will feel the pain enough to repent of my unhealthy lifestyle and receive Christ's pain-relieving forgiveness and restoration.

JERRY MUNCY

Blue Mondays

And my God shall supply all your need according to
His riches in glory by Christ Jesus. Phil. 4:19, NKJV.

CARDIOLOGISTS AT THE Baltimore VA Medical Center found that 21 percent of irregular heartbeat incidents struck on Monday mornings. Why? It may have to do with another little-known fact. Of the 25 highest risk indicators of a catastrophic health event, your attitude about your job is tied for first place.

Bad attitude about your job? Your entire life is in upheaval. A lot of stress is involved. Your digestion is affected, and probably your sleep, eating habits, interaction at home, regularity, and your walk with the Lord.

Which brings us to another little known fact: pastors are among the poorest health risks in the nation because of heart disease, strokes, and diabetes. Again it is most likely stress-related.

I am reminded of the words of apostle Paul, "I have learned in whatever state I am, to be content." "In everything give thanks; for this is the will of God." "Be anxious for nothing . . . and the peace of God . . . will guard your hearts and minds." Then consider the words of Matthew, "But seek first the kingdom of God and His righteousness, and all these things shall be added to you," and those of the psalmist, "Delight yourself also in the Lord, and He shall give you the desires of your heart. Commit your way to the Lord, trust also in Him, and He shall bring it to pass."[1]

Remember, your primary stress outlet is prayer. Don't bottle things up. God is there and will listen. He will act in your very best interests—every single time, without fail, no exceptions.

If job stress continues, the Lord may be trying to tell you that you need a change. There are two possible alternatives. The first is to change your attitude. Think of five positive things about your job and praise the Lord; then consider the most negative—and thank the Lord again. The apostle James said, "Count it all joy when you fall into various trials, knowing that the testing of your faith produces patience."[2]

The second alternative is to change your job. Impossible, you say? Remember, "With God all things are possible."[3]

The next time you have a blue Monday, let God's Word take away the stress.

E. JOHN REINHOLD

---

[1] Phil. 4:11; 1 Thess. 5:18; Phil. 4:6, 7; Matt, 6:33; Ps. 37:4, 5, NKJV.
[2] James 1:2, NKJV.
[3] Mark 10:27, NKJV.

What Is a Good Samaritan?

But a certain Samaritan, as he journeyed, came where he was. And when he saw him, he had compassion. So he went to him and bandaged his wounds, pouring on oil and wine; and he set him on his own animal, brought him to an inn, and took care of him. Luke 10:33, 34, NKJV.

YOU KNOW THE story well. The lone traveler going from Jerusalem down to Jericho; the sudden seizure by thieves who took all he had in spite of his courageous attempts at self-defense. At least, I think he tried to fight them off, for he was wounded, half dead, and naked.

The priest—one of the official intercessors between God and man especially delegated to attend to such needs—made a hasty detour to the other side of the trail. The Levite, one of those especially delegated to interpret the character or law of the Great Physician, after an evaluative look also detoured around the unconscious brother. Perhaps he had no first-aid kit. Perhaps he was late to an important conference at Jericho.

The third person that came along was shunned and looked down upon by others because he was a foreigner, but that didn't stop him from doing what he could. He dismounted his donkey, hastily checked pulse and respiration, assessed the bleeding wounds, and from his supplies took out the alcohol (wine) to control infection, and soothing ointment for pain relief.

I suppose he also dressed the half-conscious man in his own extra clothing before positioning him on his animal, and stabilized him as they walked down the trail to Jericho. Upon reaching the most suitable motel, the foreigner secured lodging for them both, and tenderly watched over his charge until morning. How do I know he did it tenderly? The account specifically mentions compassion. Wonderful word, compassion. And then, upon paying the bill, he left an additional two days wages, with the promise, "If he needs to stay longer, I'll pick up the tab the next time I come!"

Putting it in today's setting: Would you pull over if you saw a man hurt beside the road? Would you dress his wounds as best you could, put your own coat on him, and help him into your car, realizing that his blood might soak through the upholstery? Would you drive him to the nearest motel, stay with him all night to make sure he was OK, and then leave two days wages—maybe a couple hundred dollars—with the motel owner to make sure the man had a place to recuperate? Or would you just dial 911 on your cellular and keep driving?

What could you do to be a good Samaritan to someone today?

MARJORIE V. BALDWIN

Children Getting Fatter Faster

At the end of the 10 days, Daniel and his three friends looked
healthier and better nourished than the youths who had been
eating the food supplied by the king! Dan. 1:15, TLB.

ONE DAY, INSTEAD OF serving the usual hot meal, the school cafeteria handed out peanut butter and jelly sandwiches. After lunch, a satisfied first grader marched out the door and complimented the cafeteria manager: "Finally, you gave us a home-cooked meal!" Sad to say, home-cooked, around-the-table meals are now the exception in most American homes, often being replaced by engineered foods. More than half of today's high-school kids head off to fast-food eateries and snack machines instead of to school lunch rooms. And we are paying the price. American children are getting fatter faster than ever. Four to six million youngsters aged 6 to 11 have serious weight problems; the number of super-fat children has doubled during the past 15 years.

Being overweight predisposes a child to heart disease, gallstones, adult onset diabetes, hypertension, cancer, and full-blown obesity later in life. Obese children have more orthopedic problems and upper respiratory diseases. And that is only one side of the story. They often suffer major social and psychological problems. The rapid increase of serious depression, eating disorders, drug use, and suicide among teenagers is frightening.

Genes do play a role in a person's weight, but they aren't the whole answer. Environment plays a critically important role—as shown by the fact that the percentage of obese Americans has increased steadily over the past 50 years. Our gene pool can't change that fast!

The major causes of obesity in children are the same as for adults—a sedentary lifestyle, TV viewing, the Internet, the snack-and-soda habit, and the popularity and availability of highly processed and concentrated foods. Many major medical centers are developing weight control programs for children that involve the whole family. Proper eating and lifestyle habits are a family affair, and a youngster especially needs the support of the family. Even when the rest of the family is not overweight, everyone benefits from a healthier lifestyle.

Here is a spiritual analogy: Just as fast food and a sedentary lifestyle causes children to be more susceptible to obesity and other diseases; so fast devotions and a sedentary Christianity can make a person more susceptible to temptation.

Lord, help me resist temptation and do what I know I should do.

AILEEN LUDINGTON

Bishnu Rai

"He will wipe every tear from their eyes. There will be no more death or mourning or crying or pain, for the old order of things has passed away." He who was seated on the throne said, "I am making everything new!" Rev. 21:4, 5, NIV.

FOR SOME UNKNOWN reason the Asian country of Nepal has an inordinate number of cleft lip and palate victims. It is estimated that one child from each 500 births has this defect, which translates into more than 40,000 people.

Bishnu was born in a remote village near Mt. Everest. At age 16, she is the oldest child among five. All of her young life she had been ashamed of her ugly face with it's upper lip twice split, revealing deformed spatial teeth and a tunnel up into her flaring nostrils. The gaping hole in the roof of her mouth had made initial survival precarious and speech unintelligible.

When she was 5 years old, Bishnu walked 30 minutes each way to attend the nearest government primary school, where both she and another student had cleft lips and palates. Some of their classmates resented the presence of "harelips" and made life miserable for them. It was painful to have their impaired facial features ridiculed and their defective speech mocked.

After attending school five years, Bishnu quit to begin work. She needed to help earn money to help provide food for the family. At first she worked for neighbors, planting and harvesting crops or taking care of their animals. Now Bishnu's left eye continuously waters as the result of a water buffalo's kick.

In May 1999 she became an apprentice in a Kathmandu clothing business, where she is learning sewing skills. Once she completes her apprenticeship she will earn money, most of which will be sent back to her family.

In Kathmandu, Bishnu heard about ADRA Nepal's Cleft Lip and Palate Program. She made contact with the organization, which performs the repair surgery entirely free to destitute people. In September 1999 Bishnu's operation was done, creating for her the new face she had dreamed about. In Nepali village culture, 12-15 is the marriageable age. With her improved appearance, Bishnu now has hope of a normal family life with a husband and children.

Jesus said He'll make all things new. For Bishnu, this promise has already been fulfilled.

What could you do today to help someone experience God's promise of restoration and hope?   GLENN and JERRE ST. CLAIR

Feeling Good

And now abide faith, hope, love, these three;
but the greatest of these is love. 1 Cor. 13:13, NKJV.

IT IS GOOD TO feel good. We want to feel good physically. We want to feel good about family and friends. And we want them to feel good about us. There are good health principles that help us feel good physically. Faithfully serving God and our fellow humans, achieving our best, and doing the right thing at the right time will help us feel good about ourselves. It is largely within our hands to feel good physically and to feel good about ourselves. The challenging goal is to get others to feel good about us. But for this, too, there is a principle to follow.

Many years ago I was hired from outside an organization to fill a key position. A person within had expected promotion to that position. She promptly resigned. She was very close to my new secretary, who was also disappointed that I was her new boss. This secretary could contribute to my success or detract from it. She preferred the latter. I could work at keeping her or at replacing her. I preferred the former.

Could I make her feel good about me by helping her appreciate the greatness of my mind and my background? Hardly. I sought ways to help her feel good about herself. I examined her performance prior to my arrival. I let her know of her contributions to the organization, that I trusted her, and that I envisioned a bright future for her. I gave her specific reasons as to why she was special, and I acknowledged the accomplishments of her departed mentor.

The response was amazing. She became a loyal employee and a good friend. She proved that if we would have others feel good about us, we must make them feel good about themselves. We need not expend energies to make them feel good about us. Love is the key for making them feel good about themselves.

"Man is required to love God supremely, with his might, mind, and strength, and his neighbor as himself. This he cannot possibly do unless he denies himself. To deny self means to rule the spirit when passion is striving for the mastery; to resist the temptation to censure and to speak words of faultfinding. . . . It means to work patiently and cheerfully for the good of others" (Ellen G. White, *In Heavenly Places*, p. 223).

Dear Lord, help me to love others as You love me. Let me live by Your love principle today and see what a difference it will make in someone else's life.

CLARENCE E. HODGES

The Road Less Traveled

And we know that all things work together for good to those who love God, to those who are the called according to His purpose. Rom. 8:28, NKJV.

IN THE GAME of life, why is it that some people give up when they suffer a setback and others under tremendous disadvantages and hardships end up winners? When a problem looms, it's as if the road forks. You have two possible choices—the path labeled, "All things work together for bad," and the other, "All things work together for good." Everything after this point will be determined by the path you choose. Everything will be affected by your attitude.

The first is the well trodden path. We live in a world of sin, so obviously bad things happen. We think, *It can't get so bad but what it can't get worse.* Or in the words of that old baseball song, "It's one, two, three strikes, you're out." That's it. You're doomed to failure.

Those that take the road less traveled choose the opposite response. They declare, "All things work together for good," even though it may not look that way. In making this choice, they are immediately freed from debilitating worry and fret. They can rest in the Lord and find the peace He promises, even in the midst of the terrible battle between good and evil, health and sickness, or life and death.

Choosing to look at life positively is like knocking down the first domino in a row. When that goes, the rest follow. Without deliberate planning, positive thinkers begin to take responsibility for making sure that "good" does, indeed, come from the bad. Whatever the strike that is called against them, they stay in the game, doing their best.

When tennis pro Monica Seles was stabbed in the back by a crazed fan, many thought she would never be back. But fighting physical disability and the fear of another attack, Monica returned to the game. After a horrific shooting accident in which more than 40 shotgun pellets ripped through his body, bicyclist Greg LeMond, representing the U.S. in the Tour de France, beat the odds and came back to win. And Greg Louganis, after suffering a concussion when the back of his head hit the three meter board in the Olympic diving event, came back later that day to win Olympic gold.

They all took the road less traveled and made "good" out of "bad." The next time you suffer a strike against you, which path will you choose?

Lord, help me choose the road less traveled and make good out of bad.

KAY KUZMA

Commanded to Rest

He said to them, "Come aside by yourselves to a deserted place
and rest a while." For there were many coming and going,
and they did not even have time to eat. Mark 6:31, NKJV.

SITTING ON THE EDGE of the examining table, I stared with disbelief at the medical form that the doctor placed in my hands. "No work for two months." That couldn't be possible! What was I supposed to do with myself? Closing my eyes, I listened while the doctor said that if I didn't change my lifestyle I would soon be dead. "You're overcommitted. You're a workaholic."

Wayne Oats defines a workaholic as "a person whose need for work has become so excessive that it creates a noticeable disturbance in the person's health, happiness, or relationship." That definition fit me! I was addicted to work!

Now I had no choice. So with time on my hands I began to reflect on such things as George MacDonald's comment, "Work is not always required of a man. There is such a thing as a sacred idleness—the cultivation of which is now fearfully neglected."

I began to make choices that would give my life a healthy balance. In the process I discovered how all this fits together in the Sabbath. When we get together with other believers, that is socially healthy. Then we stimulate our minds with Bible study. It's good for our emotional health to share our feelings in small groups. We grow spiritually when we worship God. And finally, after a healthy meal we can go for a walk in nature or rest, whichever our bodies need.

I think when Christ created the Sabbath He must have known just how difficult it would be for some of us to slow down and rest on His holy day, so He did two things. He gave us a preparation day to start gearing down, and He made it a command. (It is one of the Ten Commandments!)

One of these days I'm going back to work. But now I see the wisdom of Christ's advice to His disciples—that if they wanted to help others they needed rest and solitude themselves.

I was very fortunate in that even though I lost sight of God's plans for my life, God never lost sight of me. He allowed my body to become totally exhausted so I had no choice but to come aside and rest. So like David I say, "It is good for me that I have been afflicted, that I may learn Your statutes" (Ps. 119:71, NKJV).

Write down all your roles in life. Did you include taking care of yourself by resting?
CAROLINE WATKINS

True Value

*Even the very hairs of your head are all numbered. So don't be
afraid: you are worth more than many sparrows. Matt. 10:30, 31, NIV.*

HOW DOES ONE determine value? Nothing is of value to you unless it costs you something. Remember the "pearl of great price" (Matt. 13:46, NKJV)?

We value education by the tuition costs or by the income that it might help us to make. When we purchase something—a house, car, appliances, clothes, or even food—its worth is determined by what people will pay to own it.

Let's talk about cars. I have a 1985 Jeep with 132,000 miles. Now, that Jeep is not worth much on the used car market; however, to me it's worth much more. Why? I have replaced the fuel system, the suspension, and the drive train. I have scars on my head and cuts and bruises on my hands to remind me of the personal effort I have put into "that Jeep" to keep it running. "That Jeep" has provided me with what seems to be more of my share of frustrations. ("Why won't it start?" "Why is it beginning to use oil?") But I also have had some wonderful trips with "that Jeep," which compensate for the frustrations. A newer Jeep may have fewer problems, but no memories!

Several years ago I provided multiple anesthetics to a young man for the surgical procedures that were part of his cancer treatment. He eventually died from that cancer. Today I anesthetized his mother; as she tearfully emerged from unconsciousness I heard her softly call her son's name and say, "I loved you so; if only I could have saved you!"

How great was that mother's love! How great the value that parent placed on her child. Whatever she could have done to have saved her son's life, she would have done it.

Because God places so much value on us we need not fear personal threats or trials. These events cannot remove us from God's love. However, this doesn't mean that God will take away all our troubles. Those that stand up for Christ in spite of their troubles have lasting value.

Our true value is God's estimate of our worth, not that of our peers. Their value of us is based upon how we look or perform, or what we achieve. God values us because we belong to Him. We may frustrate God, but as long as we belong to Him, He will care for us.

God values you so much that He knows the number of hairs on your head. How does that make you feel? Why don't you tell God?   BURTON A. BRIGGS

Overcoming the Impediments of Healing

When He saw their faith, He said to him, "Man, your sins are forgiven you. . . .
But that you may know that the Son of Man has power on earth to
forgive sins"—He said to the man who was paralyzed, "I say to you,
arise, take up your bed, and go to your house." Luke 5:20-24, NKJV.

ANNA'S JAW CLENCHED angrily when asked what had happened to her. She'd attended our emotional healing seminar at which we shared the story of the paralytic. For healing to occur, the faith of the supplicant must overcome any barriers to the healing power of Jesus. The barrier in this story was the crowd, so his friends let him down through the roof.

Jesus' first act of healing was to say, "Your sins are forgiven you." Subsequently He implied that it is easier for a person to receive healing when his sins are forgiven. We challenged the group, "Destroy any impediment that stands between you and Jesus' healing power."

Later Anna asked for counsel concerning her lawsuit against her husband's three brothers, who had raped her. She was still struggling with her own feelings of anger and shame.

"Anna, do you think you could forgive your husband's brothers?"

Anna stiffened. Her body language showed defiant resistance.

"Forgiving is almost impossible, humanly speaking," Ray continued. "But God is faithful and will give you grace if you choose to forgive." Ray asked her if she would be willing to be led in a prayer for forgiveness. She was and, at the conclusion, she heaved a great sigh of relief.

At the court hearing, Anna asked to speak before the interrogation began. She stood nervously but delivered her well-rehearsed speech. "Judge, God has been gracious to me and given me peace. I would like to forgive those who have wronged me, and withdraw my lawsuit." Forgiveness doesn't necessarily mean the offending persons should not experience legal consequences, but in her case, Anna was impressed to drop the charges. The courtroom sat stunned, then broke into applause.

The judge said, "Never in my career has anything like this happened in my courtroom."

The result? Anna's mother asked to be lead to Jesus. Her estranged husband said, "I've noticed a change in my wife. I want to return to church."

When we choose forgiveness, healing starts, because the impediment is gone. When we act like Jesus, people want to know the Jesus we know.

Is there any impediment between you and the healing power of Jesus? Why not give it up and experience the miracle of healing God has for you?

RAY and LENI PUEN

Healing Because of Sickness?

*The eternal God is your refuge, and underneath
are the everlasting arms. Deut. 33:27, NIV.*

I'VE DISCOVERED THAT getting sick with a life-threatening disease can become a healing experience if it causes you to lean on Jesus more. I used to be a Type A person who had to be up and about and doing most of the time. But that changed in May 1993 when I was diagnosed with breast cancer. Surgery immediately followed, then months of chemotherapy and radiation treatments, leaving me sick and exhausted.

I wondered, *Why me?* I had always tried to live a healthful lifestyle. My doctor reminded me that it was probably hereditary, for my mother had died of the same disease. But that didn't ease the pain or the fear of what might lie ahead for me. That's when "Safe in the Arms of Jesus" became my song. I'd sing it again and again.

Now as I look back on the ordeal, I think I know Why me? Having had cancer was actually a part of my healing—the healing that is found in *complete* dependence on Jesus. Cancer taught me I didn't have strength to get through the day on my own. Without Jesus I couldn't do anything! (John 15:5)

God kept me alive to serve Him with all my heart, *in His strength,* and that's all that matters now. The purpose of my life is to help others find Jesus—my Healer. Each day is a gift to me so that I can use it to pass on the joy of His healing to someone else.

I thank God daily there has been no recurrence of cancer—although, being quite human, it is a concern of mine. I am doubly impressed that I must trust in God totally to stay well, for trusting brings health (Prov. 3:8). In addition to following a physically healthy lifestyle, I must daily choose to think positive thoughts. "Courage, hope, faith, sympathy, love, promote health and prolong life. A contented mind, a cheerful spirit, is health to the body and strength to the soul. 'A merry [rejoicing] heart doeth good like a medicine' (Prov. 17:22)" (*The Ministry of Healing,* p. 241). On the other hand, "Grief, anxiety, discontent, remorse, guilt, distrust, all tend to break down the life forces and to invite decay and death."

I thank God for giving me a second chance for life, and for showing me the healing power of trust.

Thank You, Lord, for holding me safely in Your arms while You teach me the lessons I need to learn about the healing power of total trust.

MAY-ELLEN COLON

Making a Little Bit of Heaven on Earth

*Anyone who claims to be in the light but hates his brother is still
in the darkness. Whoever loves his brother lives in the light,
and there is nothing in him to make him stumble. 1 John 2:9, 10, NIV.*

THERE IS TOO MUCH hate in our world—racial hatred, jealousy, murder, and wars. Wars happen for many reasons—some because certain ethnic groups hate each other; some because a more powerful country wants to take over a weaker one. Every time I hear about all this hate, I think, *Isn't there enough trouble in the world today caused by accidents and illnesses? Why do we humans have to add to this misery by heaping hatred on top of our existing pile of woes?*

We may not be able to stop all accidents or illnesses, but we can stop the emotional cancer of hostility. Sometimes, we dislike others because they are different than we are or because they are irritating. However, God says we must treat everybody with respect. "Do nothing out of selfish ambition or vain conceit, but in humility consider others better than yourselves" (Phil. 2:3, NIV). Can you imagine how much more pleasant life would be if everyone would consider others better than themselves? We would be charming and gracious to others. There would be no wars. And all would help to relieve the suffering of others, as the Union College students did when a young father was dragged under a logjam and drowned. With her husband gone, Meriel, a single mother of three young boys, had no hope of finishing the home improvements her husband had been working on—that is, until the students came to her rescue, donating their time and resources.

We love to read newspaper stories about the kind deeds of others. Most likely it wouldn't make the news if you were kind to that irritating co-worker, or if you helped that pesky neighbor kid learn how to bake a cake or make something out of wood. But it would give you the same warm feeling you get when you help someone in need. Besides, you would know that you did what God would have wanted you to do, because you are treating others with respect, even those who aren't easy to like.

Inasmuch as we are hostages on this planet of sin, we must work together to make this world a better place. Only in heaven will we live in perfect peace and love. But in the meantime, let us try to make a little bit of heaven on earth by showing love and respect to all with whom we come in contact.

To whom can I show more love today?

BONNIE SZUMSKI and KAY KUZMA

The Lost Alligator

What do you think? If a man has a hundred sheep, and one of them goes astray, does he not leave the ninety-nine and go to the mountains to seek the one that is straying?. . . Even so it is not the will of your Father who is in heaven that one of these little ones should perish. Matt. 18:12-14, NKJV.

ON SEPTEMBER 30, 1997, Florida state trooper Mike Taylor bagged the "longest ever" alligator from beside a boat dock in Lake Monroe, Florida. That gator, more than 14 feet in length and weighing 800 pounds, was an ugly beast that had been hanging around the boat dock for several years. No, he hadn't hurt anyone or even slowed down the jet skiers. He had just hung around doing gator things: lying with his all-seeing eyes barely above the water, sliding silently out from under the dock, terrifying fishermen and house owners.

His presence surely made for exciting waterfront activities! Imagine waterskiing on Lake Monroe. You could do a dock start, but landing safely takes on a whole new meaning! And what if Monster Gator steals your freshly caught bass? Nobody likes—or trusts—a hungry gator.

Sheep, on the other hand, are calm bundles of cuddly wool, inviting adoption. They are so cute, winsome, and vulnerable that we can even accommodate their odor. And the gift of their wool provides us with shirts, socks, and blankets. Sheep are easy to love. Gators are easy to hate.

Maybe that's why Jesus told the story about the lost sheep and a searching shepherd rather than about alligators and a fisherman. We feel good imagining shepherds searching for, finding, holding, loving, and saving lost sheep. But imagine a tale of Christ searching for a lost gator!

Jesus used the lost sheep story to show how much God loves lost people and to challenge us to follow His example as we "search out and save" those who are "lost." That's an OK assignment when we're talking about "sheepy" people, such as the nice woman you met at Wal-mart, or the smiling gentleman who rings the bell beside the kettle at Christmas time. But what happens when "search out and save" refers to "alligator people"? Are we then still willing to serve on Christ's salvation team? Take the angry fellow who made an obscene gesture when you pulled out in front of him. Or the office worker who's always gossiping about you. Or even swindlers, child abusers, druggies, terrorists, rapists, kids with earrings, and all the others we find hard to like.

Maybe, just maybe, the original story began: "Once upon a time there was a lost alligator."

Are you at times more like a gator than a sheep? Isn't it wonderful to know God is on a "search and rescue" mission for you? DICK DUERKSEN

Hope

Not getting what you want can make you feel sick, but a
wish that comes true is a life-giving tree. Prov. 13:12, CEV.

THE DAILY ONE hour of travel to work has afforded many opportunities to muse about things simple, things esoteric, things unsolvable, and sometimes nothing. Challenges are provided by the license plates, humor by license plate frames, and insight by bumper stickers. Trying to decipher the various combinations of letters and numbers on vanity plates has been a great way to relieve the boredom of the daily commute.

This morning my attention was grabbed by the following bumper sticker: "I feel better . . . since I have given up HOPE!" I am not sure if "hope" referred to a female or a feeling! I wonder had the driver of that car been disappointed so many times with his expectations that he no longer had any goals, aspirations, or future plans? Had his marriage failed, was he overlooked for a promotion, had his only child been killed? Were his house and property inundated by a flood, ravaged by fire, or destroyed in an earthquake? Or was everything going so well for him that he was bored with life and had no further challenges? Were his expectations greater than what was realistically possible?

When I was about to enter military service, my father gave me some sage council that he had learned while serving his military obligation in World War II. He said, "I got everything that I wanted, because I only wanted what I knew I could get!"

That advice has done much to help differentiate unreasonable expectations from obtainable goals and aspirations. Hope is that desire that provides us with goals and keeps us going. In contrast to wishing, hope is active; we dream, we plan, we work toward our goals, we recruit others to participate in order that they may share in the joy and satisfaction of completing that hope.

Hope keeps you afloat when others are sinking. Hope keeps you holding on to life when others are letting go. Hope gives you the courage to try again when others are quitting.

When I read the bumper sticker about giving up hope I first smiled, but then a sad feeling came over me. Is life ever worth living without hope?

Instead, may we be able to say with David, "May your unfailing love rest upon us, O Lord, even as we put our hope in you" (Ps. 33:22, NIV).

Thank You, Lord, for the hope You have promised—for something better.

BURTON A. BRIGGS

The Great Germ-warfare Battle

I will praise You, for I am fearfully and wonderfully
made; marvelous are Your works. Ps. 139:14, NKJV.

THE MORE I LEARN about my body and how God designed it to fight germs such as microorganisms, viruses, and bacteria, the more I praise God, for we are wonderfully made!

You cut your finger. Immediately you come under attack by germs that enter the cut and rapidly multiply. They multiply exponentially (two become four; four become 16). They secrete their toxins and, if allowed to reproduce, they cause a massive infection that can prove deadly.

Your white corpuscles are ready for such an invasion. A silent chemical alarm goes off when you cut your finger. The blood in the immediate area of the wound starts to get sticky. Blood cells hop up on the capillary vessel walls and slow down the blood. New blood cells keep arriving, making the area slightly swollen and tender. This is called an inflammatory response.

Within moments of being cut, your white blood cells crawl through the capillary walls. They leave the blood vessels and head for the site of the invasion where the battle rages. The first troops surround the invading germs and fight. Your white troops that die in battle become pus. The surviving troops continue to clean up the area until they have defeated the invaders.

Most of your immune cells are like foot soldiers who will go after anything that threatens you. You also have an elite killer force called lymphocytes. The elite combat officers are white blood cells that attack specific targets. You have four main categories of lymphocytes that come from the bone morrow: T-cells, B-cells, NK-cells, and macrophages. T-cells identify the invader and send a message either to the NK-cells to kill the invaders or to the B-cells to produce antibodies to immobilize or destroy the enemy.

Do you see why it's important to keep your immune system healthy by eating nutritious food, drinking enough water, getting adequate sleep, breathing fresh air, absorbing sunlight, and exercising? Why would anyone want to continue unhealthy habits such as smoking?

Your body is marvelously designed to fight off disease—if you'll just keep your blood cell army fit for battle.

Are there some changes you need to make in your life to ensure a healthier immune system? JAN W. KUZMA and CECIL MURPHEY

A Doer of Wonderful Works

The Pharisees said to Him, "Look, why do they do what is not lawful on the Sabbath?". . . And He said to them, "The Sabbath was made for man, and not man for the Sabbath." Mark 2:24-27, NKJV.

THE BEST MODEL for kindness, thoughtfulness, unselfishness, and generosity can be found in the life of Jesus Christ. The Jewish historian Josephus wrote: "Now, there was about this time, Jesus, a wise man, if it be lawful to call him a man, for he was a doer of wonderful works, a teacher of such men as receive the truth with pleasure. He drew over to him both many of the Jews, and many of the Gentiles. He was Christ."

Ponder the significance of the statement, "He was a doer of wonderful works." This reality was at the center of the debate over Christ's Sabbath miracles. In the beginning, within a six-day process God performed a series of miracles that produced a wonderful environment for human beings! The success of this undertaking was then celebrated by the institution of the Sabbath. While Christ walked on this earth He maintained that benevolent love and attachment to His creatures by reversing the debasing and destructive evidences of sin, including on the Sabbath. His goodness and tenderheartedness was clearly documented.

What does history record of the Pharisees, who seemed steeped in systems and structures that were devoid of moral obligations such as sympathy and genuine, disinterested love? There is no record of this group doing wonderful works! There is no history of this group ever impacting the lives of the hurting and the disenfranchised!

In Mark 2:23-3:6 we have an excellent description of Christ the Creator and His noble view of the Sabbath. Here He is portrayed as having sympathy for the hungry apostles as they pluck corn to eat, and compassionate concern for the man with the withered hand. On the other hand, there are the gazers—the religious leaders. In their own minds they may be worshipping, but hunger they do not feel and a withered hand they do not see.

They are so removed from these realities by the ivory castles of their own exclusivity that they are not able to embrace with the slightest bit of interest the human need of either of these situations. Condemnation therefore pours out of their mouths. They think they are worshiping God, but they are kneeling on the Sabbath at the foot of the idols of their own making.

Next Sabbath, what will you see? What will you do?

SAMUEL THOMAS, JR.

Spiritually Handicapped

*If you bite and devour one another, beware lest
you be consumed by one another! Gal. 5:15, NKJV.*

MY FRIEND JASON rides a motorized wheelchair, but he's a deep thinker
and knows his Bible. His legs don't work, but his spirit walks with God.
Last time I saw him, he asked me to pray that his problems won't make
him grow impatient and snap at those caring for him. That momentary
lack of gratitude and an occasional slide into depression seem to stem from
his physical challenges.

What deficiency interferes with your walk with God? Perhaps you
sometimes grow impatient and say things you shouldn't. Perhaps you are
so shy that you refuse to tell the good news to those who ask. Perhaps you
have a limp called lust, and you are easily led away by pornography. Perhaps you love money and don't want to share with those in need. Perhaps
you tend to argue during Bible study for the sake of argument. Perhaps you
dislike praise songs in preference for the grand old hymns—or vice versa.
Perhaps your deficiency is biblical literalism or an inability to accept any
Bible version but the King James. Perhaps you are overcome by your appetite. Perhaps you are addicted to television, sports, hobbies, work,
housecleaning, or yard work.

These are disabilities that, untreated, lead to sin. But consider this:
Some disabilities you can overcome, such as stuttering or lisping. Some disabilities you can learn to work around, such as a paralyzed muscle. If you
learn to surmount your spiritual disabilities, you may become a role model
for others. Overcomers make good teachers. They know what works.

The primary purpose of Alcoholics Anonymous is to minister to alcoholics and their families. Alcoholics attend regularly held meetings during
which they admit their weakness and ask a "higher power" for help. They
are strengthened by the support of other alcoholics who are also determined to be free of the slavery of alcohol.

Why can't the church be a sort of Sinners Anonymous? Why can't it
be a place where people can acknowledge their spiritual disabilities and
have someone place their hands on them and pray that the Master
Physician will give them strength to overcome sin?

We all have disabilities, but the closer we as church members press
together, the less often we'll fall. The further we walk together, following
our Good Shepherd, the stronger we'll grow.

*Think about it. We're all recovering sinners. What can you do today to grow
closer to your church family?*   ED CHRISTIAN

The Power of Early Training

Train a child in the way he should go, and when
he is old he will not turn from it. Prov. 22:6, NIV.

WHILE AT OUR children's grandparents' house for a visit we wanted to eat breakfast quickly because we had special plans for the day. Grandma kindly made oatmeal, with milk, sugar, and raisins. I began eating right away so that we could go soon. Our two girls (about 4 and 2) also began to eat, but then I noticed that the older one had quit eating. With urgency in my voice I asked, "Ruthie, why aren't you eating your oatmeal? We would like to leave soon."

Uninhibited as children often are, she blurted out loudly for all to hear, "I don't like it." Unexpected and embarrassing times like these are difficult. My initial instinct was to quiet her quickly, but instead I asked a question, "Why don't you like the oatmeal?"

Without hesitation she loudly explained, "It has sugar in it!" I had eaten oatmeal with sugar many times in the past so this dish was not unusual for me. But our children had never had sugar in their oatmeal. They would use bananas, raisins, or other fruit, and did not like the taste of sugar in their oatmeal!

What a lesson for me. Our children had adopted and enjoyed a dietary habit that others might consider restrictive. There is no moral law for or against sugar in oatmeal, but the laws of health suggest that less sugar is better. Were our children deprived? Of course not!

The average person in the United States eats about 35 teaspoons of sugar per day, or about 18 percent of their total calories. Such high sugar intake should be cause for concern because sugar is associated with dental caries, obesity, decreased resistance to infection, and diabetes, which increases in a population ingesting more than 10 percent of their calorie intake as sugar.

We need to educate our children by precept and example to have the best possible quality of life. Training them in health habits is beneficial for a lifetime. Training them to love Christ is for eternity. May parents have the fortitude to lead their children from infancy to love God and His ways with all their hearts! May God help us to instill within them principles of health and morality so that the body "may enjoy good health and that all may go well," even as God desires the soul to "[get] along well" (3 John 2, NIV).

Are you living the kind of life you would be proud to have others follow?

ALBERT SANCHEZ

When Good People Die

He said to me, "My grace is sufficient for you." 2 Cor. 12:9, NKJV.

TIM AND I WERE in Mayaguez, Puerto Rico, as student missionaries. At 11:30 p.m. the phone rang. We ignored it. No one ever called us at that time! Dr. Luthas answered, then called to me, "Dick, it's for you." I recognized the voice of Walt Blehm, a good family friend: "I have some bad news for you. Your mother has been killed in an automobile accident and your father is in critical condition in a California hospital. You better come home right away." I was shocked!

I didn't sleep that night. Instead, I thought about my parents. The more I thought, the angrier I became. Why was God taking away the two people I loved the most? How could Mom be gone? Why hadn't I had a chance to say goodbye? By morning I was little more than a confused set of frayed nerves. Dr. and Mrs. Luthas loaned me money for an airline ticket to San Juan, and I gave an agent a bad check for the flight to San Francisco. He said he would hold it for me for three days, until I could get the money to cover it.

I stared out the plane window without seeing America. I dug into my bag and took out a small copy of *The Living Prophecies,* Kenneth Taylor's Bible paraphrase. I read aimlessly. Then a phrase caught my heart: "The righteous pass away; the godly often die before their time. And no one seems to care or wonder why. No one seems to understand that God is protecting them from the evil to come. For the godly who die will rest in peace" (Isa. 57:1, 2). I underlined the verses.

"Are you OK?" A TWA stewardess knelt beside me. I mumbled something incoherent, and she sat down in the next seat. I tearfully poured out the whole story. "What are you reading?" she asked as she picked up my Bible. She then read the verses I had underlined, and pointed to the phrase, "God is protecting them from the evil to come."

"I don't know your mother," she said, "but I do know God, and I know that He can be trusted. Your mom is resting in peace—where God is protecting her from the trials ahead. That's reason for celebrating." She squeezed my hand and went on about her stewardess duties.

Dad came through the surgeries well, and is still preaching, teaching, and encouraging others.

Thank You, Lord, for protecting us in Your grace, in life as well as death.

DICK DUERKSEN

The Food Everybody Doesn't Need

For everyone who partakes only of milk is unskilled in the word of righteousness, for he is a babe. But solid food belongs to those who are of full age, that is, those who by reason of use have their senses exercised to discern both good and evil. Heb. 5:13, 14, NKJV.

GOOD HEALTH IS NOT the result of following tradition or taste; it is based on cooperating with the laws of health that God established when He created us. And milk wasn't on the original menu! Milk became popular after the Flood, when God gave man meat to eat because of the lack of fruits, vegetables, nuts, and grains. This secondary diet, however, was much inferior and resulted in drastically reducing the number of years that people lived.

The U.S. Government has now rejected the American Dairy Association's 1974 statement that "everybody needs milk." There are some dangers in eating dairy products, especially for children. The ADA won't tell you that cow's milk is associated with increased allergies, iron-deficiency anemia, lowered intelligence, milk sensitivities (chronic fatigue, tension headache, musculoskeletal pain, hyperactivity, bedwetting, aggravation of allergies and congestion, ear infections, asthma, and other respiratory difficulties), early atherosclerosis, juvenile diabetes, acne, rheumatoid arthritis, dental decay, and infectious diseases. Breast milk, however, provides a baby with the mother's antibodies and white blood cells, which fight infections. It contains lactoferrin, which tends to block the growth of E. Coli in the intestine, and it's usually sterile. There's a reason God created cow's milk for calves and breast milk for babies!

Milk is a controversial food. Low-fat milk is found among some "top 10" lists of healthy foods—primarily for its calcium. But most don't know that the high-protein content of milk causes loss of calcium! Dr. Neil Nedley says in his book *Proof Positive,* "The culmination of my extensive research on the subject of milk is that there is absolutely no reason why adult humans should feel that they need the milk of another species for health."

Since Bible times the health of animals has degenerated. There have been numerous scientific warnings about milk. Just knowing that Mad Cow disease can't be killed in the pasteurization process is enough to make me shy away! Do you need to drink milk? Probably not, if you believe God's original diet is best.

Are you drinking milk when you should be having solid food? Meditate on the message of Hebrews 5:13, 14. KAY KUZMA

Golden Years? Try Golden Moments!

O God, You have taught me from my youth; and to
this day I declare Your wondrous works. Now also when I am old
and grayheaded, O God, do not forsake me. Ps. 71:17, 18, NKJV.

A FEW YEARS AGO I accepted without question the term "golden years" for describing the time following retirement. I didn't realize it was a euphemism. Along with the majority in our society, I was not consumed with a desire to consider what life was like for the old—or to become old myself. A few months ago I asked a friend in her 80s, "How are you?" She answered with a gracious smile, "I'm feeling my age." Visiting a woman in the hospital, I hinted broadly that I would be interested in knowing how old she was. "Well, age is only a number, and mine is unlisted" was her response.

Our language lacks adequate words to describe old age. Writer Mark Gerson suggests that "growing whole" is a much better way to describe aging than "growing old." The human spirit is central, not the body. Golden time is possible in retirement years for those who successfully stay "young." For those who have lost their health, the struggle for golden time can be uphill. How is it possible to have golden time when you can't hear or be heard? How is it possible to have golden time when you must call another to assist you in everything you do?

I found part of the answer when with new eyes I read 2 Corinthians 4:16: "Though outwardly we are wasting away, yet inwardly we are being renewed day by day" (NIV). This is what Mark Gerson must have meant when he suggested the term "growing whole."

I wrote in my journal that day: "God give me the grace not to talk about the wear and tear of life on my body. May I concentrate on the growth of my soul and not the decay of my body. May I focus on new experiences of grace to share with others. May I accept outward physical changes and live so as to keep decay minimal while remembering that some things are only awkward and inconvenient. May I find people to share this outlook with. May I claim Your compassion in my dealings with others. May I not minimize their aches and pains but remind them of One who will give them the grace to live above their aging bodies. And may I resolve to do more to bring golden moments into the lives of others—especially the old who are often ill and lonely.

Life will not always be golden on this earth, but I will not wear dark glasses to hide the gold that is around me.

Be on the lookout for golden moments. Recognize and claim them, and resolve to share them. JOYCE RIGSBY

Saving the Lost

The Son of man is come to save that which was lost. Matt. 18:11.

THERE ARE MANY areas in your mouth where you probably do not remove the bacterial plaque effectively when you brush or floss your teeth. That's why you need periodic dental checkups!

In between the teeth and around the gums are the places most frequently missed. Bacterial plaque especially likes to get into the gum pocket or collar of the gum tissues surrounding the teeth. This causes the gum tissue to become swollen from the irritants produced by the plaque bacteria. As the gums swell they become detached from the tooth, allowing a gum pocket to form. This pocket fills up with more plaque; even your toothbrush bristles and floss will not remove it. This is how periodontal (gum) disease begins.

Periodontal disease continues to damage your gums and teeth because you are unable to remove the plaque from the gum pocket. After a period of time the bony tissue surrounding the tooth will be destroyed. This leads to advanced periodontal disease. If enough bone is lost, the teeth start to move and can become so loose they sometimes fall out on their own!

Periodontal disease can lead to serious problems. I tell my patients that if they have lost their teeth because the bone is gone from around them, they have also lost their bone! They usually don't think about the significance of bone loss if they want partial or full dentures. But the question is what bone will they have left to support the dentures?

There are treatments for periodontal disease, but there is no cure. Only preventive maintenance by your hygienist or dentist can help prevent it. If the disease becomes advanced there are surgeries that may help save your teeth. But your dentist can't always work miracles and save that which you have lost through negligence and poor diet.

Fortunately, that's not the case when we are suffering from spiritual disease. Satan tries to be a destructive force in our life and hides his true intent for us, like the plaque hidden in the gum pocket. He does damage deep down by hurting us emotionally and spiritually, where we have a hard time reaching. But Jesus, our Savior, can restore that which we have lost through our foolish, sinful behavior. If we go to Him, He can be our prevention and cure for the sin problem.

Thank You, Jesus, for saving us! Regardless of how hopeless you may feel your sin problem is, Jesus can save you. All you have to do is ask. Why not do it now!

EDDIE C. TOWLES

What Alzheimer's Does to the Brain

You will keep him in perfect peace, whose mind is
stayed on You, because he trusts in You. Isa. 26:3, NKJV.

WHEN YOU THINK of Alzheimer's, the faces of Ronald Reagan or Charlton Heston may come to mind. Patti Davis, the daughter of Ronald and Nancy Reagan, writes that there is another way that faces tell the story of Alzheimer's: "In the early stages of Alzheimer's the eyes have a wariness, a veil of fear. It's as if the person is standing at the edge of a fogbank, knowing that in time it will engulf him and there is no chance of outrunning it. I used to see my father's eyes simultaneously plead and hold firm. It would happen when a sentence broke off because he couldn't remember how to finish it. Or when he would say, 'I have this condition—I keep forgetting things.'. . . Slowly—sometimes over months, sometimes years—the eyes stop pleading. There is a resignation, an acceptance of distance, strangeness, a life far from home. You know the look when you see it, and the only mercy is that fear seems to have subsided."

Alzheimer's is characterized by the gradual spread of sticky plaques and clumps of tangled fibers that disrupt the delicate organization of nerve cells in the brain. As brain cells stop communicating with one another, they atrophy, causing memory and reasoning to fade. The brain shrinks in size and weight, and the once-tightly packed grooves on the surface become pitted with gaps and crevices. Other than this, we know precious little about this terrible illness, which threatens to strike some 14 million Americans by 2050. But we're beginning to get a handle on it. The Nun Study, conducted by Dr. David Snowdon (who was previously involved in the Adventist Health Study), has shown that a history of stroke and head trauma can boost your chances of coming down with Alzheimer's. On the other hand, a college education and an active intellectual life may actually protect you. After analyzing short autobiographies of almost 200 nuns, written when they first took holy orders, Dr. Snowden found that the sisters who had used more complex sentence structure and concepts, and those who had, as girls, expressed the most positive emotions in their writing, lived the longest.

Inasmuch as it is through our brains that the Holy Spirit speaks to us, how important it is to protect them from injury, to keep them actively challenged—and to think positively!

I can't think of a better way to keep positive than to keep one's mind on Christ;
can you? KAY KUZMA

Get Rid of It!

You were taught, with regard to your former way of life, to put off your old self, which is being corrupted by its deceitful desires; to be made new in the attitude of your minds; and to put on the new self, created to be like God in true righteousness and holiness. Eph. 4:22-24, NIV.

THE MEMORY IS AS vivid as this morning's breakfast and brings with it a chuckle. Two newlyweds with a $50 Pontiac, the smallest enclosed U-Haul available, and all the wedding gifts and possessions we owned, traveled expectantly to our first apartment.

More than 34 years and 22 moves later the stuff in our one-car garage would fill that little U-Haul! As we have moved during our college and pastoral years, we have accumulated many treasures—our children's mementos, our books, furniture and china, wardrobe, and on and on.

On several occasions, we have endeavored to weed out unnecessary things, but that is almost a useless task. Our married daughters have inherited some of the items they cherish; we have shared with others, donated to Community Services and Goodwill, and filled the trash receptacle often.

God's counsel for this situation is: "Do not store up for yourselves treasures on earth, where moth and rust destroy, and where thieves break in and steal" (Matt. 6:19, NIV).

Many of us store up other kinds of trash—the garbage of bitterness, rage, anger, malice, brawling, slander—those items Paul counsels us to "get rid of" in Ephesians 4:31 (NIV). These feelings and attitudes become idols that we worship as if they were silver and gold. Often we accumulate people who we demand will provide us with safety and certainty, fulfilling our deepened desires. Whether it's things, attitudes, or people, we turn from God to these to fulfill our needs, and find that these desperately disappoint us.

Is the prospect of giving up your treasures frightening? Do you fear that giving up your attitudes will leave you too vulnerable to attack? Have negative tactics for meeting your needs characterized who you are, and you fear identity loss if you should give them to God?

Actually, if you are willing to dump the trash, God will replace it with the treasure of His love, which, shining out through you will become the new you.

Are you holding on to something that might be hindering you from becoming the person God wants you to be?   RON and NANCY ROCKEY

Don't Be Buffaloed Into Rejecting God's Hope Option

No test or temptation that comes your way is beyond the course of what others have had to face. All you need to remember is that God will never let you down; he'll never let you be pushed past your limit; he'll always be there to help you come through it. 1 Cor. 10:13, Message.

WHY DOES IT seem so easy to become discouraged and so hard to accept God's hope option? I think the enemy has most of us buffaloed!

American Indians used to get meat for the winter by driving buffalo off the top of bluffs. The rocks below are still littered with bones.

No, buffalo (bison) are not stupid, but the Indians were smart. The entire village would line up across the prairie, forming a giant funnel that had its small opening at the top of a cliff. A few of the braves would steal into a buffalo herd and begin a stampede toward the waiting tribe. Startled by the Indians jumping, waving blankets, and shouting, the buffalo ran faster and faster. The result was "fast food" at the bottom of the cliff.

Life today has many of us stumbling along with our herd, dashing too fast, answering too many phones, disconnected from loved ones, rushing toward somewhere and doing something that seems important at the moment. We're overwhelmed, like stampeding buffalo that an enemy has frightened away from what is meaningful. But *stop!* There is an alternative! God offers full safety from the enemy. You can find *focus* instead of *distraction, calm* instead of *frenzy, hope* instead of *death.* Listen to God. He has a hope-filled promise for you that can keep you safe from the enemy. *Listen:*

Along with every temptation, I will provide a way of escape (1 Cor. 10:13).

I am a place of protection. Good people can run here and be safe (Prov. 18:10).

"Come to me, all of you who are weary and burdened, and I will give you rest" (Matt. 11:28, NIV).

When you're down in the dumps, remember Me. I love you all day and am singing your song all night. I will put a smile on your face! (Ps. 42:5-10).

This alternative is far superior to the cliffs of discouragement and depression. In fact, accepting God's hope option is rather like standing out in the wide open space of God's glory and grace and shouting His praise! *Hallelujah!*

What should you do today to avoid being driven over the cliffs of discouragement?

DICK DUERKSEN

Thinking Right

And do not be conformed to this world, but be
transformed by the renewing of your mind. Rom. 12:2, NKJV.

INTERESTING RESEARCH has been done on the cerebral lateralization of the brain. Scientists have found that the two sides of the human brain function differently from each other. The left mode is generally analytical, verbal, factual, logical, scientific, temporal, and punctual. The right mode is more visual, spatial, nonverbal, intuitive, color-conscious, emotional, nontemporal, nonpunctual. The way we think affects many things, including our actions and our ideas about politics and religion. Some people are more right-brained, others are more left-brained.

There's an old Chinese saying, "He who has imagination without learning has wings but no feet." Can you see the left and right mode function in this? "He who has imagination [R] without learning [L] has wings [R] but no feet [L]."

To be right-brained, creative, artistic, musical, and imaginative is wonderful. It's thinking the way an artist thinks. It's doing your own thing, but it's not everything. A bird may fly, glide, and soar with his wings, but when he gets hungry, without feet he'd have a difficult time in landing and getting food. We need balance. Both sides are good and useful.

Now let me take this concept a step further. I propose that *proof* is to the left mode what *conviction* is to the right. *Facts* are to the left what *faith* is to the right. *Doctrines, proof texts,* and *logical persuasions* are to the left what *experience* and *experiential knowledge* are to the right.

For what did the martyrs die? The facts, proof texts, doctrines of their faith, *and* their experiential relationship with Jesus Christ. They never would have died for facts and doctrines alone. We need a balance. We need that good old disciplined training: texts, history, doctrines. But we also need a living, exciting relationship with the One the Scripture study is all about.

Here's an interesting thought: "He who places himself unreservedly under the guidance of the Spirit of God will find that his mind expands and develops. He obtains an education in the service of God which is not one-sided and deficient, developing a one-sided character, but one which results in symmetry and completeness"(Ellen G. White, *Selected Messages,* book 1, p. 338). That should be our goal.

What could you do to become a more balanced thinker? ELFRED LEE

Rightly Dividing the Book of Nature

*Study to shew thyself approved unto God, a workman that needeth
not to be ashamed, rightly dividing the word of truth. 2 Tim. 2:15.*

TEN-YEAR-OLD JULIE had been to the doctor more than 20 times since the age of 1, taking numerous rounds of antibiotics, mainly for earaches. The doctor bills were overwhelming. Since cold weather began, Julie had seen the doctor one to three times a month. In January, the pediatrician said Julie had to take another round of antibiotics and then have tubes put in her eardrums because of the thick secretions behind the drums.

Julie's mother felt she needed a second opinion and called me. I suggested she keep Julie's extremities clothed well, avoid sweets, have her drink plenty of water to keep the secretions thin, and avoid milk products. Milk gives many children secretions too thick to pass from the middle ear through the eustachian tube to the throat, causing the fluid to build up behind the drums.

For weeks we heard nothing. Then in May, the mother called to say Julie had gone for five months with no earaches! She exclaimed, "Such simple things with such good results!"

Three months later Julie contracted a bad case of poison ivy. When the pediatrician saw her she exclaimed, "Why, I haven't seen Julie since January. That last course of antibiotics must have cleared up the germs causing all those earaches."

"No," her mother answered. "I felt uncomfortable with Julie taking antibiotics so often, so I called for a second opinion, and the physician recommended she stop drinking milk. Since then Julie has not had a single earache." The doctor seemed pleased and remarked, "Yes, that can do it." And added, "Milk sensitivity is probably the commonest cause of middle ear infections in children."

If a child has more than two colds in one winter, we suspect milk sensitivity. Replace milk with greens, whole grains, legumes (beans and peas), or fortified soy milk. Children quickly adapt to the change, and love the freedom from colds and earaches.

Being a Christian parent leads one into a relationship with God that opens up lines of study into two important books—the Bible and God's book of nature. Both must be read prayerfully and carefully to discern truth and find healing. Soon the world will be healed of all sin and disease—and children will have no more earaches! Oh, glorious day!

Thank You, wise God, for providing two important books to help us find healing truth. AGATHA THRASH

OCTOBER 15

Energized by Eating the Word

Your words were found, and I ate them, and Your word was to me the joy and rejoicing of my heart; for I am called by Your name, O Lord God of hosts. Jer. 15:16, NKJV.

NOTHING COULD BE more mundane and universal than eating. Yet everyone loves it! If only we loved the eating of the Word as well!

Eating is a fine art in the Orient, where the proper balancing of different kinds of foods is important: salty, sweet, spicy, sour. M-m-m, what might the Word look like as a sample menu? Piquant Proverbs Appetizers; Fragrant Genesis Soup; Kings and Chronicles Fiber-rich Salad; Isaiah Sweet-and-Sour; Four-Gospel Casserole; Revelation Rhubarb Pie; Creme Brûlée à la Galatians; Philippians Sparkling Beverage! Have you eaten a healthy balance today?

What it takes to enjoy eating the Word is similar to what it takes to enjoy food.

"Your words were found." Real food preparation requires personal effort. "Finding" entails seeking, and seeking takes time. Food preparation demands time, with appropriate tools and a strong flame. You've got to put yourself into the cooking before you put the cooking into you! Do you see the parallel to Bible study?

"I ate them." To eat means to put food in your mouth, chew, and swallow. Fiber-rich food yields only to patient mastication. Preparation remains unfulfilled purpose until the food touches your tongue, teeth, and stomach. And just as physical digestion can be hindered by distractions, trying to do too many things at once also hinders the digestion of the Word.

"Your word was to me the joy and rejoicing of my heart." You can't taste how good a dish is until your nose, lips, and tongue have done their work. Only then can a deep savoring sigh and a smile emerge. Real joy is a whole-body experience.

Ingest the Word; put the Word in you as you put yourself in the Word. For example, put your name into Psalm 91:14-16 and experience the energizing effect. "Because [your name] has set [her] love upon Me, therefore I will deliver [her]: I will set [name] on high, because she has known My name. [Name] shall call upon me and I will answer [her]: I will be with [name] in trouble; I will deliver [her], and honor [her]. With long life will I satisfy [name], and show [her] my salvation" (NKJV).

Did you feel energized after reading yourself into Scripture? That's what eating the Word is all about!   RUTH E. BURKE

Promises to Keep

I sought the Lord, and He heard me, and delivered me from all my fears. Ps. 34:4, NKJV.

"ABRAHAM! ABRAHAM!" "Who are you?" "It's the Lord." "What do You want?"

"Leave your country, your people and your father's household and go to the land I will show you" (Gen. 12:1, NIV).

Abraham grabbed hold of God's stupendous promises and took off on a life detour as the most colossal dare-taker in salvation history. He never imagined he'd spend the next 115 years existing on nothing but promises.

Then the critical act in the drama: "Abraham!"

"Yes, God?"

"Take your son, your only son, Isaac . . . Sacrifice him there as a burnt offering" (Gen. 22:2, NIV). As Abraham trudges toward Moriah in obedience to God, his mind flashes back to his fears when he first got to the Promised Land. *Famine. Pull up stakes. Move down to Egypt. Live by your wits. Lie to Pharaoh to save your neck.* His fears got him into trouble. Then he remembers another night when he threw Molotov cocktails at Chedorlaomar and the Palestinian border patrol. He came home quaking so badly God had to appear to him in vision (see Genesis 15). And now Satan presses, "Abraham, you're no man of faith. Remember your tryst with Hagar? You trusted righteousness by virility. Salvation by sperm. This trip to Moriah? You're going to offer a human sacrifice after all these years you've preached to the heathen? No, Abraham. Go home." Abraham was scared.

Have you ever been so frightened you were paralyzed? For me, it was June 1978. I was 31 years old. The dreaded words: Cancer . . . Melanoma . . . Fourth level. I'll never forget Jeannie and me slumping to our knees and crying out, "O God, no! We're scared. Am I going to die? Lord, speak to us!" And more recently an AVM (arteriovenous malfunction). For nine months I had a terrific pounding inside my head. Doctors couldn't find the problem until specialists at Loma Linda University Medical Center diagnosed a rare "dural fistula"—just in time to save my life. We wrestled with God. I claimed Psalm 34:4, and we found God was faithful.

You know the end of Abraham's dilemma—he raises his dagger and begins to bring it down on his son when an invisible force stays his arm. Then the voice: "Abraham! Stop! It is enough!" And God Himself provided a lamb! He had a plan, just as He had one for Abraham—and for me.

God has a plan for you, too. Don't be afraid. Believe Him when He says, "Trust Me."
LONNIE MELASHENKO

What You Can Tell by the Handwriting

Jesus continued to develop physically, to increase in wisdom and to mature in His relationships with God and man. Luke 2:52, Clear Word.

ADVENT HOME IN Calhoun, Tennessee, is a live-in school for 12- to 16-year-old boys with learning difficulties, often termed attention deficit hyperactivity disorder (ADHD). In general, these boys are brighter than the average but, for different reasons, they are usually one to four years behind in basic skills such as math, spelling, writing, and reading.

Steve was 12 years old when he came to the Advent Home. He was behind in his social and academic skills. He was a glutton, his hygiene was poor, he got into fights, and did poorly in school. After three months in the program, his parents observed that the letters he was sending home showed improved handwriting. His mother told me she appreciated the fact that we were teaching her son good handwriting skills. I told her that the quality of Steve's handwriting reflected his emotional state of mind rather than training.

If a child is anxious, stressed, fearful, or depressed, it could show up in handwriting (as well as behaviors such as accident-proneness, untidiness, tardiness, and poor eating habits). As a general observation, the more anxious a person, the more terrible his handwriting might become.

Children who are abused or over-disciplined by too strict and inflexible parents tend to get discouraged; their initiative is stifled. Excessive and continuous loud music, habitually staying up late, long hours on computer games, indulgence in idleness, are symptomatic of emotional problems.

At the Advent Home, one way we help students develop mental health is to provide them a minimum-distraction environment. Home should be peaceful, happy, interactive, and safe. It should be free from excessive noise from radio or TV and overindulgences in eating, interactive games, or internet access. Steve's handwriting was improving because he had found a place where he could talk, express his feelings, ask questions, and get answers. He was given meaningful work and chores to do. He interacted with adults who role-modeled proper adult behaviors.

Jesus' growth was a harmonious development of all His faculties. This should be the model for every parent-child relationship.

How emotionally healthy is your home environment for growing children? Could you envision Jesus growing up there?   BLONDEL E. SENIOR

True Source of Healing

And in the thirty-ninth year of his reign, Asa became diseased in his feet,
and his malady was severe; yet in his disease he did not seek the Lord, but
the physicians. So Asa rested with his fathers. 2 Chron. 16:12, 13, NKJV.

ONE OF MY MORE humbling days as a physician came from reading the nursing notes in the chart of one of my patients: "Dr. Wise in to see patient. Appears confused." I never had the courage to ask the nurse if the subject of the second sentence was the patient, or myself!

Certainly medicine has become increasingly complex and sophisticated. Many people think that with today's wonderful technology virtually no one should die prematurely. The danger that doctors and other healthcare professionals face is to become seduced into believing that it's the pills and the machines that save lives, not God. Medical students and residents commonly state on rounds, "We gave the patient antibiotics, and he's responding well." They sometimes fail to recall that for thousands of years before the discovery of antibiotics, patients often recovered from pneumonia. The body's natural healing power and God's intervention are rarely considered.

Physicians may come to believe that their "M. Deity" degree is a substitute for faith and prayer. Likewise, patients may pour more faith, trust, and money into the quick fix promised by expensive machines and magic pills than they do into right living, healthy lifestyles, and divine power.

King Asa was the great-grandson of the wisest man who ever lived, Solomon, but he paid the consequences of misdirecting his trust away from God. Admittedly, in his day the practice of medicine was rudimentary at best and fatal at worst. Not so very long ago physicians were treating patients with "state of the art" techniques such as bloodletting, purging, strychnine, and leeches. Although medical science has advanced markedly in recent years, all will eventually sleep with their fathers. Even Lazarus died a second time. Science has not changed the final fact that we are all mortal.

God is our only source of peace in this life and security of immortality in the next. Because of sin, bad things do happen to good people. Despite the "slings and arrows of outrageous fortune" that may befall us our confidence in God's love and care must never be shaken. May we remember to give all praise, honor, and glory to the true source of our healing and comfort—the Great Physician.

Father God, we praise, honor, and glorify You as the true source of our healing and comfort. GREGORY R. WISE

OCTOBER 19

How God Helped Me Fight Depression

I prayed to the Lord, and He answered me. He delivered me from all
my fears. . . . Taste and find out for yourself how good God is.
Happy is the man who takes refuge in the Lord. Ps. 34:4-8, Clear Word.

LOOKING BACK, I think I was mildly depressed from the time I was 16 years old. I was always very quiet and didn't know how to chit-chat with friends; I didn't know what to say to people.

This problem became compounded with the extreme stress I came under at my job. My depression started escalating about seven years before I was laid off. During the last year I was on the job I became extremely depressed. I could hardly function. I could not make decisions—when I went out on a business call it would take me several minutes to decide if I should turn left or right to get out of the parking lot. I felt very alone; my heart felt empty, even while playing with my grandson. I didn't want to be around family or friends; I cried a lot; I had no motivation.

When I was laid off I was actually relieved to be getting away from my stressful job. I saw the Lord's hand in it because a doctor had told me shortly before, "Don't be afraid to lose your job." I decided to listen to that advice and to trust in God. By doing so, I saw miracles happen in my life. As I packed up my desk my coworkers told me I was "glowing."

I helped in my own recovery by getting out more with my friends and reaching out to help others. At times I still experience moments when I forget to trust in the Lord to help me, and I slide into depression over some disappointment. I will feel as though life is hopeless and I am alone. But after a day or so I sit down and read my Bible and pray to the Lord to lift my burden. When I allow myself to let go of my problem, it seems He always leads me to the right Bible verse that will give me comfort or suggest a solution.

Now I praise Him for all things, including the depression I went through. I am a very happy, outgoing person. God has changed me. I'm a living example of the fulfillment of Isaiah 40:31: "Those who hope in the Lord will renew their strength. They will soar on wings like eagles; they will run and not grow weary, they will walk and not be faint" (NIV).

So, "Do not be afraid or discouraged, for the Lord is the one who goes before you. He will be with you; he will neither fail you nor forsake you" (Deut. 31:8, NLT).

God changes things—even you and me!   DIANE BURRIS

A Second Chance

The road to life is a disciplined life; ignore correction
and you're lost for good. Prov. 10:17, Message.

AT AGE 55 CONNIE was in bad shape. She had coronary heart disease, gout, hypertension, diabetes, depression, and was overweight. She had been told by her physicians that there was nothing more they could do for her. She had received a triple coronary bypass and then, four years later, an angioplasty. She was taking 27 pills and 60 units of insulin each day. She couldn't walk more than 100 yards without popping nitroglycerine pills. Her heart was so fragile her cardiologist forbade her to fly—which meant canceling her plans to spend the winter in Florida. She was so depressed and felt like such a drag on her family that she asked her husband to put her into a nursing home.

Instead, he enrolled her in the Coronary Heart Improvement Project's (CHIP) 40-hour lifestyle change seminar. Grasping at any straw of hope, Connie began living a natural, plant-based nutritional lifestyle. No more meat, dairy products, eggs, and soda. She substituted fresh fruits and vegetables for refined sugars and processed foods, and upped the consumption of grains.

Six months later she was down to three pills a day, her insulin had been cut in half, and she was walking three miles a day and swimming regularly. Her weight had normalized. Instead of being depressed, she went on a health cruise to Alaska. Most of her pain was gone. Instead of $490 a month for medications, her bill was now $80 a month.

Asked how her physician reacted, Connie said, "My doctor was very skeptical at first. Later his eyes widened in disbelief, and he began to inquire about the nutritional and lifestyle aspects of the program. Some of my specialists are quite excited and have even referred some of their patients to me in hopes that I might be able to motivate them and provide some education."

Ten years later Connie is still healthy and strong. Last Christmas she and her husband sent a postcard from Perth, Australia. "We're just leaving for Hong Kong, and not by boat. We're thankful to God for leading us to a new lifestyle and giving us a second chance at life."

The restorative power that God has put into the human body is incredible; if only we would treat it as God designed!

Do you agree that "the road to life is a disciplined life"? If so, is there any area *in your life that could use a little more discipline?*　　　HANS DIEHL

Big Brother

*Greater love has no one than this, than to lay
down one's life for his friends. John 15:13, NKJV.*

I BENT PAINFULLY low in order to look directly into the dirty, Kool Aid-stained face. "Hey, big guy! What's your name?" I asked. No reply. His wide, green eyes told me enough.

My monstrous 73-inch frame had intruded into his fragile world beneath the brown card table. Softly I said, "My name's Adam."

A testy voice interrupted. "His name Jordan; he my cousin." I turned to face the speaker, a skinny 7-year-old girl. She told me a little about the boy beneath the table and her role in watching out for him.

"Jordan. That's a really cool name," I said, turning back to him. His fear-stricken eyes continued to stare at me as I plopped myself down in front of him. Nothing I said seemed to breach Jordan's frightened speechlessness. I reached into the depths of my boggled mind in an effort to say something that would elicit response. He gave no audible reply then, but little by little I earned his trust. Then one day I succeeded in drawing him from his shelter. As I read to him, he began to scoot closer to me. I extended my hand to him, and I felt his short, grubby fingers grasp it apprehensively. I hesitated a moment before pulling him close, then I draped my arm around him, and he timidly snuggled into the contours of my body. Over the course of several weeks he began to trust me more and more, but never completely.

To see Jordan laugh and smile was a great relief, but I often felt an overwhelming sense of anger and frustration. I was incensed with the individuals who would allow a young child to be denied what he yearned for most—love, understanding, and a gentle touch. My personal problems with calculus, and my need for a car seemed so trivial. Jordan's life had been emotionally devastating. He had been neglected, abused, ignored.

Interacting with Jordan led me to reason that nothing I would achieve in my life would be of any worth or meaning if I was not prepared to use it to help end such appalling wrongs. Fifty years from now I will be able to look back with gratitude upon my accomplishments only if I have used my education and acquired skills to help eliminate human suffering.

What could you do today to help eliminate the suffering of one of God's children? (They come in all sizes and ages!) ADAM DAVID GETCHELL

When Hurting, Help Others

Is it not to share your bread with the hungry, and that you bring to your house the poor who are cast out; when you see the naked, that you cover him, and not hide yourself from your own flesh? Isa. 58:7, NKJV.

ONE OF THE SUREST hindrances to the recovery of the sick is the centering of attention upon themselves. Many invalids feel that everyone should give them sympathy and help, when what they need is to have their attention turned away from themselves, to think of and care for others. . . .

While we offer prayer for these sorrowful ones, we should encourage them to try to help those more needy than themselves. The darkness will be dispelled from their own hearts as they try to help others. . . .

The fifty-eighth chapter of Isaiah is a prescription for maladies of the body and of the soul. If we desire health and the true joy of life we must put into practice the rules given in this scripture. . . .

Good deeds are twice a blessing, benefiting both the giver and the receiver of the kindness. The consciousness of right-doing is one of the best medicines for diseased bodies and minds. When the mind is free and happy from a sense of duty well done and the satisfaction of giving happiness to others, the cheering, uplifting influence brings new life to the whole being.

Let the invalid, instead of constantly requiring sympathy, seek to impart it. Let the burden of your own weakness and sorrow and pain be cast upon the compassionate Savior. Open your heart to His love, and let it flow out to others. Remember that all have trials hard to bear, temptations hard to resist, and you may do something to lighten these burdens. Express gratitude for the blessings you have; show appreciation of the attentions you receive. Keep the heart full of the precious promises of God, that you may bring forth from this treasure, words that will be a comfort and strength to others. This will surround you with an atmosphere that will be helpful and uplifting. Let it be your aim to bless those around you, and you will find ways of being helpful, both to the members of your own family and to others.

If those who are suffering from ill-health would forget self in their interest for others; if they would fulfill the Lord's command to minister to those more needy than themselves, they would realize the truthfulness of the prophetic promise, "Then shall thy light break forth as the morning, and thine health shall spring forth speedily" (Isa. 58:8, KJV).

ELLEN G. WHITE—*The Ministry of Healing*, pp. 256-258.

305

Fresh-air Addiction

*Hear me, O Judah and you inhabitants of Jerusalem: Believe in
the Lord your God, and you shall be established; believe
His prophets, and you shall prosper. 2 Chron. 20:20, NKJV.*

A COMMON BELIEF in the 1800s was that fresh air was harmful to one's health. Windows were shut tight at night, and the sick were kept indoors. That's when Ellen White, inspired by God, started debunking many of the "health" practices of her day. She wrote: "Air is the free blessing of heaven, calculated to electrify the whole system. Without it the system will be filled with disease and become dormant, languid, feeble" (*Testimonies for the Church*, vol. 1, p. 701).

"The lungs are constantly throwing off impurities, and they need to be constantly supplied with fresh air. . . . To live in close, ill-ventilated rooms, where the air is dead and vitiated, weakens the entire system" (*The Ministry of Healing*, p. 274).

I believe it is vital to be exposed to oxygen-laden air even at night, summer and winter. It's amazing how quickly the air in a room becomes "electrified" when a window is open just a crack.

Without fresh air our bodies would be filled with disease and become dormant, languid, and feeble. Why? Impure air, in which the ions are positively charged, restricts the absorption of oxygen, so essential to life. Without oxygen not a cell of our bodies can live. Without it we cannot have healthy blood, clear thinking, or good circulation.

An excess of positive ions causes overproduction of a stress hormone, serotonin. Too much of it in the bloodstream causes anxiety, insomnia, migraine headaches, and sudden mood changes. Recently it has been discovered that a lack of oxygen in the blood causes the platelets to stick together, which can contribute to heart attacks. Pure air is the first of the eight laws of health written about by Ellen White.

Is it any wonder that man's first home was outdoors, where life-giving oxygen, the gift of our Creator, was free and abundant? Since the earth is always negatively charged, it is good to live away from inner cities, and to have health resorts located near waterfalls, seashores, forests, and mountains. Even a small concentration of negative ions can kill airborne bacteria that cause colds, flu, and other respiratory problems. Daily exposure to pure fresh air will supply the oxygen so vital to radiant health. It's one of heaven's richest blessings.

Have you breathed deeply of God's good fresh air today?

MARCELLA HARROM

Death on Highway 285

God is our refuge and strength, a very present help in trouble. Ps. 46:1.

TERRY AND I WAVED goodbye to family in Michigan and headed west in our 1970 Chevy Nova to attend college in Gunnison, Colorado. Married just one week, we were excited as we anticipated facing the world together, along with our little kitten, Small Fry.

Northeast of Denver we heard a noise from under the car. Terry stopped and reattached the exhaust pipe. A few miles later it fell off again. By this time it was dark, and I begged Terry to stop and take a motel. In the morning, with the tail pipe attached once again, we drove past Denver and onto Highway 285 to wind our way up the mountain. Rain had started to fall so we rolled up the windows. Little did we know that that simple act would almost cause our demise.

Soon Terry complained of a terrible headache and was sick to his stomach. He asked me to drive. I, too, was beginning to have a headache, rare for me. Terry became violently ill, throwing up, passing out, coming to, throwing up again and passing out. Frantic, I pulled over to flag down help. No one came! Terry was turning blue and stopped breathing. My strong husband was dead!

With no help available, I headed for the nearest town. Small Fry also was acting strangely, jumping up on the seat and onto me. I pushed the cat away and kept driving. "Lord, I don't know what's happening. Save my husband. Help me find someone who can help us!" An hour later I drove into a gas station in Buena Vista, nearly taking down the pumps. I jumped out of the car and yelled at the attendant, "My husband is dead in the front seat. I don't know what's happening to us!" A doctor and his wife, a nurse, who were paying for their gas, immediately recognized the symptoms of carbon monoxide poisoning. They carried Terry inside and began administering oxygen. It took more than 30 minutes for Terry to respond. Then they gave oxygen to me and Small Fry.

The miracle of the story was that I had passed up five stations on my way into town and stopped at the only one that had oxygen available—with a physician and nurse paying for their gas at the exact moment of my arrival.

The devil is just like that odorless, tasteless poisonous gas that attaches to the red blood cells, preventing them from carrying oxygen to the body, causing people to fall asleep and die without realizing what's happening. He's trying to plot our demise without us realizing it!

Never forget, regardless of what the devil might throw at you, God is in charge.

NANCY NELSON

Wounded Hands

Babylon will suddenly fall and be broken. Wail over her! Get balm for her pain; perhaps she can be healed. . . . "The Lord has vindicated us; come, let us tell in Zion what the Lord our God has done." Jer. 51:8-10, NIV.

WHEN I WAS 7 years old, my brother and I were watching my dad burning brush in the backyard and throwing grass and sticks into the flames.

Eventually one of us found a long pipe and put one end of it into the fire to see if smoke would come out the other end. Sure enough, after a while smoke started curling out of the end that lay in the grass.

Not understanding the laws of physics—that if one end of the pipe was hot the other would be too—I picked up the end lying in the grass. I firmly grabbed it with both hands. The pipe was so hot it literally fried the palms of my hands and the insides of my fingers. I experienced the most vivid sensation of pain I had ever felt, and I let out a scream that must have been heard down the block!

Mom and Dad came running and tried to relieve my suffering. Dad put salve on my hands and assured me that everything would be all right. Sure enough, the pain of that experience is now but a distant memory. What mattered most to me as an injured child was that my daddy was there to reassure me and soothe my wounded hands with salve.

Pain is an ever-present reality on this planet. Like our shadow, it follows us wherever we go, sometimes making itself more felt than at other times. As we mature, we discover new kinds of pain that go much deeper than our surface skin, that penetrate our innermost souls and wring out our hearts! Divorce, death, racism, abuse, loss of employment, and disease—all strike at the very heart of human optimism and dare us to find joy in their presence.

When we are in pain it's comforting to know that our heavenly Father surrounds us with His wounded hands. Lovingly He assures us, whatever the hurt, that one day it will be just a distant memory. He doesn't tell us to stop crying. Instead He gives us a shoulder to cry on and covers our wounds with His healing balm.

Is there something in your life that is causing you pain? Let your heavenly Father soothe it with His healing balm. RICH DuBOSE

Praise the Lord!

I will praise You, O Lord, with my whole heart; I will tell of all Your marvelous works. I will be glad and rejoice in You; I will sing praise to Your name, O Most High. Ps. 9:1, 2, NKJV.

"HURRY!" IT WAS just a couple hours before flight time, and we still had to pick up a satellite dish to take back to Tennessee. I had the address, but we had difficulty finding the place; finally we found it, only to discover the dish wasn't packed for shipping. Frantically we created a makeshift box and taped it all together. At the ramp onto the freeway we encountered a major traffic jam. We chose to take an alternate route—but hit all red lights.

Breathlessly we ran into the terminal just 15 minutes before flight time, but there was a long line of passengers waiting to be checked in. I stepped to the front of the line and asked, "Can we still make the 10:20 flight to Nashville?"

The harried agent looked up and sighed, "It's been canceled."

"Praise the Lord!" I exclaimed.

The agent smiled faintly and said to the disgruntled passenger she was trying to rebook, "You see, what's bad for one is good for another."

Later, when our turn came for rebooking, the agent said, "I really appreciated your comment, because the person I was helping was very angry until you said, 'Praise the Lord.' After that, there were no more complaints. Now, let's see what I can do for you."

Right away she pointed out a problem: "Your cat travel carrier is too big to fit under the seat, and because it's summer we can't let pets travel in the baggage compartment."

I groaned, "Oh, no! What will we do with Felix? We're trying to fly him to Nashville, where his owner can pick him up."

"Well, let me see," she said. A few minutes later she returned with a smaller cat carrier. "You can have this one. And because you've been so helpful to me, I'm not going to charge you the $50 pet travel fee. And I've got a couple first class seats available if you want them. You'll have more room for the cat that way!"

I couldn't believe what I was hearing. Later I commented to my husband, "Isn't it interesting how a simple 'Praise the Lord' brought so many blessings!"

Why not try praising the Lord today and see if it doesn't make a difference?

KAY KUZMA

The Need to be Sick

Give your bodies to God. Let them be a living and holy sacrifice—the kind he will accept. When you think of what he has done for you, is this too much to ask? Rom. 12:1, NLT.

"ANOTHER LOUSY COLD. I might have known—it's the first week of January!" I muttered as I opened the medicine cabinet filled with cold remedies. This pattern might have continued for the rest of my life if a friend hadn't asked, "Cec, what's going on that makes you need to be sick?"

"What a stupid question," I said. "Why, I caught a virus and . . ."

"Are you sure that's the reason? If your head doesn't have enough sense to slow you down, your body will eventually do it for you."

I didn't like the idea that getting sick had been my fault! Then I thought about the hectic weeks of December. I pastored a thriving church, and we had something going on almost every night. I loved the adult-class parties (with all that rich food), the carol sings, visits to shut-ins, and three Christmas Eve services. Despite my efforts to rest after Christmas, something always clamored for attention. "I'd rather burn out than rust out," I said once, in my own defense.

Like countless others, I lived a lifestyle of racing down the fast lane. Because I have a lot of physical stamina, I deluded myself into thinking I didn't need to rest. To get sick, however, was an honorable way to temporarily stop the activity cycle. Who would expect me to be out there giving myself 100 percent if I was lying in bed with a 103-degree temperature?

I finally learned how to avoid colds and illness. Not only did I begin to observe a weekly Sabbath, something I had never done in my life, but during each day I learned ways to relax, to stop and watch the world rush by instead of running with it.

Today, whenever I sense the threat of any physical downswing, I ask myself, "What's going on that makes me need to be sick?" Often, it's my cue to slow down. But sometimes it's more complicated, such as fulfilling a request or forgiving someone who has wounded me. Sometimes I don't know the answer, but I still pull out of the fast lane and park. Taking that reflective time is usually enough to stave off impending colds or minor illnesses. I want to live a lifestyle where I don't need to be sick.

Caring God, help me live a life that honors You—the kind where I don't need to be sick, because I listen to You and know when to slow down. Amen.

CECIL MURPHEY

Just Another Drink?

*Delight yourself also in the Lord, and He shall
give you the desires of your heart. Ps. 37:4, NKJV.*

I WAS ONLY 12 when I became addicted to one of the most common legal drugs in the world, caffeine. Every day after school I worked at my dad's manufacturing plant. After putting down my books and greeting the workers, I'd go to the jar of quarters that my dad kept for me, put one in the vending machine, and get myself a Dr. Pepper. I knew Coke and Pepsi were bad for you because of the caffeine, but no one told me Dr. Pepper was also caffeinated—and I never thought to read the label. (Did bottles have labels in those days?)

Anyway, by the time I learned the truth about Dr. Pepper it was a real struggle to give up. Grape soda just didn't give that afternoon pick-up that I had been getting from caffeine. I now know that what I was experiencing was "borrowed" energy that I'd have to pay back by living with a lower energy level later—just about the time I needed to do my homework!

When you ingest caffeine it shocks your system by doubling the level of adrenaline that causes your liver to dump glucose into your bloodstream, resulting in that borrowed energy boost!

When my husband and I were building our house I was amazed at the number of cans of caffeinated soda the workers went through each day. I wondered if they would drink it if they knew it unbalanced their autonomic nervous systems, which controls the function of every major organ in their bodies. The sugar boost aggravates hypoglycemia, increases blood pressure, stimulates the central nervous system, causes irregular heart beat, increases urinary calcium and magnesium losses, constricts blood vessels, and increases stomach acid secretion, which aggravate stomach ulcers. It can also cause tremors, irritability, nervousness, anxiety and depression, and heightened symptoms of PMS. (Most of them didn't have to worry about that!)

What makes me most upset is when I see children drinking caffeinated sodas. Children up to 5 years of age are the heaviest consumers of caffeine per body weight. For a 7-year-old, three cans of Coke are equivalent to an adult drinking eight cups of coffee!

God wants to give us the natural high that comes from a close relationship with Him. He doesn't want us self-medicating on an addictive drug that harms the bodies He created for us!

Are you self-medicating on caffeine drinks to get that borrowed boost of energy? How much better to go for God's natural high! KAY KUZMA

The (Lost) Wages of Gambling

Work with your own hands, as we commanded you, that you may walk properly toward those who are outside, and that you may lack nothing. 1 Thess. 4:11, 12, NKJV.

IT'S ONLY A $17.95 *processing fee and I might win the sweepstakes—I'm not gambling, am I? What's wrong with a lottery ticket? Gambling's a harmless entertainment. No problem!* The statistics say otherwise. In the U.S. alone, with more than two thirds of the population playing the odds and more than 15 million problem and pathological gamblers, the impact is huge. What's wrong with gambling?

Cigarettes, alcohol, and narcotics are addictive; they trigger a mind-altering connection between the substance and the reduction of pain, feelings of pleasure, or the excitement of an adrenaline rush. It feels good! And *bingo!* (Excuse the pun.) Before the person realizes what's happening, they've got to have another—and another. But second or third doses don't quite bring on the same "high," so the next doses are sooner and/or larger—and the user begins sinking into an addiction that willpower alone usually can't overcome. Not every person succumbs to this chemical connection. But until you're trapped you don't really know if you have the at-risk gene or not!

It's the same with gambling. Casual gambling often triggers an obsession and addiction similar to that of drugs. Compulsive gamblers report an adrenaline rush from the anticipation and excitement of "throwing the dice." And the stage is set for associated evils: bankruptcy, theft, drugs, family violence, divorce, suicide, and criminal activities. In the words of George Washington: "Gambling is the child of avarice, the brother of iniquity, and the father of mischief."

Gambling is a "legitimated theft" that takes from the poor and makes a few people rich—a selfish principle completely at odds with Jesus' call for mutual love and support. Early Christians shared their material possessions (see Acts 2:45). "Thou shalt not covet" means not wanting to have what belongs to others—which is exactly what gamblers want! Ephesians 5:5 reminds us that no covetous person has an inheritance in the kingdom of God. And putting one's trust in a random chance contradicts the Christian's trust in God as the giver of all good and perfect gifts.

The counsel of Charles Simeon, a nineteenth-century American clergyman, still rings true: "The best throw with the dice is to throw them away."

Lord, help me to be a good steward of the time and money that You have given me. Amen.   JOHN GALLAGHER and KAY KUZMA

For Such a Time as This

For if you remain completely silent at this time, relief and deliverance will arise for the Jews from another place, but you and your father's house will perish. Yet who knows whether you have come to the kingdom for such a time as this? Esther 4:14, NKJV.

QUEEN ESTHER WAS my favorite Bible story. When I was a child my father read it to me so many times that he had it memorized. I believed that if I lived my life in harmony with God's plan that He had a role for me like Queen Esther had in saving many lives. But years went by. . . .

I finished college and medical school. I had always wanted to go into surgery but did not match any surgery residencies. "God," I cried, "what are You doing? This is such a disappointment. I want to excel at something difficult and show that women can be important in medicine."

Just prior to starting my family practice residency I was asked to teach a stop-smoking class. That's when I learned how tough it is to quit the tobacco habit. When I returned to Loma Linda University I considered reapplying to general surgery. But a small voice said, "Linda, you can now see the big picture. Get a Masters in public health. You will find your niche in prevention."

While working as the medical director of the Addiction Treatment Unit at the Loma Linda Veterans Administration Medical Center I felt called to address the number one cause of preventable death and suffering: tobacco! Nicotine gum was not effective enough, so I started to search for solutions and found that depression and smoking were highly associated. Realizing that nicotine is an antidepressant, I searched for a non-addictive antidepressant that would act like nicotine on the human brain. That's when I discovered bupropion (Zyban). It was more effective in helping smokers quit than the patch. In eight months more than 2 million prescriptions for Zyban were written, saving at least 300,000 people from a premature death.

I believe this discovery was from God. He knew just what He was doing by placing me in a primary care residency when it was not "fashionable." That broad background is just what I need now for my current challenges in preventing tobacco-related diseases.

You are unique and precious to God. Use all the resources He places in your hands, and be grateful for where you are. If you ask God to direct you, you'll never be disappointed in the outcome. God doesn't make mistakes.

Have you considered that you too may have "come to the kingdom for such a time as this"? LINDA HYDER FERRY

Meeting the Creator at His Gates

*Yet your love for us, O Lord, is as high as the heavens and your faithfulness
extends to the universe. Your righteousness towers up like the mountains, and
your justice is as deep as the oceans. You provide for the needs of man
and beast. How priceless is your eternal love! Ps. 36:5-7, Clear Word.*

KEN RINGLE, IN the March 1999 issue of *National Geographic,* described
a dive into one of northern Florida's aquifers. The force of the current
threatened to shoot him back up the chimney he had just pulled himself
down through. "The tunnels down which I shone my light were empty of
anything but water, yet the power of the current surging from them gave
the eerie, pulsing sense of geologic life. It was like crouching at the aorta
of the world."

I'm at the other end of the continent, up against the Rocky Mountains,
but I feel this life force, too. It's a physical pulse in the thundering chinook
winds and mountain storms. It's a force that demands respect—as much as
your life is worth. You can't mess with the mind of a mountain.

But I can also feel this pulse on the balmiest days, when the mountains
seem most friendly and serene. Their massive bulk rises in sheer cliffs and
rocky turrets. Short grassy meadows shear away in abrupt drop-offs as if the
rest of the alpine valley were cut off with a butter knife, leaving the creeks
and rivulets from the mountain peaks to drop off hundreds of feet into space.

The physical evidence of Creation and the tremendous tumult of
earth's rearrangement during the Flood are in my face. The bigness of God,
the raw power He has to do as He wishes, is larger than life. The laws He
gave Creation to follow are being worked out in finite and infinite spheres.

I can't help but notice that all nature keeps those laws without pause, but
I don't. Nature wasn't created with a choice, but I, a human, was. Despite
God's overwhelming intelligence and power and goodwill and energy, I
have the power to choose to turn my back on Him and do my own thing.

It strikes me that this power to choose is bigger than the mountains!
It's the most awesome force He has put into action, for it has threatened
His universe and caused Him ultimate sacrifice. I'm awed that the
Monarch of the universe would purposefully design and strictly protect the
sovereignty of my will at such a price! There is a largeness to His charac-
ter at which the mountains can only hint.

*Lord, I am awed at the forces You built into nature. May I use the powerful
force of choice to always choose You as my Savior and Lord. Amen.*

CHERYL WOOLSEY DESJARLAIS

If Only Blanche Had Known

If you diligently heed the voice of the Lord your God and do what is right in His sight, give ear to His commandments and keep all His statutes, I will put none of the diseases on you which I have brought on the Egyptians. For I am the Lord who heals you. Ex. 15:26, NKJV.

THE UNITED STATES has the highest rate of degenerative diseases of any nation. The more fat and refined carbohydrates eaten, the more degenerative diseases. This fact brings to mind a story. Tucked away in the trees by the side of a road in Verdigre, Nebraska, is the three-room log house where I was born. This old house has a special place in my heart and is also a historical legend in Knox County, dating back possibly to the mid-1880s. Several years ago my cousin's wife, Blanche, painted this old house on a plate for me. However, this treasure has turned out to be a sad reminder of the devastating results of diabetes. In recent years, Blanche has suffered severely from it.

First there was the amputation of her lower leg. (Each year more than 56,000 amputations are performed on diabetics.) Soon after, she began losing her eyesight and had to give up her artistic gift of painting. (Each year, approximately 24,000 people lose their sight because of diabetes.) About three years ago Blanche had to have her other lower leg removed. She now lives in a nursing home.

What causes this terrible disease? The problem revolves around insulin, a pancreatic hormone, a kind of chemical messenger that enables glucose in the blood to enter the cells. In order to unlock the cell "door" to let glucose in, insulin has to connect with these receptors.

Why won't the cells open their "cell doors" and allow the glucose to enter the cell? Excess fat decreases the number of insulin receptors and/or deactivates them, which causes the pancreas to produce more insulin. After years of this overwork and abuse the pancreas often suffers "burnout" and fails. Then the body has no insulin to notify the cell to take in the glucose.

Is there hope for those who have this disease? In recent years thousands have experienced dramatic results in the recovery from various degenerative diseases by making simple lifestyle changes. Lifestyle programs such as the Weimar Health Institute's NEWSTART offer hope in maintaining and restoring health by promoting eight basic laws of health: N-utrition, E-xercise, W-ater, S-unlight, T-emperance, A-ir, R-est, and T-rust in divine power.

If only Blanche had known!

How best can I share these lifestyle principles so others can enjoy the blessing of good health? MARCELLA HARROM

The Hawaiian Lifestyle

My son, do not forget my teaching, but let your heart keep my commandments; for length of days and years of life and peace they will add to you. Prov. 3:1, 2, NASB.

WHILE LIVING ON the island of Kauai, Hawaii, I was medical director of Kauai Care Center, a small nursing home in Waimea. The oldest resident was a sweet little Japanese woman of 110 years, still up and walking. Many of the other residents were also close to their hundredth birthday and in great health for their age.

Hawaii (specifically Kauai) has been documented to have the longest life expectancy in the United States. Why? It must have to do with the moderate climate, the fresh salt air, sunshine, fresh fruits and vegetables available year-round, the relaxed Hawaiian lifestyle, and the aloha spirit.

There is a paradox here because while Hawaii is statistically the healthiest state in the United States, the Native Hawaiian people have the worst health in the nation. Careful analysis indicates that those people who are most long-lived are not Native Hawaiians but more recent immigrants—Asians and Caucasians—who seem to have lower rates of many chronic diseases.

The Native Hawaiians were the healthiest in the world until the Islands were discovered by Westerners. Their diet consisted of taro, poi, sweet potatoes, taro greens (cooked), mountain apples, fish, and seaweed. When the tropical paradise was discovered, processed foods and diseases were introduced. Now the Native Hawaiians are plagued with heart disease, hypertension, arthritis, asthma, allergies, cancer, diabetes, stroke, gastritis, and many other chronic conditions that are reaching epidemic proportions.

More than 100 years ago, when Ellen G. White wrote *The Ministry of Healing,* she mentioned eight natural laws for health: "pure air, sunlight, abstemiousness, rest, exercise, proper diet, the use of water, trust in divine power" (p. 127). She then made this statement: "Those who persevere in obedience to [nature's] laws will reap the reward in health of body and health of mind" *(ibid.).*

As I read through the list of eight natural laws I was amazed at how closely it resembled the factors that we believe have contributed to people living longer and healthier in Kauai. I wonder what would happen if the rest of the nation would start living this lifestyle?

Lord, help me to learn something from those who live healthy and long, that can help me make better choices. KEVIN CLAY

A Book Full of Blessings

And God is able to make all grace abound to you, so that in all things at all times, having all that you need, you will abound in every good work. 2 Cor. 9:8, NIV.

OVER THE PAST three years I've become an expert at recognizing blessings. In fact, I write them all down. Three years ago my 13-year-old daughter, Lana, was diagnosed with a rare neurological disease called Rasmussen Syndrome. Lana endured constant seizures, and eventually had to undergo a very risky brain surgery.

Desperate to understand these awful events in our lives, I determined to be positive, and I started to record blessings: Things like being provided with nurses who turned out to be prayer warriors, and being blessed with parking spaces that enabled Lana better wheelchair accessibility. I was on the lookout for anything and everything that would indicate to me that God was paying attention to our prayers for Lana's healing and recovery.

Strangely enough, I've become so enthusiastic about my blessings that I've found myself praying that God would give me an opportunity to be a blessing to others. A few hours after praying for the first time to be a blessing to someone else, I was waiting for Lana to complete rehab at an in-patient facility, and I encountered a young mother. She had traveled quite a distance to bring her 12-day-old baby to the clinic. She literally had only the clothes on her back and a five dollar bill. She asked me if I could give her change for her five, so that she could buy detergent and wash the clothes she was wearing. I was able to provide her with my room and something to wear, while I washed and dried her clothes for her. I was so excited about being a blessing to her. And I was astounded at how fast God had answered my prayer.

Now I have even more blessings to write down—the blessings God sends my way, and the ways that God allows me to be a blessing to others. Writing in my blessing journal has had a tremendous effect on how I view things that happen to me and my family. I've noticed that God is involved in the most minute details of our circumstances.

When I feel discouraged I read my blessing journal and I get so excited about all the things the Lord has done that it's impossible to continue feeling discouraged! Writing down blessings makes me feel so hopeful. I've discovered that the more you look, the more blessings you find.

Why not start a blessings book today and see what a difference it will make in your life?   GAYE HENRY with MICHELE DEPPE

God's Cuddle Time

Behold what manner of love the Father has bestowed on us,
that we should be called children of God! 1 John 3:1, NKJV.

LUNCH WAS OVER. Michael, my just-barely toddler, announced it quite emphatically by mashing and spewing macaroni and cheese all over the high-chair and floor. It was definitely nap time! I sat down with him in the rocking chair. He snuggled up against my neck and lay his head on my shoulder.

I proceeded to tell him a story about God, our heavenly Father, who created a wonderful world for us. I talked about each day of Creation, of how God made the warm sunlight he enjoys, and the soft green grass, and the beautiful flowers with every color imaginable. Then God decided the oceans needed flower gardens, too, so He made the incredibly exquisite coral reefs.

Michael raised a sleepy little head in a small show of excitement when I told him that God created dogs. I told Michael how God made Adam and Eve, and that everything was perfect.

On the seventh day God rested. I explained to Michael that God didn't rest because He needed it. After all, He is all-powerful and He doesn't need rest or sleep . . . and then suddenly I stopped the story. How was I going to explain the Sabbath to my sleepy little 14-month-old?

Perhaps God helped me finish the story. "You see, Michael," I said, "God didn't need to rest, but He knew that people did. Just as sleepy little boys need naps, big people need breaks from all the running around they do all week. So God made a special, quiet, rest time for everyone. And just like little boys need their mommies and daddies to spend time with them, to go for walks with them, to tell them stories, and to cuddle them, God knew that all people needed a special cuddle time—even grownups. Sabbath is that special time for God to be with the people He loves and cuddle us."

By this time Michael was fast asleep, so I don't know how much he got out of the story. But I got something. As a young person, I had been warned not to bring God down to my level. I needed to keep Him at a slight distance to fear, respect, and revere Him. But in the Creation story I suddenly saw a heavenly Father who loves His children. From now on, I think I will always associate Sabbath with cuddle time.

Thank You, heavenly Father, for Your Sabbath. DAWN JAKOVAC

Good Night, Sleep Tight . . . ?

I will both lie down in peace, and sleep; for You
alone, O Lord, make me dwell in safety. Ps. 4:8, NKJV.

ACCORDING TO THE National Sleep Foundation, Americans are not getting enough sleep. About one in five struggle nightly with insomnia. Research indicates that America's sleep problems have reached epidemic proportions, and may be the country's number one health problem.

Sleep deprivation affects us in a variety of ways. For example, those who sleep fewer than six hours a night don't live as long as those who sleep seven hours or more. But sadly, among most young people the longevity issue doesn't seem that relevant. Their attitude is, "Who cares?"

Lack of sleep is expensive. The National Commission on Sleep Disorders estimates that sleep deprivation costs $150 billion a year in higher stress and reduced workplace productivity.

And it's risky! An article in the *Journal of the American Medical Association* points out that in the morning after 24 hours of sleeplessness, a person's motor performance is comparable to someone who is legally intoxicated! You take unnecessary risks when you get too little sleep.

According to Dr. Russell Rosenberg, Director of Northside Hospital Sleep Medicine Institute in Atlanta, "The most common problem with sleeplessness, or not getting enough sleep at night, is stress." Anxiety, stress, and worry never take time off. Sleep problems following the death of a loved one or a traumatic experience are pretty normal. But chronic, long-term anxiety, stress, or a nagging disposition to worry results in long-term, chronic sleep difficulties. This can easily become a vicious cycle, with stress causing sleeplessness and not being able to get to sleep causing stress.

There are thousands who wish that as nighttime rolls around they could become a little more phlegmatic and "who cares" all their troubled thoughts away. One answer to the sleep problem is change—especially change in thought patterns, lifestyle, and dependence on God rather than yourself.

It helps to stop your busy activities an hour or so before bed. Walk around the block, relax in a hot bath, and divert your mind with a good book. But Dr. Rosenberg also recommends that you take 20 or more minutes before bedtime to write down your worries. Then write down what you can do about each one. This will show you what you can change and what you should leave to others. Then pray, giving each specific worry you can't do anything about, to God—who can!

Journaling is good for sleep—and your soul. Write down your worries and give them to God. RISË RAFFERTY

The Message of the $2 Bill

It is more blessed to give than to receive. Acts 20:35, NIV.

COOL EVENINGS IN the winter of 1997. The health evangelism class is ready to pass through the baptism of fire. Ten scared students ready to give their first stop-smoking clinic. Will it be a success? How many will come? How many will *keep* coming? How many will truly quit the habit?

The first night. Only seven show. Failure? Prejudice? Whatever, let's get started! The students, learning the fine art of persuasion through lectures, short movies, group discussions. The addicts, a small dose of fear, a big one of hope. New resolutions. Excellent feedback. Lots of excitement on both sides. "Hey, this thing really works!"

Finally the key night. "Folks, this is your evening. We're going to take all your cigarettes, matches, lighters, ashtrays. Just let them fall in this bag. You don't have to worry anymore; we're going to burn them. From now on you are free." Some of them have tears in their eyes—that stuff was for them like a child. And now it's gone. Forever? "And don't forget, folks, for every 24 hours you stay away from nicotine, you will get a brand new $2 bill."

Night after night brand new $2 bills are handed out. Maggie, a young woman in her 30s, is ahead of all the others. She carries a newborn baby, sleeping in a car seat. One night toward the end she is diligently arranging her pile of $2 bills as though working on a puzzle. "Hi, Maggie, what are you going to do with that big pile of money? Going to buy a new car, or what?"

You can see she is very proud of her treasure. She puts her arms around her money. "No car," she says in her super Southern accent. "I'm gonna frame them and hang them on my kitchen wall. And then, when my girl will be old enough, I'm gonna tell her, 'Honey, this is the price Mommy paid so that you could grow up held in arms that don't smell like nicotine.' Yes, sir, that's exactly what I'm gonna do."

That evening Maggie makes me feel that I am *doing something* worthwhile on this planet. I can still feel the thrill. It's still worth giving stop-smoking clinics. It's still worth helping others become *free*. Yes, it's still worth taking Jesus at His word: "It is more blessed to give than to receive."

How can you experience the thrill of really doing something worthwhile on this planet?   CEZAR R. LUCHIAN

Questions, Questions, Questions

So the Lord God caused the man to fall into a deep sleep; and while he was sleeping, he took one of the man's ribs and closed up the place with flesh. Gen. 2:21, NIV.

THERE ARE OTHER texts in the Bible that refer to a "deep sleep," but none are related to anesthesia and surgery. After Adam named all of the livestock, all the birds, and all the beasts, no suitable helper for Adam was found. It was time for surgery. The operative report was very brief:

Preop diagnosis: No wife	Wound: Healed
Postop diagnosis: Wife	Blood administered: None
Anesthesia: General	Condition of patient: Healthy
Specimen removed: Rib	Pain Medications: None

We need not wonder as to the "why" of the surgery. God saw the need and Adam explains it: "This is now bone of my bones and flesh of my flesh; she shall be called 'woman,' for she was taken out of man" (Gen. 2:23, NIV). The Bible goes on to say, "For this reason a man will leave his father and mother and be united to his wife, and they will become one flesh" (verse 24, NIV).

It is the "how" that intrigues me. First, how did God anesthetize Adam? Did Adam breathe some special gas, or did God give him something to swallow or something through the vein, or acupuncture?

Modern anesthesia began in 1846 with the use of inhaled ether. Subsequently many different agents have been developed and used. In spite of more than 150 years of modern anesthesia, we do not understand completely how it works. But it works! There are several theories, but no theory explains all situations. How did God do it?

How did God make the incision? Was it with a sharp object like a knife, did He use His finger, or did He use a cautery or laser type of device so there was no blood loss? How did He close the wound? Did He use sutures, surgical glue, or staples? Was there a scar? Our concepts and techniques are inadequate to explain what happened.

However God provided the first anesthetic and performed the first thoracic surgery, the results speak for themselves. When I get to heaven my skills of providing anesthesia will not be needed, but I have many questions I want to ask. In fact, I want God to show me how He did it!

God does not ask that we understand Him, only that we trust Him. Will you trust Him with your life?   BURTON A. BRIGGS

NOVEMBER 8

Lessons From a 12-Year-Old

So it was that after three days they found Him in the temple, sitting in the midst of the teachers, both listening to them and asking them questions. And all who heard Him were astonished at His understanding and answers. Luke 2:46, 47, NKJV.

WHAT HAPPENS WHEN someone hits you with angry, bitter, hurtful words? Do you react in kind or do you give a thoughtful response and avoid an emotional collision?

Picture this scene: Mary and Joseph had just spent the Passover week in Jerusalem. Jesus was 12 years old, a man now by Jewish standards, and they had just celebrated His coming of age. Now they are returning home to Nazareth. After a day's journey with their friends and relatives Joseph sees Mary traveling with the women and asks, "How is Jesus doing?"

"What do you mean?" she replies. "He's with you, isn't He? After all, He is a man now!"

"No, surely he's with you!" Joseph responds.

Can't you just imagine how panicked these parents are? Not only have they lost their son, but they have lost God's Son as well! This is serious! Immediately they head back to Jerusalem. There they begin searching frantically. After three days, Mary comes into the temple and sees Jesus across the courtyard. Overcome with emotion she cries, "Why have you done this to us? Your father and I have been half out of our minds looking for you!" (Luke 2:48, Message).

Now consider for a moment how a normal 12-year old would respond to an irate mother who blames him for something he didn't do, especially in front of important people. Can't you hear a kid react by saying something like this: "What do you mean, what have I done to you? You're the ones who left me!" Or, "Mom, chill out! You're embarrassing me!" But had He reacted to his mother's out-of-control concern it would have been a collision of emotions, causing hurt and more accusations. Instead Jesus calmly said something like this: "Mom, since I was a baby you've told Me who I was. You should have known I'd be doing My Father's work."

He didn't have to blame His mother just because she blamed Him. He didn't have to embarrass her just because she embarrassed Him. At 12 years of age Jesus gave us an example of how to respond when someone hits us with uncontrolled emotion so that the confrontation will be defused, rather than igniting more damaging emotions.

Thank You, Jesus, for teaching not only the teachers in the Temple—but us as well! KAY KUZMA

Winning the Cold War

War broke out in heaven: Michael and his angels fought with the dragon;
and the dragon and his angels fought, but they did not prevail, nor
was a place found for them in heaven any longer. Rev. 12:7, 8, NKJV.

WITH THE FIRST CHILLY winds of fall, it's time to guard against colds, flu, and infections. Start with exercise. Walk briskly out of doors for a mile or two each morning. Exercise elevates your white blood cell count, increasing resistance to germ invasion. Be careful with strenuous outdoor exercise (such as jogging) in the winter, for cold air hitting your lungs may actually lower resistance. Also, even a moderate amount of sunshine will increase the action of the white blood cells.

When outside or if you sleep in a cold room, keep your extremities and exposed skin warm. Prevent heat loss by wearing a cap if your hair is thin (or gone), and a neck scarf or high collar.

Always be sure that there is some air circulating throughout the home. Open your bedroom window at least a crack at night. Crisp winter air and the freshness of a circulating breeze is a valuable aid to health and a prevention of many wintertime illnesses. But avoid sitting in a draft where a chilly wind blows on your neck, face, or other exposed body parts.

Don't sabotage yourself during the cold winter months by eating candy, ice cream, and extra helpings of sweet desserts—even natural ones! Excessive intake of sugar will decrease your white blood cells' ability to destroy invaders. Even an excess of fruit juice can be hazardous because of the refinement and concentration of soluble nutrients, including sugar. Instead, eat plenty of protective foods such as vegetables, fruits, and whole grains, which are high in necessary vitamins and minerals and add bulk for proper elimination.

The kidneys play an active role in the elimination of body toxins. To help them do their job, drink plenty of pure water between meals—at least 8 to 10 glassfuls daily, even though you aren't thirsty. Water is a great internal and external cleanser. Wash your hands frequently with soap, and enjoy a hot bath followed by a cold shower. It does wonders to the circulatory system.

Armed with exercise, sunshine, a good diet, water, and fresh air, you can win the "cold war." But what are you doing to win the cold war for your soul? Satan is blowing up a storm!

Lord, help me to exercise my willpower, stay in your Son light, eat the Bread of Life, drink from Your Word, and avoid the draft of evil. YEW-POR NG

Little Things Matter

Well done, good and faithful servant; you have been faithful over a few things, I will make you ruler over many things. Enter into the joy of your Lord. . . . For to everyone who has, more will be given, and he will have abundance. Matt. 25:23-29, NKJV.

EASTERN RELIGIOUS LEADERS often remind their disciples that even a little poison can cause death, and that a tiny seed can become a huge tree. Buddha, for example, taught that even tiny drops of water eventually will fill a huge vessel.

And Jesus said, "If you have faith as small as a mustard seed, you can say to this mountain, 'Move from here to there' and it will move. Nothing will be impossible for you" (Matt. 17:20, NIV). The practical application of Jesus' teaching is that the "mountains" of life—our heavy burdens, dashed hopes, crushed dreams—can be transported or transformed when we exercise faith, however small.

An inspiring example of this is the case of James R. Jeffreys. When he was born in 1932 with osteogenesis imperefecta (brittle bone disease), doctors held out no hope for the family, predicting the infant would not live more than a year. If by some miracle he survived the first 12 months, they said, he would be so totally disabled that he could never live a productive life.

Yet James Jeffreys did live. He rolled his wheelchair two miles a day to and from high school. By the age of 21 he had opened his own cabinet shop. Jeffreys was also a prize-winning drag racer. Using a car equipped with special handheld controls, he won 14 racing awards.

He married a nurse. They had two children and then adopted seven more when they learned there was a 50 percent chance that their own off-spring could inherit brittle bone disease. One of their adopted children is blind, one was crippled by polio, one has a spinal disorder, one was born with no legs, and one suffers from diabetes. Four of the children are bira-cial and two are Korean. In 1977 Jeffreys was named Outstanding Adult of the Year by the American Brittle Bone Society. The governor of New Jersey (the state where Jeffreys was born and lives) proclaimed a James R. Jeffreys Day, declaring that "the life and career of James R. Jeffreys serves as an inspiration and a source of strength to all persons afflicted with phys-ical handicaps." Jeffreys is a glowing example of someone who made great gains by taking small steps.

Regardless of how big your "mountain" of difficulty, faith can keep you hammer-ing away at it, little by little, until one day you realize that you've tunneled through.

VICTOR M. PARACHIN

Will You Come and Talk With Me?

Perfume and incense bring joy to the heart, and the pleasantness of one's friend springs from his earnest counsel. Prov. 27:9, NIV.

THE PHONE RANG. Bad news! Maryanne's pained voice faltered: "I just found out Joey's hooked on drugs. I've suspected it, but I've lived in denial for months." Abruptly she hung up while I was still catching my breath, working on something to say. Joey was Maryanne's good-looking, intelligent, charming 20-year-old son.

I fumbled through breakfast. What am I supposed to do? Maryanne is only a friend—she isn't family. She isn't even my *best* friend. What does she want from me? Should I go over to her house? Call back? Write a note? But then, maybe she deserves this. She spoiled Joey. He seldom had to face the consequences of his bad behaviors. Now she's reaping the consequences.

Then I remembered something. I flipped through *Sons and Daughters of God,* one of Ellen G. White's devotional books. On page 161 I found these words: "Things will go wrong with everyone; sadness and discouragement press every soul; then a personal presence, a friend who will comfort and impart strength, will turn back the darts of the enemy that are aimed to destroy. Christian friends are not half as plentiful as they should be."

I mused, "How modern those words sound—even though written a hundred years ago!"

The passage continued, "In hours of temptation, in a crisis, what a value is a true friend! Satan at such times sends along his agents to cause the trembling limbs to stumble."

I mumbled to myself: *Satan is in on this! And he's over there working on Maryanne now!*

"But the true friends who will counsel, who will impart magnetic hopefulness, the calming faith that uplifts the soul—oh, such help is worth more than precious pearls."

These words are for me, I thought. *It's not about what Maryanne did or didn't do. I can scatter pearls in Maryanne's path. No, I can be even better than a pearl to her.*

Mental health personnel will often use three common terms to describe a person who is de-energized, perhaps even suffering depression: "The person feels helpless, worthless, and hopeless." So I ask: When I'm in a crisis, down and out, distraught and damaged, will you come to my house? Will you talk with me? Will you be more than a precious pearl?

Is there someone who needs you to be their friend today?

TOINI HARRISON

From SAD to the Son

Do not fear therefore; you are of more value than many sparrows. Matt. 10:31, NKJV.

I was feeling like a sad country song. I still had my wife, my dog, my truck, my kids, my job, and all those things usually mentioned in melancholy country songs, but I was depressed. My life hadn't fallen apart. No, I'd simply tried for a promotion I shouldn't have expected, and failed.

I did everything I could. I took the tests, did the interviews, and presented my barren resume. After the dust had settled I was left out. Now I had a deep, empty feeling inside that made me want to hang my head and quit.

I'd read in the paper about a condition called SAD (seasonal affective disorder). Basically, during the winter months, people with SAD get depressed, presumably because they aren't getting enough sunlight. Maybe that's me, I thought. Maybe this feeling would vanish if I just got out in the sunshine. There are no windows in the factory where I work but the weatherman said it was supposed to be an unseasonably warm January day, with plenty of sunshine. At break I'll go outside and take a walk. That might help.

At 3:00 p.m. I hurried outside to take my walk but was disappointed when greeted by a cool, cloudy day. *Oh well,* I sighed, *exercise is good. I'll take this walk anyway, because exercise also makes one feel better.*

As I walked briskly around the building I saw a shaft of sunlight racing like a giant spotlight across the landscape toward me, illuminating different parts of the field. The light passed over me and seemed to pause on a nearby brush pile. As the hole in the clouds closed I noticed tiny sparrows flitting about, busying themselves with whatever sparrows do. It was as if the sunbeam was God's finger trying to make me notice those tiny birds.

I paused for a moment to envy their carefree life. God pointed those sparrows out to help me realize that He cared about how I felt. Barely 10 minutes after leaving the building with a heavy heart, I returned to work feeling downright invigorated. I realized it wasn't sunlight I was missing, but Son light. When you sense that your life is in God's control there is no reason to be depressed over things beyond your control.

Thank You, Lord, for lighting up my life with the thought that I am far more valuable to You than sparrows. And You care for everyone! Amazing!

STEWART T. PEPPER

The Dental Cripple

I will give you a new heart and put a new spirit in you; I will remove from you your heart of stone and give you a heart of flesh. Eze. 36:26, NIV.

HAVE YOU EVER heard of a "dental cripple"? I see them all the time! People are trying to eat with so many teeth missing that their chewing ability is significantly diminished.

For one reason or another a lot of people have had their teeth removed and have not had them replaced. The other teeth can drift and lean into the void. If allowed to remain that way for a period of time the teeth that are left will move, causing the bite to collapse. Collapsing of the bite can cause problems with the jaw joint. If this is coupled with the stress of clenching the teeth or a head or neck injury, the result could likely give a person tempromandibular dysfunction (TMD)—which is extremely painful. TMD is a condition involving the joint in front of the ear where the lower jaw hinges with the upper jaw.

Removing a tooth can become a serious problem for many people!

Dentistry today can prevent many of these problems. If you have had a tooth removed it is important to replace it so your teeth will not drift. You can replace it with a fixed bridge that fills in the void. Another choice is to replace the tooth with a dental implant, which is placed directly into the bony tissues where the tooth was. There are ways to prevent future problems caused by the loss of a tooth if you should have no choice but to have an extraction. You don't have to be a dental cripple!

Talking about "dental cripples" reminds me that people can also become spiritual cripples. We let sin create a void in our life like that formed by the removal of a tooth. We continue to let this gap damage our spiritual integrity until our life is in total dysfunction.

We are thankful that God has a solution for this void. He has defeated the enemy through the blood of His Son so that we can have victory over the problems that sin causes. The solution is to claim the result of Jesus' victory and to let Him have control of our life. Let Jesus bridge the void that sin has created. Let Him implant into your heart and life what you need to be spiritually healthy.

Lord, thank You for Your promise to remove my stony heart and give me a new heart and spirit.   EDDIE C. TOWLES

Religion Is Good for Your Health

Blessed are those who dwell in Your house; they will still be praising You. Ps. 84:4, NKJV.

DID YOU KNOW that going to church, studying your Bible, and praying is good for your health? In 1998 Dr. David Larson reported that those who attended a religious service once a week and prayed or studied their Bible once a day were 40 percent less likely to have high blood pressure than those who didn't! Another study stated that older people who take part in church activities tend to have lower blood pressure than those who are less active church members.

Researchers have found that monthly church visits improved the mental health of elderly people. Other researchers found that adults who attended church at least once a week were less likely to have high levels of interleukin-6, an immune system protein associated with age-related diseases. More than half of the study subjects attended church at least once a week and prayed at least once a day. Most (75 percent) tuned in to religious TV or radio at least once a week.

The *American Journal of Psychiatry* reported that psychiatrists who have active spiritual lives consider prayer and Bible study a more effective treatment for many mental problems than medications.

According to a review of the medical literature conducted by Dr. Dale Matthews at Georgetown University School of Medicine, religious commitment may help prevent physical and mental illness and aid recovery from illness. Analysis of published studies shows that more than 75 percent of people want their physician to consider spiritual issues in relation to their care and almost 50 percent want their physician to pray with them.

Dr. Matthews' review showed that religious commitment was shown to have an effect on specific health concerns. For example, religious commitment appears to protect against depression and suicide, substance abuse, cancer, and cardiovascular disease. Many studies are also concluding that people who are actively religious may cope better with illness by relying on their beliefs.

Following open heart surgery, elderly patients who reported strong faith and depended on that faith to help them cope had a mortality rate one third lower than patients without a sense of faith.

The evidence is convincing! Perhaps the best health insurance in the world is making sure your connection to God is healthy.

Thank You, Jesus, for continuing to heal Your people.   GERARD MCLANE

Think Healthy

Finally, brethren, whatsoever things are true, whatsoever things are honest, whatsoever things are just, whatsoever things are pure, whatsoever things are lovely, whatsoever things are of good report; if there be any virtue, and if there be any praise, think on these things. Phil. 4:8.

NORMAN VINCENT PEALE once told about speaking to the Chinese owner of a tattoo shop. One of the designs read: "Born to Lose." Peale asked why anyone would want those words permanently imprinted on himself or herself. The man responded, "Before tattoo on chest, tattoo on mind."

The way you think will have a powerful effect on your health. When you're positive you can better resist stress and ward off cardiovascular disease and gastrointestinal troubles. Your immune system is less likely to break down and may even work harder to protect you against allergies, arthritis, and cancer. Your brain manufactures natural pain-relieving chemicals so that you feel better. When you think of yourself as losing weight or getting well, the chances are greater that you will! It's self-fulfilling. Cultivate these five positive-thinking patterns:

1. *Think "This will pass."* When you face problems this technique is vital. Most upsetting situations are insignificant. Tell yourself, *In five years I won't even remember this incident.* When suffering, don't think of this as lasting a lifetime. Instead, focus on getting through one day at a time.

2. *Think God thoughts.* This can only happen if you put God's Word in your mind. Memorize Bible passages that will challenge and inspire you.

3. *Think love.* It has tremendous potential for improving health. Poet Elizabeth Barrett Browning, best known for "How Do I Love Thee?" was an invalid because of a childhood accident and was confined to the house by a domineering father. When she found love in the person of poet Robert Browning, he rescued her from an atmosphere of control and took her from England to Italy. In an atmosphere of love her health improved so much that she gave birth to a son.

4. *Think affirming thoughts about yourself.* Jan's wife, Kay, wrote the following self-talk statement in the flyleaf of her Bible: "I will not allow my self-worth to be influenced by others' perceptions of me, but by my own perceptions of whether or not I am living with integrity, being humble, knowing what to take credit for, and what is a gift from God."

5. *Think positive for 21 days.* Yes, that's how long it takes to establish a new habit.

Discover the truth that, with God's help, you can become that which you believe.

JAN W. KUZMA and CECIL MURPHEY

The Battle of the Bulge

*See if there is any offensive way in me, and
lead me in the way everlasting. Ps. 139:24, NIV.*

"TAKE YOURSELF IN hand, guy. If you keep eating like this you're not going to make it in your career." The words stung. A straight-A high school student, intent on being the very best attorney in the state or perhaps the nation, was facing a taste-bud battle that would likely escalate into the battle of the bulge! He questions, "Should I heed the warning, or down another double cheeseburger and a can of soda?" Unfortunately, too many succumb to the temptation of taste. "Just one more time—and then maybe I'll change!"

Maybe you can relate to this scenario. Your conscience may be a little uncomfortable. Good. The truth is, the longer you eat junk foods, too much food, or get too little exercise, the greater the chance that you will not make it to the top of your career. There are two reasons for this: (1) You will be at greater risk for cardiovascular disease, diabetes, arthritis, coughs and colds; and (2) despite your academic achievement, the obese prospective employee is shunned in favor of the equally able person of normal weight. Employers want healthy, cost-effective employees!

Now is the time for action. Science has given you plenty of reasons to keep excess fatty foods and empty calories out of your system, and even more reasons to put on your walking shoes!

Approximately one fourth of the school children in the United States are obese. In 1993 that was estimated to be approximately 11 million children—and things are worse today. During childhood, the greater the obesity and the more unstable the weight, the more likely a child will end up as an obese adult.

Research shows that obese children are spending more time doing the comfortable, minimal energy-consuming activities of watching television, reading, and playing video games than other children. They also find it hard to make friends, which may lead them back to food for comfort.

The good news is that if you are young (and even if you're not) and you are overweight, you don't have to stay that way. It is treatable. Decide to take the problem in hand. Make some changes in your eating habits and start an enjoyable exercise program. If you do, you'll find lasting benefits to your career, your social life, and your self-esteem. Determine today to win the next taste bud battle!

When you face your next taste temptation, ask God to give you the willpower to make a healthy choice. TABITHA ABEL-COOPER

What Value Is Man?

What is man that you concern yourself with him? Of what value is he that you continue to care for him? Ps. 8:4, Clear Word.

BACK IN THE DISTANT eons of time when God was considering the kind of beings He would design to populate planet Earth, it might be He thought that surely if He made them multidimensional, much like Himself, there would be great joy! They would have high intelligence and eager response. They would have the boon of individuality, the power to think, to imagine, to creatively experiment—to go in any direction their minds could devise!

The gift God values most highly would be theirs—total freedom of choice! What excitement! The dimension of completeness. Each healthy body would exult in the ability to direct itself, to be equal to any challenge, to run with speed and power, to move gracefully and with discipline, and to sit quietly in contemplation of the surrounding beauty.

In the light of truth with which God would surround them, each mind would perceive truth—how they were loved—and they would recognize the lofty plans God had for them. They would respond with wonder at the possibilities for intellectual understanding and pursuits open to them.

In addition to all these gifts they would have the gift of procreation, the possibility of entering more fully into the experience of God. The responsibility for a life brought into existence by one's own choice and desire would be an introduction to the attitude of the divine Creator toward His creatures.

The birth of a child would bring the dimensions of nurturing, caring, and the capacity for delight in each stage of development. God must have chuckled with pleasure as He visualized a baby's first lopsided smile, the first hesitant steps, the first words: "Abba, Daddy!" How happy God's earthly family would be in the enjoyment of each child.

These children, conceived in love, would turn in trust and dependence to God and to their parents—trust and interdependence between themselves, God, and other created beings. Together they would develop ideas, learn concepts, and share understandings. The uniqueness of each personality would bring great diversity in loving relationships.

What delight God must have had as He designed His earthly family! Holy fun at its best!

We are so wonderfully made—why is it that sometimes we don't like ourselves?

ROSE NELL BRANDT

God's Honor Guard

*Beloved, do not think it strange concerning the fiery trial which is to try you,
as though some strange thing happened to you; but rejoice to the extent
that you partake of Christ's sufferings, that when His glory is revealed,
you may also be glad with exceeding joy. 1 Peter 4:12, 13, NKJV.*

TRAVIS WAS DYING. He had been anointed, but the leukemia only worsened. At first he lamented, "Why me?" One night the Holy Spirit impressed him with the idea that of all the gifts heaven can bestow, suffering with Christ gives the highest honor. He said to himself, *If God needs someone to go through this experience and still trust Him, why not me?*

But in spite of having peace about his eternal destiny, Travis would sometimes awaken his mother at night. "Mom, I'm scared. I don't want to die at 18."

She would say, "Son, you'll just go to sleep and next thing you know, you'll be looking into Jesus' face. Just visualize that."

Near the end, Travis rallied and went home. Monday he woke up and said, "I'm not doing well." They put him in the car and started for the hospital. He said he had to go to the restroom, so they stopped at Denny's. The restroom had only two stalls. Both doors were open; no one was there. As Dad was trying to help, Travis said, "I can hardly breathe. You'd better call 911." At that moment a voice from the other side of the partition said, "Travis, it is all right; you are going to be OK." Dad then noticed shoes and the trousers of a dark blue silk suit.

As Dad left to call, Mother came in. The voice continued, "Travis, it is all right; I am here." Paramedics put Travis on a stretcher. At this point the stranger from the other stall came out, went to the head of the stretcher, and looked into Travis' face. Travis, who had been looking at his mother, riveted his eyes on the face of the stranger. The paramedics asked, "Are you his father?"

"No, I am his friend." He continued to lean over Travis as they took him to the ambulance. When they got to the hospital Travis was unconscious and the stranger was gone. No one had seen the stranger's face except Travis. They even asked the receptionist at the restaurant if she had seen someone in a dark blue silk suit. She replied, "People in silk suits don't come into Denny's."

Could it be that Travis' angel called heaven's 911? "Lord, this is a special case. Could You spare five minutes for one of Your honor guard?" And that He did?

Lord, give us faith enough to trust You even when things do not go right.

MORRIS VENDEN

Diet and Destiny

Whatever you eat or drink or whatever you do,
you must do all for the glory of God. 1 Cor. 10:31, NLT.

IN 1863, ONLY a few months after the organization of the Seventh-day Adventist Church, God gave Ellen White a vision about the importance of health. At first it may have seemed a deviation from the gospel commission. What does eating a good diet, exercising, and getting enough rest have to do with preparing people for the second coming of Jesus?

The fact is, our spiritual perceptions are at risk when we fail to follow God's plan for our bodies. Here is how Ellen White put it: "Those who overcome as Christ overcame will need to constantly guard themselves against the temptations of Satan. The appetite and passions should be restricted and under the control of enlightened conscience, that the intellect may be unimpaired, the perceptive powers clear, so that the workings of Satan and his snares may not be interpreted to be the providence of God" (*Counsels on Health,* p. 574).

Fact No. 2: What we eat and drink affects our ability to be used by God's Spirit in the work of reaching souls. "In all our work we must obey the laws which God has given, that the physical and spiritual energies may work in harmony. . . . Ministers should be strictly temperate in their eating and drinking, lest they make crooked paths for their feet, turning the lame—those weak in the faith—out of the way. If, while proclaiming the most solemn and important message God has ever given, men war against the truth by indulging wrong habits of eating and drinking, they take all the force from the message they bear" (*ibid.,* p. 575).

And No. 3: Control of appetite is the first step in controlling other temptations—and can determine one's eternal destiny! "The controlling power of appetite will prove the ruin of thousands, when, if they had conquered on this point, they would have had moral power to gain the victory over every other temptation of Satan. But those who are slaves to appetite will fail in perfecting Christian character. The continual transgression of man for six thousand years has brought sickness, pain, and death as its fruits. And as we near the close of time, Satan's temptation to indulge appetite will be more powerful and more difficult to overcome" (*ibid.,* p. 574).

Lord, I give You my life today, which includes my taste buds and stomach. Help me to glorify You in everything I choose to eat or drink.   JIM BRACKETT

Whatever It Takes

Then I will give them a heart to know Me, that I am the Lord:
and they shall be My people, and I will be their God,
for they shall return to Me with their whole heart. Jer. 24:7, NKJV.

"WHATEVER IT TAKES, Lord, to bring me back into a saving relationship with You, let it happen. Thank You, Jesus, for knocking again at my heart's door, and for giving me time to get my life back together. Whether I live 10 years or 10 months, I give You my heart once again. May I be a loving and faithful witness for You, Lord, as I go through this valley, and may the remainder of my life, however long it may last, be used to lead others to You."

This was the heartfelt prayer of my dear friend and neighbor, Socorro, when she was diagnosed with breast cancer and was facing surgery. For 15 years I have loved her like a sister. I have been with her on mountaintops and in valleys—and this, perhaps the lowest valley of all!

As she prayed, my heart responded, "Yes, Lord, whatever it takes to burn away the dross of earthliness and sin in our lives so that we may reflect Your loving character to others—let it happen."

Jesus longs to come soon; indeed, all the signs that are thickening about us shout that He is near, even at the door! Jesus is not waiting for the wicked to grow more wicked. He is waiting for His children to lay hold of the mighty power of the Holy Spirit to reflect loving, Christlike characters to the world around them.

He wants to fill each one of us with the Water of Life , which quenches our thirst so that we can make others thirsty for Him, the Fountain of Living Water.

How we need to be interceding for our loved ones! Perhaps you have children who have strayed from Jesus and from the principles they were taught when they were young. Keep praying! God will send His mighty angels to answer every sincere prayer. He has promised to give them new hearts that long to know Him. They will return to Jesus and serve Him with their whole hearts! Pray that God will refine and purify their lives—whatever it takes.

When Jesus comes in the clouds of glory and we are taken home to be with Him forever, the trials of this life will fade into insignificance. Whatever it takes, it will be worth everything to be in the presence of our Lord and Savior throughout all eternity!

In your valleys of life, have you been able to pray Socorro's prayer, "Whatever it takes, Lord"? Why not submit your life totally to Him and pray that prayer now?

KAY COLLINS

The Master Diver

*When you pass through the waters, I will be with you; and
through the rivers, they shall not overflow you. Isa. 43:2, NKJV.*

THE WIND WHIPPED my hair into my face as the roar of the dive boat's engine filled my ears. Time had forsaken me and fear gripped my heart as I realized my destiny. Outwardly, I faked the smiling cool exterior of a Jacque Cousteau-experienced diver. But inside I was thinking, *I must be crazy—not knowing anything about scuba but planning to dive onto Australia's Great Barrier Reef.*

My only hope for survival was Rod, my dive master. I listened diligently as he gave me a crash course in buoyancy, how to clear my mask, and the most crucial rule: "Don't hold your breath."

What happened next was one of the most memorable experiences of my life. Rod jumped into the water first, and I followed. Panic bubbled feverishly behind my green eyes. Like a robot I followed instructions to put my regulator in my mouth and start breathing. Rod adjusted all the confusing buttons and buoyancy devices attached to me. I was going under water. Terror devoured every cell in my body, and I gestured for Rod to take me back to the boat. Rod assured me that my fear was natural. I clenched his hand with Olympic strength, and he promised to not let go.

Underwater I started to relax. I continued to focus on my breathing and began to discover a fluorescent underwater paradise. The Australian sun penetrated the crystal clear water, exposing colorful groups of fish and random formations of multicolored coral. Forever changed by the experience, I thanked God for this amazing and unexpected gift of hidden beauty. The sun's golden rays beckoned me as I swam through thousands of small cobalt blue fish that parted in perfect choreography. Picture books can only give a suggestion of the true splendor I experienced that day.

I was vividly reminded of our involved Creator. This same Jesus has promised never to leave our side. He has vowed to hold our hand through the deep waters of our lives.

How much more fulfilled we could be if we would let Jesus be the dive master of our lives. He will hold our hand when the rough waters of life are pushing us under. With Him as our guide we will be safe. When we trust Jesus we can relax and begin to enjoy the beauty and splendor of the incredible journey God has planned for our lives.

Precious Lord, take my hand and hold on tightly so that I can go places and do things for You that I'd be scared to do alone. BONNIE YAW

Don't Let It Sneak Up on You

*You yourselves know perfectly that the day of the Lord so comes as a thief
in the night. . . . But you, brethren, are not in darkness, so that
this Day should overtake you as a thief. 1 Thess. 5:2, 4, NKJV.*

OSTEOPOROSIS KILLED my mother. It's taken me a while to reach this conclusion, but now I'm almost sure. The final blow to her body came because of a terrible head-on collusion. But, I wonder, would her injuries have been so many and so ultimately fatal, if it weren't for osteoporosis?

Mom was only 78 when she died. She was in perfect health except for osteoporosis. The accident tore my foot off my leg bone, but the seat belt saved me from crashing into the steering wheel. The seat belt, however, didn't save my mother. Instead, it may have killed her by breaking so many of her bones and causing so many internal injuries. I'm positive I had a couple cracked ribs in that same accident. My mother's rib cage was shattered, causing respiratory distress, internal injuries, and septicemia.

Mom was always healthy, but osteoporosis sneaked up on her. We began to notice when she was about 65 that her back was more humped, and she complained that even though her eyes were still blue, she was no longer five-feet-two!

She began treatment to prevent more bone loss. She walked on a treadmill each day for 30 minutes because physical, weight-bearing exercise builds bones. She got at least 15 minutes of sunlight each day for Vitamin D, which builds strong bones. She also faithfully ate all the milk products her physician prescribed so that her body would get the required amount of calcium. She had no idea that too much protein can actually cause calcium loss—not gain! It would have been better if she got her calcium from green leafy vegetables.

Osteoporosis affects 25 million people (most are women) in the United States, and yet most doctors don't screen for it. Calcium loss in bones begins around age 30, but it accelerates after menopause when the body quits producing estrogen—that's why many physicians recommend replacement therapy.

The scary thing is that osteoporosis sneaks up on you. Therapy can help rebuild remaining bone, but the intricate honeycomb pattern that makes bones both light and strong can never be restored. I wish my mom had known all of this years before.

Don't let osteoporosis or Christ's second coming sneak up on you like a thief in the night!   KAY KUZMA

You Are What You Eat

God said, "See, I have given you every herb that yields seed which is on the face of all the earth, and every tree whose fruit yields seed; to you it shall be for food. Gen. 1:29, NKJV.

"YOU ARE WHAT you eat." That's a scary thought, especially after Thanksgiving dinner. If the aphorism holds true, I have now been transformed into an eclectic collection of our friend Beth's delicious gluten steaks, home-made mashed potatoes, perfectly cooked veggies, the best bread rolls I've eaten for years, and pumpkin pie that was truly to die for. Too much of all.

"You are what you eat." I do not know anyone who would like to become a gluten steak, so if I had my druthers, I'd like to become the pumpkin pie!

"You are what you eat." I think it's a statement about cholesterol, fat cells, sugars, quantity, and follow-through on all those desperate promises to exercise. If I eat half the box of See's chocolates, I will be sick. Or at least sicker. On the other hand, if I balance my plate with "at least three colors each meal" I will be healthier! Let's see, the chocolate counts as a "dark," the corn is a yellow, the peas a green, and the tomatoes a red. That's sort of balanced.

"You are what you eat." More than a commentary on nutrition, it's a challenge to be alert to what's happening to my body, to analyze the options and make wiser choices. Too often I just wallow through the day, grabbing food that is available and easy to eat while doing three other things. My "diet" pays little thought to planning or preparing. Unfortunately, I often work right through the time when I should be eating . . . and then suddenly realize I'm hungry and tired.

There is another interesting truth about eating: All food has greater nutritional value if it is taken while in conversation with others at the table. Good friends can make even pizza and popcorn into a healthy three-color meal! Good friends make a simple meal a banquet!

I think that's what God had in mind on the sixth day of Creation. First He created all of the mammals, except humans. Then He made Adam and Eve. And almost the next thing He did was to give them dinner. (See Genesis 1:29.) I think God stayed around for the meal. They talked about the animals, about the trees, about fish, birds, sun, stars, and kangaroos. He showed them what to do with walnuts, wheat, peaches, lettuce—and pumpkins. They laughed a lot and said "thank you" a gazillion times. 'Twas the first Thanksgiving dinner!

Every meal can be "Thanksgiving" with your Creator. Invite Him to eat with you today.   DICK DUERKSEN

The Sound of Silence

Then, because so many people were coming and going that they did not even have a chance to eat, he said to them, "Come with me by yourselves to a quiet place and get some rest." So they went away by themselves in a boat to a solitary place. Mark 6:31, 32, NIV.

IT HAD BEEN A doozy of a day. I collapsed onto the couch beside a pile of laundry that threatened to topple to the floor before I could fold it. Dirty dishes were stacked in the sink and covered every grubby counter top. A puddle of orange juice had congealed on the kitchen table. I couldn't remember the last time the place had been vacuumed, let alone dusted. I had at least 24 hours of work ahead of me and it was, technically, my bedtime.

Panic overwhelmed me. There was no way I could do it all. I wasn't Superwoman. I was just super tired. All day, every day, people in my life took, took, took. No one replaced anything. At the end of each day I was dry as dust. Not only wasn't there anything left to give, there wasn't anything left. Period. My insides were shriveled up.

The worst part was that I knew I was going to leave most of the work undone, drag myself to bed, and repeat the whole process tomorrow. And the day after that. And the day after that.

"Help, Lord," I cried silently. "How do You expect me to do all this?"

"I don't" was the simple reply.

"You don't?" It came slowly. Realizing what He meant. I didn't get it at first. It wasn't until I looked at Jesus that it finally snapped into place. Jesus was tired too. Everyone around Him made demands, night and day, day after day. They didn't let Him rest.

But that never stopped Him. He took the initiative. He went off by Himself, He crossed lakes, He climbed mountains. All in the name of solitude. And He came back refreshed, energized. Ready to meet the new demands of each day. Because He met God there.

So, I did too. I went on long runs. I climbed a mountain. I found my quiet places away from the crowds. Oh, the dishes are still there, the demands still come, but my quiet place, my solitude, gives me a new perspective on things. It's there He speaks to me the loudest. Buried thoughts surface and we deal with them. Letting go of them gives us the energy to face the next crisis.

Where do you go to find a solitary place away from the "crowds" where you can find God? Have you been there today? Share how this time of silence energized you.

CÉLESTE PERRINO WALKER

Something You Shouldn't Do in the Dark

Light is sweet, and it is pleasant for the eyes to behold the sun. Eccl. 11:7, RSV.

BEFORE I MOVED to Maryland nearly seven years ago to become *Vibrant Life* editor, I spent virtually all my life in southern California. So I've had a lifelong love of sunshine. In southern California, getting outside and enjoying the sun's warmth on your face is a year-round pleasure.

Believe me, life in Maryland can sometimes be jarring for a sun lover. As I'm writing this, I can look out my office window and see a beautiful blue sky and what looks like a wonderful sunny day. Just one problem—the wind chill outside is 22° F. Twenty-two! Even after seven years this Los Angeles native can't get used to those numbers on a weather report. But recently an interesting item crossed my desk, one that has caused me to think that maybe I need to just bundle up and head outside anyway.

A researcher at the University of California at Irvine recently surveyed a number of college students who are concerned about their weight or dieting, trying to lose excess weight. He found that darkness can serve as a trigger for binge eating. It seems that low light levels make dieters feel less self-conscious, which leads to more uninhibited eating habits. The study also found that those who spent more of their waking hours in daylight were less likely to show binge eating tendencies. This isn't an insignificant finding—at any given time more than half of American women are on a diet, as are 25 percent of American men.

It has long been known that shorter winter days can cause depression in some people. But this study puts a whole new spin on that New Year's resolution you made to lose some weight. Spending more of your waking hours in darkness puts that goal at a high risk for failure.

Many years ago a very wise man made an observation that could have predicted the results of this new research: "Light is sweet, and it is pleasant for the eyes to behold the sun." God gave us the sunlight, and it's free to everyone. It's important to get out and enjoy the sunshine every day possible.

Hey, I'm not saying I'm perfect. I enjoy warm Krispy Kreme doughnuts in the evening as much as anyone. But, pushed to make a choice, I like shooting hoops with my boy on a warm sunny afternoon better.

Have you had your daily dose of sunshine today? If not, get up and get going!

LARRY BECKER

Playing Chicken With Sin

Therefore submit to God. Resist the devil and he will flee from you. James 4:7, NKJV.

WOW! I THOUGHT as I picked up *Time* magazine's January 21, 2002, issue and read Christine Gorman's article, *Playing Chicken With Our Antibiotics.* "I'm glad I'm a vegetarian!"

The article begins: "A few of the birds in a so-called grow-out building have started snickering—the chicken equivalent of coughing." It appears that the problem is a respiratory infection that could spread to the 20,000 other birds in the chicken house in a matter of days. But since it's impractical to treat the sick birds individually, the vet recommends the antibiotic enrofloxacin (the animal version of Cipro) be put into the drinking water of the entire flock of chickens. Five days later the birds are doing fine. Disaster has been averted.

But it's not OK! "While enrofloxacin kills the type of bacteria that sickened the chickens, it doesn't quite eliminate a different strain, Campylobacter that lives in the intestine. The surviving germs, which don't cause any poultry diseases, quickly multiply and spread the genes that help fend off the antibiotic. Six weeks later, when the broilers are carved up at the slaughterhouse, resistant bacteria spill out everywhere." It is pointed out that even with the best sanitary controls "some *Campylobacter* is shrink-wrapped along with the thighs, breasts, and drumsticks that are delivered to your kitchen counter."

Campylobacter is a major cause of food poisoning if you don't properly wash your hands or you eat undercooked meat. The antibiotic, Cipro, is so closely related to human Cipro, that any germ that survives the chicken antibiotic will not be killed by the human one! Here's the problem: The more antibiotics used, the more drug resistant germs become and the less effective antibiotics are in conquering such illnesses as pneumonia, tuberculosis—or anthrax.

It's a lot like the sin problem. The more you dabble in worldly things that compromise your health (spiritually and physically), the less sensitive you become to the danger. It looks good, it feels good, and you begin to think it *is* good, whether it's over-the-counter-drugs, pornography, overeating, or gossiping. My advice? Don't play chicken with sin! It dulls your conscience, and you become resistant to the Holy Spirit. Jesus is the only answer!

The Bible promises that if you submit to God and resist the devil, he will flee from you. Why not ask Jesus, right now, to give you the strength to say no to harmful habits?
KAY KUZMA

Midnight Meditations in ICU

Woman, where are those accusers of yours? Has no one condemned you?"
She said, "No one, Lord." And Jesus said to her,
"Neither do I condemn you; go and sin no more." John 8:10, 11, NKJV.

IT STARTED BY my shoveling snow. I knew I shouldn't be doing it. Because of my heart disease, a kind and dutiful doctor friend had warned me. Nevertheless, it seems as though those laws that are given for our own best good are the ones we transgress far too easily. In temporal matters we call it a lack of judgment, disobedience, or defiance. In spiritual terms we call it sin.

Halfway through my snow-shoveling task I felt as though giant hands were grabbing hold of my chest with unbelievable force. Gasping for breath, I barely managed to get inside the house before everything went black. A doctor gave me injections. The ambulance took me away. Before I knew it, I was lying in the Intensive Care Unit. Here definite laws governed. Efficiency and cleanliness prevailed. Personal attention, thoughtful care, and love were given priority. These life-savers, these marvelous servants of mercy, moved quietly and efficiently. I felt a hand on my shoulder; I got a comforting word. Fear was banished and replaced by knowing that I was in safe hands.

Here I was in an ICU bed, decidedly a physical "sinner." I had been shoveling snow contrary to my doctor's orders, and now I was reaping the full consequence of my disobedience. It would have been quite natural to expect words of condemnation. But I didn't experience a single negative syllable from those who were doing their best to save my life.

In the hospital the primary concern is to save life. Isn't that also what ought to be the all-prevailing interest of the church? Why do so many sinners in the church—those who in one way or another have gone contrary to the will of God—feel condemned, even rejected? What makes it so hard to come back if one has failed? Could it be we are lacking in love?

Now I am back home, trying to apply the lessons gained from this experience. Every church member is in need of a private intensive care unit. I like to remember that Jesus calls us to give time, sympathy, and understanding care in service to others. Saving lives is still the primary thing.

The words that were left with me as I left the hospital were uttered firmly and decidedly, but with a sympathetic smile by the doctor in charge. In their practical simplicity, they reminded me of the words of Jesus to the sinner: "Now, go home, but shovel snow no more."

Do you hear the Savior saying something similar to you? Isn't it about time to go home?   ALFRED C. BERGER

341

The Praying Hands

Give, and it will be given to you: good measure, pressed down, shaken together, and running over will be put into your bosom. For with the same measure that you use, it will be measured back to you. Luke 6:38, NKJV.

ALBRECHT DÜRER'S masterpiece, "The Praying Hands," has changed my life. But it's the story behind the picture that brings those hands to life—and has given me an understanding of what it means to sacrificially give to others.

The story unfolds in the fifteenth century in a village near Nuremberg where there lived a family of 18 children. The father, a goldsmith, worked 18 hours a day to keep food on the table.

Two of the brothers, Albrecht and Albert, had a dream to study art in Nuremberg. But there was no money. The boys agreed to toss a coin. The loser would go into the nearby mines and work to support his brother. In four years when the winner completed his studies, he would support the other. Albrecht won the toss.

Almost immediately Albrecht was a sensation. His etchings, woodcuts, and oils were far better than most of his professors, and by the time he graduated he was beginning to earn considerable fees for his commissioned works.

When the young artist returned to his village, his family celebrated with a festive dinner. Albrecht rose to propose a toast to his brother who had made it all possible, "And now, Albert, it is your turn. Now you can go to Nuremberg to pursue your dream, and I will take care of you."

"No, no, no!" cried Albert, tears running down his cheeks. "It is too late. Look at what four years in the mines have done to my hands! The bones in every finger have been smashed at least once, and I suffer arthritis so badly in my right hand that I cannot even hold a glass to return your toast, much less make delicate lines on parchment or canvas with pen or brush."

To pay homage to Albert for his sacrifice, Albrecht painstakingly drew his brother's hands with palms pressed together and abused fingers stretching skyward—the famous praying hands.

Now as I look at Dürer's drawing I wonder, do I really know what it means to sacrificially give? To give until it hurts? To give my life for another? Am I missing the promised blessing in Luke 6:38 by not giving as God has given to me?

Lord, You sacrificed Your life for me. What can I give sacrificially in return?

CAROLYN TOWLES

God Forgets More Than Dented Cars

Hide Your face from my sins, and blot out all my iniquities. Create in me a clean heart, O God, and renew a steadfast spirit within me. Ps. 51:9, 10, NKJV.

ONE DAY AS I was driving my husband's new dream car to work, I dented the back fender. When I realized I couldn't get it fixed before my husband found out, I asked my small children to be sure to let me be the one to tell their daddy what I had done. At about 5:30 that evening they stopped him as he turned into the driveway. "Daddy, you won't believe what Mommy did!"

"What has she done?"

"Daddy, it's so terrible that she doesn't want us to tell you that she dented the Mercedes!"

So by the time my husband gave me a welcome kiss, he already knew about the dent. I felt terrible and wanted to get it fixed immediately. But he was so understanding. "Sweetheart, I don't see why we need to get it fixed right away. Maybe you'll dent it again, and then we'll just get both dents fixed at the same time!" We laughed. He kissed me again, and as far as I know, he not only forgave me, but he also forgot—he chose not to recall! He never again mentioned the dent.

Did you know that God also forgets? Remember all the terrible things King David did? He committed adultery, then murder to try to cover up his affair, and . . . well, if we really knew, he probably broke every one of God commandments. But in 1 Kings 14:8 there is an interesting reference to King David. Here's the background: After David, his son Solomon reigned, and then the kingdom was divided, and Jeroboam, who was not of the house of David, became the king of the 10 tribes of Israel. When Abijah, the son of Jeroboam, got sick, Jeroboam told his wife to ask the prophet, Ahijah, what was going to happen. Here's the message God told Ahijah to tell Mrs. Jeroboam: Even though God took the kingdom away from the house of David and gave it to Jeroboam, "yet you have not been as My servant David, who kept My commandments and followed Me with all his heart, to do only what was right in My eyes" (NKJV).

"Wait a minute, God. What do You mean, David kept all Your commandments and never did anything wrong? He committed adultery and murder, and—"

When God forgives, apparently He also forgets! Now that's good news!

If God forgives and forgets, shouldn't we also forgive and forget those who wrong us? KAY KUZMA

God Says It With Flowers

The steadfast love of the Lord never ceases, his mercies never come to an end;
they are new every morning; great is thy faithfulness. Lam. 3:22, 23, RSV.

THE GREATEST NEED in the world is to be loved; loved because you exist, not because of what you do or how you look. God loves us that way, but so few realize it! They may sing, "Jesus Loves Me" or quote John 3:16, but do they really feel His love enough to wake up every morning with a love song in their hearts?

I believe God is trying to remind us of His awesome love through the gift of nature. To me, God says it best with flowers.

As I write, I am marveling over several cyclamen blossoms that I couldn't resist picking from hanging plants outside. The petals are a delicate magenta brushed with white, an exquisite living watercolor. With my glasses on, I can see a wondrous shading of color and texture that brings tears to my eyes. Cyclamen are a special wintertime gift from God, blooming bravely and beautifully through unbelievably cold California weather when so few other flowers can be found. The individual blossoms last for one to two weeks, a tiny foretaste of the New Earth. Each winter cyclamen, in vibrant shades of purple, pink, lilac, and magenta, brighten our deck and bring joy to our hearts. But what means infinitely more to me is the message that God has written upon each petal—if only we have eyes to see it: "I love you, I love you, I love you!"

" 'God is love,' is written upon every opening bud, upon the petals of every flower, and upon every spire of grass" is the way one inspired author put it! (*Patriarchs and Prophets,* p. 600).

Why is it that so many miss these messages of love that God has written upon every living thing? I believe the answer is simply that we need to see with our heart as well as with our eyes. Anyone can enjoy a lovely flower, but only those who believe the Bible truth of God's steadfast love for each one of us can see His "secret messages" written across earth and sea and sky. This, I believe, is the secret of living a life filled with joy and peace in a sin-spoiled world—the abundant life that only a loving God can give.

My prayer is that you, too, have seen an "I love you!" from God today.

What is it in nature that reminds you most of God's love for you? Thank Him for sending you His love message.   RUTHIE FLYNN

When You've Missed
Out on Fame and Fortune

I said, "I have labored to no purpose; I have spent my strength in vain and for nothing. Yet what is due me is in the Lord's hand, and my reward is with my God." Isa. 49:4, NIV.

YEARS AGO I HAD a dear friend who constantly moaned that no one appreciated her work. She felt she was laboring in vain, and my attempts at helping her to feel worthwhile were useless. One day I read Isaiah 49:4 and shared it with her, and she was able to unload her guilt at feeling unproductive.

When Keats was dying he said, "I have written my name in water." He didn't realize at the time, nor would he have cared, that it was written in marble. This is true of many while they live; they have no idea of the influence and the beauty they will leave behind. During life their love and hopes were not reciprocated nor their mistakes vindicated, so they feel they have disappointed God and others. Especially those who have aimed high, feel the crash of disappointment.

Elijah mourned, "I am no better than my ancestors" (1 Kings 19:4, NIV); Moses lamented, "I cannot carry all these people by myself; the burden is too heavy" (Num. 11:14, NIV); and David felt like giving up: "One of these days I will be destroyed by the hand of Saul" (1 Sam. 27:1, NIV). And then there was Jesus, who was crucified. To many onlookers, His life must have seemed like a failure.

But God sees all this in a very different light. Instead of comparing our work with that of others, let us defer it to His fair judgment. "My reward is with my God," not with individuals. It's impossible for us to estimate our life's work. Even the Messiah became disheartened: "All day long I have held out my hands to a disobedient and obstinate people" (Rom. 10:21, NIV).

God judges by motive and mission. Many a noble effort slips past coworkers, relatives, and friends, but God sees and knows all. If we keep in mind that our Brother, Jesus, missed out on fame and fortune while on earth, then we can forget about reward. For His unceasing kindness, Jesus was rewarded with the ultimate cruelty of being nailed to a cross. In perspective, our treatment is so much better than what Christ received, why should we worry or complain about what we receive or don't receive on earth?

Lord, on the days I feel unproductive and unappreciated, let me remember that my fame and fortune is in Your hands. PAT NORDMAN

The Romanian Potato Miracle

*Then Isaiah said, "Prepare a poultice of figs." They did so
and applied it to the boil, and he recovered. 2 Kings 20:7, NIV.*

SHE SAID, "GOD has put your tonsils there. Who are you to take them out?" I had never thought of it that way! I had just been scheduled for an urgent tonsillectomy at the best hospital in Bucharest. My doctor had said, "Your throat is a mess. Come tomorrow and we will take out your tonsils. If we don't, the strep will go to your heart!" And now this tiny old woman was telling me that no one should take out of my throat something that God put there!

She continued, "First of all, no more sugar, white flour, refined salt, or cheese. Eat only three meals a day, nothing fried, and make sure you have salad at every meal. Every evening take a raw potato, cut two cone-like pieces, and stick them in your ears. Grate the rest of the potato and apply it around your neck. Tie a piece of cloth around your neck and ears to hold the potato in place. Ask your wife to drop three drops of freshly squeezed lemon juice on your tonsils. Then pray and go to sleep. I will pray too."

Don't ask me why, but I gave it a try. For one week I went to bed with raw potato around my neck and in my ears. I smelled like a farm and messed up the bedding with raw potato juice.

Exactly one week later, when I looked at my throat in the bathroom mirror I was shocked! My tonsils were back to their normal size—they had not been like that since my childhood. Both of them had a bright rose color and, what was more important, all the infection was gone.

The next day I went to my doctor. When I stepped into his office he declared me at once insane, irresponsible, and a public danger. I said, "Doc, don't you want to have a look in my throat?"

"Only from behind a glass wall," he said.

"Come on," I urged, "just once."

He covered his mouth with the corner of his lab coat and came closer. I (proudly) opened my mouth. He was stunned and said, "It's impossible! Take a seat and tell me everything."

I said, "Doc, you take a potato, don't boil it. It has to be raw. It will smell awful and it will mess up your pillow, but . . ."

In the Bible God has given us hints of natural remedies, such as the application of a poultice. Do you know why a poultice works—and when to use one? Maybe it's time to find out!   CEZAR R. LUCHIAN

Please Don't Pass the Chocolate

See, I have set before you today life and good, death and evil. . . . Therefore choose life, that both you and your descendants may live. Deut. 30:15-19, NKJV.

I'M A CHOCOHOLIC! I'm addicted to chocolate. I don't just like it, I love it. The creamy taste of chocolate cherries . . . Yum! For nibbling, there are M&M's. And on a chilly evening there is nothing as pleasant as a cup of hot chocolate. Put me in front of 31 flavors or a variety of cookies, and you can bet I'll choose something with chocolate in it.

I've always known chocolate contained caffeine (actually, it's theobromine—a relative of caffeine). From Dr. Neil Nedley's book *Proof Positive,* I learned that men who ate 20 mg or more of theobromine a day doubled their risk of prostate cancer—and it doesn't take too much chocolate to reach that level! One ounce of Cadbury milk chocolate has 44 mg; 2 tablespoons of chocolate syrup has 89 mg; and 2 to 3 heaping teaspoons of chocolate flavor mix in 8 ounces of whole milk has 120 mg.

But, I rationalized, "I'm a woman. What's wrong with a little chocolate? Everyone eats it!" (I tried to overlook the fact that chocolate also contains the carcinogen alpha-methylbenzyl alcohol.) I had tried to give up chocolate before just because it's loaded with sugar—and calories. But when someone passed the truffles, I always took one.

Then came that fateful day in July 2001. . . . I was holding a women's retreat and extolling the virtue of self-discipline. "It's the key to good mental health!" Then I added with some hesitation, "But then there's chocolate!"

After my presentation Joan Misener challenged me. "I was addicted to chocolate, too. My son bet me $50 that I couldn't go without it for a year. I took the dare—and did it." Then without thinking she said, "I'll do it for another year if you will do it, too."

I was trapped. I couldn't say no. And now I've done it! Giving up a bad habit is all a matter of choice. God said He will not allow us to be tempted more than we're able to resist. But I've learned that when making a habit change it sure helps to make a commitment to someone you respect—and then ask God to help you honor it.

Is there some nagging habit you know you should give up? Take the challenge. Give it up for a year, and chances are you'll have the self-control to continue saying no.   KAY KUZMA

Developing a Beatitude Attitude

Blessed are the meek, for they shall inherit the earth. Matt. 5:5, NKJV.

THE WORD *BEATITUDE* is defined as "blessedness" in the dictionary, and blessedness is a concept Jesus taught in His sermon on the mount in Matthew 5. Webster defines "attitude" as a "position assumed."

As a child, my grandmother reminded me more than once that I needed to change my attitude. The truth was, my outlook on any given situation leaned far too frequently toward the negative. It was God's intervention in my life that helped me combine meekness and blessedness of mind, eventually leading me to what I call a "beatitude attitude."

No single encounter can be credited for the evolution I have experienced through the years. It has been a cumulative shaping of character through a myriad of experiences, with innumerable individuals. One such person, however, shines forth as a prime model to illustrate my testimony.

I sized her up from our first meeting and decided I disliked her just because of the way she looked. Beyond her looks was her brash, bold, and loud speech. She was opinionated, had a ready solution for every problem, and, in my estimation, lacked every social grace I had been taught. I determined to cross her off my candidate-for-friend list and decided to avoid her as much as possible. That was not an option, however, because we were thrown together frequently.

Things I didn't know about her at first were revealed to me gradually, through our almost daily encounters. As I learned about the circumstances that shaped her life I began to understand why she did what she did, and I began to change in the way I related to her.

She and I will never be the "soul mates" that some of my other friends are, but by the same token our friendship is much more than casual. Had I continued on the same course I was intent upon at our first meeting, I would never have really known her. It would have been my loss had I not allowed God to alter my attitude. And she is only one in a long list of individuals I would not have known without this heart change.

The "beatitude attitude" has enriched my life mentally, physically, and spiritually in developing healthy relationships with a variety of personalities. Solomon was right! "A merry heart does good, like medicine" (Prov. 17:22, NKJV).

Do you at times have an attitude problem? Why not start developing a beatitude attitude?   FERYL E. HARRIS

Liars and Those Who Believe Them

Lying lips are an abomination to the Lord, but those
who deal truthfully are His delight. Prov. 12:22, NKJV.

EVE BELIEVED THE lie of Satan, "If you eat this you won't die!" but that didn't save her from the penalty of her sin. Eve blamed the serpent for not telling the truth, but was her predicament really his fault?

Just because we are gullible and fall for a lie, whether it's a get-rich scheme or the latest food fad doesn't mean we won't suffer the consequence of losing money or compromising our health. That's why we must use our heads and get the facts rather than believe everything we're told.

In Proverbs 22:3 is this warning: "A prudent man foresees evil and hides himself, but the simple pass on and are punished" (NKJV). A simple person is foolish, an ignoramus, or one who is intellectually slow. None of us want to be "simple," yet a lot of bright people are acting like fools when it comes to believing claims such as "The stuff in this bottle will cure all your ailments." Today there are many unproven health care ideas being promoted: blue green manna, weight control methods, cancer cures. The claim is made that all the good of many vegetables and fruits can be had in a few pills! But that's simply not true. Nothing can take the place of God's original diet of a good balance of fresh fruits and vegetables, grains and nuts.

Why are we being told half-truths about many health cures? It makes money. This is the greatest reason quackery exists. A slight dishonesty can result in someone becoming a millionaire.

Why do we believe? Because of the promise that we'll get good results quickly, without any effort. Just as many fall for "get rich quick" schemes that don't require any work, so people fall for "get thin" schemes that don't limit caloric intake or require exercise. Take, for example, the lie that you could lose weight by having a balloon put into your stomach so that you feel full all the time and can't eat much. The price for the procedure was high. But in the end it was admitted that once the balloon was removed, the patient had to learn how to eat properly to keep the weight down. The truth is, a proper weight reduction program takes discipline.

Many would rather have a quick fix than to change their lifestyle. Just remember, in the end the foolish perish!

Lord, help me to love and search for truth, both for my physical health and my spiritual well-being. JOHN A. SCHARFFENBERG

God Meant It for Good

God meant it for good, in order to bring it about as it is this day,
to save many people alive. Now therefore, do not be afraid; I will
provide for you and your little ones. Gen. 50:20, 21, NKJV.

PARENTING CAN BE painful. Little did I know! It had been years since I had crumpled into my mother's arms, sobbing. We were sitting in the family waiting area outside the Neonatal Intensive Care Unit (NICU). My wife, Laura, was still hospitalized 80 miles away, where Allison had been born nearly 24 hours before. A vacuum extractor delivery had left her severely injured—two skull fractures and four hemorrhages, one in the right frontal lobe of her brain. So much had happened so quickly! The images spun in my head.

Seeing my new little daughter, only hours old, struggle to breathe and then stop breathing and turn blue while a physician worked to keep her alive. Waiting patiently for the CT scan and then, like in the movies, being asked to sit down before they explained the seriousness of her injuries. A night spent with a little person struggling to live, her tiny hand gripping my finger. Finally, when her little body started convulsing with seizures, I fell apart.

Laura was released and arrived that evening. It was a night of weeping, but then a light in the darkness. My mother shared a scripture with me that brought hope: "But God meant it for good, in order to bring it about as it is this day, to save many people alive" (Gen. 50:20).

It's been a long journey. Four weeks in the NICU. Thousands of prayers lifted up by brothers and sisters in Christ, and brain surgery under the gifted hands of Dr. Ben Carson. Did God keep His word?

The answer comes in a collage of images engraved in my mind. Nurses and other parents stooping to read the little scripture verses hung on Allison's hospital crib. Sharing with another struggling parent about God's power to cope. Charles Gibson, 20/20 anchor, who presented Allison's story nationwide, along with a warning about the risks of vacuum extractor deliveries. Judy Frobes, recently baptized into our church family, holding up Allison, gazing earnestly into her little eyes, and exclaiming, "You'll never know what a blessing you have been to us!"

Given the extent of her injuries, it is remarkable that Allison survived. Even more miraculous is the fact that today she shows no evidence of residual problems from her injury.

Praise God! He is so good! DAVID WESTBROOK

A Body Is a Terrible Thing to Waste

Do not crave his [the rich man's] delicacies, for that food is deceptive. Prov. 23:3, NIV.

RECENT REPORTS ARE chilling. Increasingly, type 2 (adult onset) diabetes is turning up in children, and health experts fear an impending health crisis. So far, all studies have pointed to obesity as a factor.

Adult onset diabetes has long been considered a disease of middle age or later. Obesity in later life increases the risk. However, until recently it was not considered a disease of childhood (in contrast to type 1 diabetes). But American children are getting fatter faster than ever. "Since the early 1960s, the general health of adolescents has declined," says the American Academy of Pediatrics. "Today's kids are flabby. They don't have proper cardiovascular tone. They are not physically fit."

Exercise physiologist Kate O'Shea warns that "the junior couch potato of today is the fat farm candidate of tomorrow." Diabetes isn't the only concern. "Heart disease begins in childhood," reports the National Institutes of Health. An examination of 360 randomly selected youngsters aged 7 to 12 revealed that 98 percent of the children already had three or more risk factors.

We now have an environment that supports obesity. There was a time when children raced home from school to change clothes and go outside to play. They climbed trees, rode bicycles, skated, and played games. Today's children spend five to eight hours a day on the internet, watching TV, or playing video games.

By advertising processed foods high in sugar, fat, and salt, television significantly influences the food preferences of children from their earliest years. Time spent in front of the TV set is largely time taken away from body-building, calorie-burning physical activities. Another concern is the rising interest of children and adolescents in the Internet. Sedentary pursuits set the stage for excessive weight gain that is also a risk factor for high blood cholesterol and heart disease.

In the first two chapters of the Bible we find that God gave Adam and Eve the responsibility of caring for the garden in which they lived and for the living creatures that He had created. Theirs was to be an active, outdoor life.

"Fitness can be fun," says Arnold Schwarzeneggar, who was President Bush's spokesman for the Council on Physical Fitness and Sports. "Stay away from junk food, get off the couch, unplug the Nintendo, turn off the TV, and go out and get some exercise. A body is a terrible thing to waste."

Lord, habits are so hard to change. Give me strength to keep going in the right direction. AILEEN LUDINGTON

Here's to Water—and Your Health!

He would have given you living water. . . . Whoever drinks of the water that I shall give him will never thirst. John 4:10-14, NKJV.

THOREAU ONCE SAID, "Water is the only drink for a wise man." That statement has now been confirmed by the Adventist Health Study at Loma Linda University Medical Center. Jacqueline Chan, chief researcher on the project, said that sufficient water is as important to heart health as other factors such as diet, exercise, and abstinence from smoking. Healthy men who drank five or more glasses of water every day had a 54 percent decrease in the risk of fatal coronary heart disease compared with those who drank only two glasses of water. Women who drank five glasses of water lowered their fatal heart attack risk by 41 percent. Researchers believe that drinking a high volume of plain water works to thin the blood, thus lowering the risk of blood clots. People who replaced some of the water with other fluids, such as fruit juice, milk, or soda, did not receive the same protection.

Five glasses of water will also decrease your risk of colon cancer by 45 percent, breast cancer by 79 percent, and bladder cancer by 50 percent.

Therese Allen, a quadriplegic, said she began drinking 14 glasses of water each day after she suffered a serious kidney infection. Here's her story: "Talk about pain! I never wanted to go through that again. My doctor, however, told me that in my situation I could expect some kind of complication every two to four years. How could I prove this doctor wrong and avoid more infections? I decided to increase my water intake. Since that infection 18 years ago I've had the flu once, three colds, and only two infections. Water works!"

But the sorry fact is that 75 percent of Americans are chronically dehydrated, and in 37 percent the thirst mechanism is so weak that it is often mistaken for hunger. Want to lose weight? Drink more water. Mild dehydration will slow down your metabolism as much as 3 percent. Lack of water is associated with daytime fatigue, back and joint pain, fuzzy short-term memory, trouble with basic math, and difficulty focusing on the computer screen or printed page.

Until we can drink that Living Water Jesus promised to every one of us, may I make a toast? Here's to water, your health, and soon, a life in which we'll never be thirsty again.

Lord, give me a thirst for Your Water of Life, and for at least eight glasses of $H_2O!$ KAY KUZMA and THERESE ALLEN

People Need People

The King will reply, "I tell you the truth, whatever you did for one of the least of these brothers of mine, you did for me." Matt. 25:40, NIV.

DR. KARL MENNINGER was once asked, "If you knew a person was heading for a nervous breakdown what would you suggest?" Everyone expected that the famous psychiatrist would say, "Make an appointment with a psychiatrist as soon as possible," but he didn't. Instead he said, "Lock your door, go across the railroad tracks, and help someone in need!"

This answer is profound. It's the outgrowth of God's second greatest commandment, "Love your neighbor as yourself." It is the essence of what separates the sheep from the goats at the final judgment when the King says, "When I was hungry you fed me; thirsty, you gave me something to drink; a stranger, you took me in; naked, you gave me clothes; sick or in prison, you visited me." It's the gospel in action—the Good Samaritan helping the hurt man on the highway.

God designed the human operating system to function best when serving others. We are wired for relationships. Basically, people need people if they want to be healthy!

Research supports this. If physical habits such as eating breakfast, keeping a proper weight, not smoking or drinking, sleeping adequately, and exercising affect longevity, what about social habits? In a survey, there were four items on the questionnaire that might give an indication as to a person's social health: if married, having close family and friends, membership in a church, or belonging to a social club. The results were startling. Those individuals who had these strong social networks lived longer than even their physical health habits would predict.

People who complain about being lonely are often people who are depressed. They may be married or single but they keep to themselves; they don't join into social activities; they're not outgoing. Instead, they're self-centered.

If this description fits you—and you want to avoid the blues and live a little longer—volunteer your services to a nursing home, community service, or soup kitchen.

Isn't it ironic! The hardest thing to do when you're depressed is the very thing that can help you most: Get up, get out, and get busy helping others.

What can you do today to strengthen your social network—and your health?

WANDA CHIPEUR and KAY KUZMA

The Amazing Snap,
Crackle, and Pop of Your Brain

Praise Him for His mighty acts; Praise Him according to His excellent greatness! . . .
Let everything that has breath praise the Lord. Praise the Lord! Ps. 150:2-6, NKJV.

OF ALL THE ORGANS and systems of the human body, nothing compares to the marvel of the mind itself. It has a hundred billion neurons (nerve cells), all in the right place. How signals travel from one cell to the next to make up our thoughts and emotions is beyond comprehension.

Even today, after thousands of generations of gradually decreasing brain power, our brains still appear to remember virtually everything! This fact was demonstrated more than 40 years ago when physicians, looking for a way to prevent seizures, inserted a probe into the brains of patients, using only local anesthesia. At measured intervals they turned on a small current to "excite" a tiny portion of the brain with the tip of the electrode. They were astonished to learn that, rather than causing a seizure, memory was triggered. The patient would remember some event as though it was happening in real time. They could hear the orchestra, and see the musicians, their instruments, their clothing—all in living color and sound!

Our brains have so much memory capacity that the Lord, when He comes again, isn't going to have to do a brain transplant. We have brains enough for eternity.

Not only does the mind remember everything, it is also marvelously creative. It has imagined and created an astonishing array of "things," as well as ideas, philosophies, art work, and literature.

Yet with all our advanced knowledge, we still don't know how memory works or understand the process of thinking. What's truly astonishing, however, is that the brain accomplishes all this with binary signals. In other words, the nerve cells don't carry complicated information, only an on or an off. There isn't a cell somewhere that carries a signal that means "blue" or one that sends "love." The only thing the nerve cell does is send an electrical "snap." It's not audible, but if the electrical snapping were amplified and connected to a speaker it would sound like a tiny snap or pop.

How does God create thoughts and emotions from a hundred billion snapping nerve cells? Scientists don't have the foggiest idea. How can snapping create love, fear, interest, and inclination? But the Master Designer holds the answer, and someday, after He's restored our brains to their original condition, He'll explain it to us—and maybe, just maybe—we'll be able to understand!

What else is there to say but "Praise the Lord!"   JIM BRACKETT

Giving Good Gifts

Every good gift and every perfect gift is from above, and comes down from the Father of lights, with whom there is no variation or shadow of turning. James 1:17, NKJV.

OUR CHILDREN LOVE to receive gifts all wrapped with pretty paper and ribbon. The highlight of their birthday is unwrapping their gifts. Each year they carefully study the presents under the Christmas tree to find out which are for them, and they eagerly anticipate opening them.

Recently, however, I was thinking about another kind of gift. I am giving these gifts to my children daily, but they don't particularly look forward to them nor do they always appreciate them. One of the gifts is the healthful lunch I try to pack each day. Another is that after school I send them outside into the fresh air and sunshine to get some exercise. Another: we teach them that it is not good to eat between meals. They must wait until mealtime for food. And when their bedtime hour arrives they are reminded to go to bed so that they will get a good sleep.

But when they open their lunch at school and pull out a sandwich with a low-fat vegetarian patty, whole-wheat bread with some lettuce tucked between the slices, some carrot sticks, a pear, and a homemade oatmeal cookie, no matter how tasty it is they look around with envy at others. They longingly eye the white bread and cheese, chips, and some sugary goodie. They don't appreciate the lunch they were given.

When all their friends are talking about the TV program my kids missed while playing outside, they don't appreciate the exercise, fresh air, and sunshine they were given.

But I know I'm giving them good gifts: the gifts of strong healthy bodies, self-control, a taste for healthful food. The blessing of not having the habit of eating all day long, and gaining excess weight. The gift of well developed muscles and a strong cardiovascular system, and a lower risk of degenerative diseases such as cancer, high blood pressure, diabetes, and heart disease. Even though my kids don't always appreciate the gifts they are being given, I know that someday they will.

Are we, too, not a little bit like children in not appreciating God's gifts of healthful guidelines? But someday we will appreciate the gift God has given us in providing us with instruction and counsel that will preserve our health.

Lord, help me to appreciate the gift You've given me in your health guidelines—and the willpower to keep them. JEANNE EKVALL

You've Got to Sleep to Get the Work Done

I will both lie down in peace, and sleep; for You alone,
O Lord, make me dwell in safety. Ps. 4:8, NKJV.

THE LIGHTS WENT OUT, and a quietness descended. Only the soft chirping of cicadas in the deep night broke the silence. As the day guard relaxed, the defense crew slowly began its nightly tasks, careful not to awaken the guard. Soundlessly, a central control system ordered workers to their stations. They brought in supplies and medicines and quietly repaired the ravages of the day's battles. All workers operated skillfully, efficiently, and without interruption.

Eight hours later, when the clanging of the alarm clock aroused the day guard, the others had finished their assigned tasks. For them, it had been a good night. The guard, now alert, was ready to fight for another day; the defense crew would return once again at nightfall to heal the day's wounds.

You have just read about sleep. You are the day guard. While you're awake, you use your energy as you move through the activities of your day. You're probably unaware that you're also causing wear in certain parts of your body. But while you asleep your "defense crew" repairs the wounds, heals the sore places, and prepares you for the next day.

The principle is this: You need to sleep well to stay well. Yet millions of Americans either don't understand that principle or they consciously violate it. It has been estimated that as many as 30 percent of fatal automobile accidents happen when drivers fall asleep. One expert suggests that every day 100 million sleep-deprived Americans are driving, operating hazardous machinery, administering medical care, monitoring nuclear power plants, and even piloting commercial jets!

Your body has built-in rest cycles. For example, your heart contracts in about one 10th of a second. The remainder of that second it rests. During the resting period, oxygen and nutrients nourish the heart. Your kidneys function in three equal shifts: action, rest, and preparation for action. In addition to all the internal built-in rest systems of your body, God designed that one third of each day should be sleep time.

Sleep and rest are part of God's plan for your life. Sleeping isn't a waste of time. This nonworking period is time for your body and mind to restore energy and re-create health.

What a blessing to be able to say, "I will both lie down in peace, and sleep."
Thank You, Lord.   JAN W. KUZMA and CECIL MURPHEY

What I Wish I Had Done Differently

Train up a child in the way he should go, And when
he is old he will not depart from it. Prov. 22:6, NKJV.

NOW THAT THE kids are gone . . .

I wish I hadn't bought so much candy. My mom always had candy around the house—so I fell into the same "motherly" pattern. The temptation to nibble is far less when it's not around. Dried papaya, pineapple, or apple slices make great desserts. A nut-filled prune or date can satisfy a sweet tooth. Cookies are just a lot of empty calories, unless they are healthy, homemade ones. I wish I hadn't bought so many and had baked healthy ones instead.

I wish I hadn't served so much cheese. I was aware of the counsel that cheese could be a problem, but I loved cheesy foods—so I rationalized that things have changed since the nineteenth century when Ellen White wrote "cheese should never be introduced into the stomach" (*Testimonies for the Church,* vol. 2, p. 68). Cheese is now processed under more sanitary conditions, but the high-fat, high-protein, and high-sodium content hasn't changed. And I've been told that the aging process doesn't kill viral and bacterial agents (which is a little scary).

I wish I hadn't served soda. I knew there was nothing nutritious about these drinks and that they contained a lot of sugar, but I didn't realize that a 12-ounce-can of soda could contain as much as 12 teaspoons of sugar! And it doesn't help to drink diet sodas because most contain aspartame, which may be worse than sugar. But the real problem is the chemical additives, some of which interfere with bone metabolism and set us up for osteoporosis later in life. I could just as easily have served a glass of water seasoned with a little lemon, pure fruit juice, or a yummy slushy made with frozen bananas, strawberries, and other fruits whizzed up with some orange juice.

I wish I had learned to cook without milk and eggs. Although most consider these nutritious foods, there are some negatives, such as cholesterol and mad cow disease. I now know that substitutions can be made quite easily if you know how—and many times your family won't even know the difference. I should have taken a good vegan cooking class.

It's too late for my kids to benefit, but I can encourage others to live up to all their knowledge so that they'll have no regrets.

Are you living up to all the knowledge you have about health? What about Bible knowledge?   KAY KUZMA

Nobody Knows the Trouble I've Seen

Never will I leave you; never will I forsake you. Heb. 13:5, NIV.

THE DETERIORATION OF the mind is a terrible thing. People look the same but they're not. What makes a person unique is personality, and when a disease such as Alzheimer's strikes it destroys memory and thoughts that make up who you are. It's your personality that sustains relationships. When something destroys a person's ability to think, the essence of that person is destroyed. The person must still be cared for with love, but he or she can't reciprocate. That's why caring for a family member with Alzheimer's is so draining. As the disease progresses, it becomes more and more a one-way relationship—the caregivers give but there is no recognition for their efforts.

Tommy was the first person I met who had been diagnosed with Alzheimer's. His wife, Betty, often spoke about the loneliness of being his caregiver. A few months before Tommy's death she wrote, "I feel so alone. Tommy demands all my time and strength. I'm not complaining about that. I love him, and I'll stick with him 'for better, or for worse.' I know he'd do the same for me.

"Yet I feel no one understands what I'm going through. Even the children aren't here enough to see the drain and the demand. Most of all, they can't understand the isolated world I live in. I can never go anywhere.

"Today I was really low. I stood at the sink, and the tears flowed. Just then I became aware of the radio in the background. They were playing a spiritual I hadn't heard since I was in school: 'Nobody Knows the Trouble I've Seen.'

"I began to sing along. As I stumbled through those long-forgotten words, I felt strengthened with the realization that 'nobody knows, but Jesus.'

"After the song finished I thought, *That's true. Nobody knows what I'm going through but Jesus.* As peace came over me I understood that at times all of us have to bear part of our pain in private. Nobody really grasps what another person goes through. But we can be comforted by the realization that Jesus understands."

As I reread Betty's letter I resolved to be more understanding of the caregivers in this world. What a wonderful service they provide. But who fills their needs? Who cares for the caregivers?

Lord, is there anyone You need me to minister to today? Help me to be more understanding when others are in trouble and lonely.   CECIL MURPHEY

Walking for the Lord

The people were amazed when they saw the mute speaking, the crippled made well, the lame walking and the blind seeing. And they praised the God of Israel. Matt. 15:31, NIV.

LIFE WAS GOOD to me. I had a wonderful wife and new daughter, and a job I loved, selling Christian books. One night I was calling on families when I drove down a road where, unknown to me, a huge hole had been dug. Construction workers had left a bar across the road to keep people out, but some children had removed it.

Suddenly my car was airborne. The next thing I knew, it slammed to the bottom of the pit so hard that the front cross members on each side of the engine ripped off!

The fall resulted in pain in my back, and neck pain so severe that for three years I was in and out of the hospital many times. I had no control of my legs. I was stuck with pins to see if I could feel them. Nothing! It appeared that I would be confined to a wheelchair for the rest of my life.

The physicians gave me three different nerve relaxants. One day I was on such heavy doses that, thinking I could do anything, I somehow managed to get into the car to pick up the mail at the bottom of our hill. I made the first curve but totaled the car on the second one when I ran into a tree to keep from going into a lake, where, probably I would have drowned.

Back in the hospital I was told I would never walk again. Ever!

I yearned for healing. God had caused the lame to walk; couldn't He do the same for me? When I heard that Pastor Glen Coon, a godly man, was going to be at camp meeting, I determined to ask him to anoint me and pray for my healing. When the time came, friends carried me up into Pastor Coon's travel bus, and he and two or three others knelt and prayed for me.

I went back to my room and fell asleep. The next morning, forgetting about my useless legs, I thought I should get up and help Donna get the car ready for our trip home. Yes, amazingly, I got up and walked! We drove home, where I loaded and unloaded 300 concrete blocks. I have never again had a backache! Praise God, I have been walking for Him ever since.

As I read the Gospels, miracles of healing are recorded on almost every page. Why aren't more happening today? I don't know, but one thing I do know: I'm living proof that God is still a God of miracles. Trust Him. And I pray that He will work one in your life, too!

Thank You, Lord, for Your healing of body, mind, and spirit!

GARY PARKER

Sabbath Appetizers

Give us this day our daily bread. Matt. 6:11, NKJV.

MOST CATERED MEALS include appetizers before the main course. Webster defines an appetizer as something that excites or whets the appetite. Appetizers are one of the favorite parts of a meal.

Sabbath Bible study time might be thought of as an appetizer before the main meal, the divine worship service. After putting a lot of creative and careful preparation into the items served, the chef (superintendent) would be very disappointed if very few guests came for the gourmet foods that are meant to stimulate the taste and add to a sense of satisfaction.

This weekly Bible study event provides an atmosphere of warmth, belonging, and love for friends and family members as all the guests dine and fellowship together. The opening prayer is a blessing upon the food that the guests are about to receive. Appetizers usually offer something special, perhaps a surprise to create a bit of excitement—a special feature or mission story.

Music is a refreshing drink. It quenches the soul's thirst for a cooling, delightful energizer—like a sip of heaven. It creates a longing to hear the angels sing and to participate in the heavenly choir.

The Bread of Life is eaten by the participants of the Bible study classes. It is chewed, digested, and assimilated according to each diner's respective ability to absorb nutrients.

What if the guests came only for the main course (the divine worship service) without first partaking of the appetizer? The diners who attend church only have missed half of the meal. Such diners will probably not starve to death, but they will not be as healthy as they would be if they ate all the nutrients provided "free" yet with much thoughtful preparation.

Ellen White gave some healthy advice when she wrote: "Let not the precious hours of the Sabbath be wasted in bed. On Sabbath morning the family should be astir early. . . . Fathers and mothers should make it a rule that their children attend public worship on the Sabbath, and should enforce the rule by their own example" (*Child Guidance,* p. 530).

Lord, help us to whet the tastes of all family members during the week so they will look forward to the delicious Sabbath appetizers and aromatic main meal that has been so richly prepared for them.

Are you getting all God wants you to get out of His Sabbath?

FONDA L. CHAFFEE

Twists and Turns

Walk in all the way that the Lord your God has commanded you, so that you may live and prosper and prolong your days in the land that you will possess. Deut. 5:33, NIV.

OFTEN IT IS IN times of crisis that we learn meaningful lessons for life. It was in a medical crisis that I came to understand the body's response to injury or surgical invasion. During the 1997 Christmas season I became the proud owner of a stainless steel knee. On the third post-operative day I returned home to enjoy my family for the holidays, but the enjoyment was to be short-lived.

When the anesthetizing nerve block wore off, excruciating pain set in! I tried everything my nurse's mind knew and every suggestion my surgeon offered, with no relief except with heavy medication. Three weeks later my husband and I set out in our motor home for a busy seminar schedule. My husband did everything possible to ensure my physical comfort with special props for my leg. But nothing helped.

When we came back home five months later, I visited my doctor and pleaded for some help to relieve the agonizing pain. He suggested physical therapy. When my therapist noticed the scars on my abdomen, I told her of the many times I had had surgery. She concluded that they had been a major factor in my need for a knee replacement. "What?" I gasped. "How can that be?"

She explained that the fascia, a supportive fishnet-like tissue in the body, forms scar tissue or adhesions from surgeries or injuries. In my case, multiple adhesions had twisted and turned the fascia, pinching nerves and hampering blood flow to the knee. This predisposed it to bone degeneration. These adhesions can be broken by pressure applied in strategic places, which releases the stranglehold on fascia.

Since that revelation, I have come to realize that emotional injuries or neglects coming to us in our character-forming years can form scars that twist and turn our thoughts and feelings, affecting our behavior. Just as a gifted therapist releases tight and twisted fascia and muscles, a loving heavenly Father instructs us how to release the emotional pain we've carried far too long.

Oh, that we would come to Him, acknowledge our hurts, follow His instruction, feel our pain relieved, and go on to lead peaceful and productive Christian lives.

Do you have some scars from your past that may be twisting your thoughts and feelings? Isn't it about time to let the Master Therapist release the pain?

NANCY ROCKEY

Win by Walking Away From Stress

Glory to God in the highest, and on earth peace, good will toward men. Luke 2:14.

IN 1999 DAN REEVES was head coach of the National Football League's Atlanta Falcons. Going into playoffs, he and his team were riding a 12-2 record. A many-time loser in Super Bowl games as coach of the Denver Broncos, Reeves was eager to have another chance to win big.

However, after defeating the New Orleans Saints, 54-year-old Reeves felt a burning sensation in his chest and throat. Team physician Charles Harrison checked him out and sent him to the emergency room, where he underwent a four-hour quadruple-bypass heart surgery.

Dr. Harrison said there was no heart attack and no heart damage, and that Coach Reeves was planning to return "for the NFC playoffs and the Super Bowl."

OK; where's sanity?

Reeves had been highly successful as an NFL head coach, one of the most stressful jobs in the world. He got angry, he shouted; he commanded and demanded 24/7. He stayed up all night mapping out the details of hundreds of football games. He demanded performance, obedience, and allegiance from all his staff and players. He drove himself and everyone else ferociously. Now with a winning team, he was determined to include a Super Bowl win in his career. To him it was a "must do!" And Reeves' heart was shouting, "Are you sure this is what you want to do?" What makes the drive for success so compelling that a person is willing to risk even life itself in order win?

It's possible that you, too, are facing life-or-death decisions. No, you're not an NFL head coach, but chances are your home/work/exercise situation may be moving you toward "fourth and long." Don't wait for your heart to shout at you. Make some moves right now: (1) Visit your doctor for a full checkup. (2) Have your doctor help you design a regular exercise and nutritional program. (3) Do a stress analysis on your work situation. (4) Do a love analysis on your family situation. (5) Fix what needs to be fixed.

The greatest Christmas gift you can give your family (and yourself) is health. It is the only gift that truly "keeps on giving." Instead of "winning" this season, glorify God and enjoy peace and goodwill among your family and friends.

Is the drive to win keeping you under too much stress? What would you win by walking away from it?   DICK DUERKSEN

The Big "C" Battle

Thanks be to God, who gives us the victory
through our Lord Jesus Christ. 1 Cor. 15:57, NKJV.

WITH THE BEST minds in the world trying to conquer cancer, and billions of dollars of research funds poured into finding a cure, this disease is still active, by far the most feared disease in history. Its threat holds no regard for race, color, sex, age, or size of bank account. It takes lives in the U.S. at the rate of one per minute. Science has determined that about a third of the cancers are nutrition related—we just don't get the right nutrients to keep our immune systems healthy. Toxic chemicals in our environment account for another third. Then there's stress. It compromises our immune systems so that we're not as effective as we should be in fighting cancer cells.

Cancer cells are similar to embryonic cells (like that in a fetus), and are believed to arise from a single cell that has mutated. They have a greater potential for growth and can divide an infinite number of times, compared to mature cells, which have a finite life span. They also express many proteins and carbohydrates found only on the surface of embryonic cells. We also know that there are at least three or more mutations that usually occur before cancer develops. Mutant cells are continually being developed and are usually eliminated by the immunologic army of macrophages, lymphocytes, and killer cells. How unfortunate that this army does not always win its wars, and we must fight cancer with outside help, such as radiation and chemo!

Wars are a series of attacks and counterattacks. The Big C war is no different. At the same time that our immune system army is trying to protect us against an invading tumor, the tumor cells devise ways to counterattack. One trick is the withdrawal of proteins from a cell surface so that the cancer cell looks like a normal cell. Another trick is to coat its surface with mucins (glycoproteins) to camouflage itself. A third scheme is to send out surface proteins that act as decoys to confuse the immune system. Our immune systems are better designed to protect us from outside invaders than from a cancer cell enemy that arises within us.

How similar to the battle between good and evil. In the beginning sin started with one mutation—Lucifer—until it took over a third of the angels and all of us here on earth. Satan is now trying to trick us into lowering our defenses by making bad things look good and by weakening our resistance. Let's strengthen our defenses! And isn't it about time for some radical surgery?

Lord, help us to keep our defenses against cancer—and sin—strong and healthy!

KAY KUZMA

My Battle With Chronic Fatigue

*Depart from me, all you workers of iniquity; for the Lord has
heard the voice of my weeping. The Lord has heard my
supplication; the Lord will receive my prayer. Ps. 6:8, 9, NKJV.*

THOSE WHO KNEW me as a child considered me to have endless energy.
All this changed after my father died and I was laid off from my job in 1994.
My new job required working for two bosses, 10- to 14-hour days and
weekends, with no overtime compensation. I had always been fairly healthy,
but I soon found myself regularly succumbing to flu-like symptoms: sore
throats, severe headaches, and colds. In 1995 I made a career change and my
energy drastically decreased. I found myself taking naps after minor activities
such as making the bed or taking a shower, until I was barely functioning.

After spending more than 700 dollars on lab tests, with everything coming back normal—except the Epstein-Barr virus test—I finally had a diagnosis: chronic fatigue syndrome (CFS). I soon found that most doctors don't
know what to do for CFS so they treat the symptoms, order bed rest, and
hope for the best. I took a leave from my job and for the first three weeks
slept 20-22 hours a day. I was still exhausted and suffered night sweats, severe
headaches, sore throats, muscle spasms, and fevers. One day I found I couldn't
lift my legs to get out of bed. I fell to the floor and sobbed uncontrollably. I
prayed, "O God, no one should have to live like this. What have I done to
deserve this?" I crawled, then rested, and crawled again until I reached the
kitchen. I had always been positive, but now I saw only obstacles before me.

Slowly my body gained spurts of energy. A few months later I was diagnosed with fibromyalgia syndrome (FMS), a disease that shares similar
symptoms with CFS. I felt as if a truck had run over me. I felt bruised even
when toweling off after a shower.

As I tried to fall asleep one night I realized that the devil was working
to break me. I told God I would depend on Him for the strength I needed
to survive. I have had many frustrations with CFS, including a recurring case
of shingles, but instead of seeing all this as punishment, I see it as God's opportunity to teach me some lessons. First: too much change means too much
stress! Second: there's a time for everything. The long work hours with little or no breaks for my physical and mental well-being had taken their toll.
I had ignored the warnings my body had tried to send me. Third: the Lord
used this disease to slow me down and teach me to depend totally on Him.

*Take time for yourself today. Be good to your body. Breathe deeply and praise
Him. Trust!*
JOYCE L. KEELER

Turning Sorrow Into Joy!

To give them beauty for ashes, the oil of joy for mourning. Isa. 61:3, NKJV.

WHEN I WAS 8 years old a most despairing crisis occurred. My 6-year-old sister ripped the string out of the back of Chatty Cathy, my one and only talking dolly. To my horror I discovered that she could no longer "chat." My life was devastated, for to me it was as if a real live person had just died in my arms.

My sweet mommy came to the rescue with the perfect remedy. No, she couldn't fix my darling dolly, but she knew someone who could—Santa Claus. She creatively wove a story so convincing that hope filled my aching heart. She wrapped Chatty Cathy in wads of tissue paper and placed her gently in a large cardboard box, telling me that she would send her to the North Pole for Santa to fix and return in time for Christmas. Three months later, on Christmas morning, I awoke to find my precious Chatty Cathy, clothed in a new red velvet dress, unwrapped and perfectly restored. I didn't need any other gift for she was all that I had hoped and prayed for.

I'm grown now and have learned that there is no Santa Claus, except in the loving acts of other people. Instead, we have something much better—a God who deeply cares for His children and has promised to give us beauty for ashes and the oil of joy for mourning.

Robert Fritz, author of the book *Creating,* describes this excruciatingly painful transition from sorrow to joy as a creative process. As humans we experience sorrow as a negative tension within our bodies. It becomes an internal crisis that demands emotional, physical, and spiritual resolution. A positive metamorphosis will occur when the sorrow within us is brought to life in something outside of us.

This has been my experience. I have felt the exhilaration of sorrow transformed to joy when, burdened with sadness, I have sat down to write, only to arise moments later with yet another poem. It has come through the painting of a bouquet and in the gift of speaking out.

God has a purpose for your life no matter what has happened or will happen in the future. Take up your pen, your paint brush, your voice, and discover firsthand that God is much more than Santa Claus and that He takes great pleasure in turning your sorrow into joy!

"Let everything that has breath praise the Lord" (Ps. 150:6, NKJV).

CATHY O'MALLEY

Modern-day Leprosy

A man who was full of leprosy saw Jesus; and he fell on his face and
implored Him, saying, "Lord, if You are willing, You can make me clean."
Then He put out His hand and touched him, saying, "I am willing;
be cleansed." Immediately the leprosy left him. Luke 5:12, 13, NKJV.

WHAT LEPROSY WAS to the world 2,000 years ago, AIDS is to the twenty-first century. Although we don't make victims shout "Unclean!" many still go out of their way to avoid them! Even church members! The leper said to Jesus, "If you're willing" when he prostrated himself and pleaded for healing. I wonder how many times he asked for help and found people unwilling? After the healing, where did Jesus send him? Back to his church family who had rejected him! Interesting!

Carol Grady tells of a young AIDS victim, Scott, who came home to die. She quotes Scott's mom: "One of the hardest things for us to bear was the reaction of our church family. Now I realize the reason our friends avoided us was that they didn't know what to say. Even when I asked them to come and see Scott, very few came. Oh, how much it would have meant to have someone just to listen and share our sorrows. And of course people were afraid they would catch AIDS. Scott wanted so much to play the organ and piano at church one more time, but it wasn't permitted."

Scott asked the pastor to anoint him but the pastor said, "I don't think it would be appropriate. Do you really think the Lord would heal you?" Scott had the grace to say, "Well, that's all right. But could you please pray for my parents, and pray that I'll be able to endure the pain?" "You know, Mom," Scott told his mother, "I think I can understand what it must have been like for Jesus to die on the cross. He was totally abandoned by those who said they loved Him. I'm sure He felt bad that His church family wasn't there for Him."

In a "caring" church, how can we allow this type of rejection? People don't get AIDS from sneezes, coughs, touching, or dry kissing. Nor can you get it from public restrooms, saunas, showers, pools, shared towels, eating utensils, mosquito bites, urine, sweat, or by being friends!

Discriminating against people who are infected with AIDS or anyone thought to be at risk of infection violates individual human rights and endangers public health. Every person infected with and affected by AIDS deserves compassion and support, regardless of the circumstances surrounding their infection. Let's give a healing touch to today's "lepers" as Jesus did!

At this special season, Lord, show me whom I should reach out to and touch for You!

KAY KUZMA

Honesty

Truthful lips endure forever, but a lying tongue lasts only a moment. . . . The Lord detests lying lips, but he delights in men who are truthful. Prov. 12:19, 22, NIV.

FOR MORE THAN 30 years I have stressed that the bottom line to real Christianity is having a personal, intimate relationship with Jesus. I have consistently worked at this—I spent three hours daily with Jesus in morning devotions; attended prayer meetings and church; taught the clients at the Drug Alternative Program about Jesus; walked two miles, five days a week; and even became a vegan—all in an attempt to connect with Jesus. But something was missing.

And then it happened. On a 10-day trip to Belgium, I found the missing link—honesty! A personal, intimate relationship with Christ isn't possible unless you are completely honest with yourself—and God. For the very first time I cried out "honestly" to the Lord, begging Him to rid me of every sin in my life. I thought I was a pretty good person until the "little skeletons" started falling out of my closet—and then the big ones. My soul was crushed, yet I begged God more and more to show me what I needed to do to "come clean" in my relationship with Him.

A part of my reaping took me back 15 years ago to a friend whom I had hurt. The Holy Spirit impressed me to call and apologize. She welcomed my apology, forgave me, and said, "I needed this call today." She prayed for us both, and we promised to meet each other in heaven if not on earth again. I can't tell you how good I felt about the healing that took place between the two of us.

What has this experience done for me? As I have recognized how my Father has blessed me "over and beyond measure" despite my sinfulness—not holding me in captivity but showering me with so many undeserved gifts—the question comes to my mind, what will He do now that my heart is totally surrendered to Him and ready to receive His grace? The thought just blows my mind!

Second, I now try to see people through the eyes of Jesus. I see what they are becoming, not as they are now! Gone is the legalism. The whole world looks different!

My plea is don't just "play" church and miss eternal life, as I almost did. Be honest with yourself and God. As Martin Luther King, Jr., said, "I'm free at last; I'm free at last; thank God Almighty, I'm free at last. And it feels so good."

Have you been honest with God—or are you harboring some secret sin in your life? Ask God what it will take to "come clean" and see what skeletons fall out of your closet! FREDDIE HARRIS

The Miracle and the Mystery

She brought forth her firstborn Son, and wrapped Him in swaddling cloths, and laid Him in a manger, because there was no room for them in the inn. Luke 2:7, NKJV.

I ONCE SAW A painting by Julius Gari Melchers entitled simply, *The Nativity*. The longer I gazed at it the more it seemed to tremble with the mystery of that "starry, starry night" long ago. Perhaps it was the way the artist captured the brooding face of the husband–not–father as he leans forward and pensively stares at the newborn at his feet in that crude box of hay. Or maybe it was the utter "spentness" of the young mother, exhausted, now prone on the cold floor, save for her slumping shoulders propped against the stable wall, her tired eyes at half mast, her weary face resting upon the side of her husband. It makes you wonder: What is it the husband broods upon? What thoughts are his? And what thoughts are hers, the young mother? Do they wonder that the "infant lowly" is the "infant holy"?

Ellen White writes, "The work of redemption is called a mystery, and it is indeed the mystery by which everlasting righteousness is brought to all who believe. The race in consequence of sin was at enmity with God. Christ, at an infinite cost, by a painful process, mysterious to angels as well as to men, assumed humanity. Hiding His divinity, laying aside His glory, He was born a babe in Bethlehem" *The Seventh-day Adventist Bible Commentary*, Ellen G. White Comments, vol. 7, p. 915). Can we ever know the depths of His "painful" descent from heaven's resplendent glory to our drab gloom?

Brennan Manning tells the heartwarming story about little 7-year-old Richard Ballenger in Anderson, South Carolina. It's the day before Christmas. Richie's mother is busily wrapping some packages and asks her young son if he'd please shine her shoes. Soon, with the proud smile that only a 7-year-old can muster, he presents the shiny shoes for inspection. His mother is so pleased she hands him a quarter.

On Christmas morning as she put on the shoes to go to church, she felt a strange lump in one shoe. Taking it off, she shook the shoe and out dropped a quarter wrapped in a small piece of paper. And on the paper in a child's scrawl were the words, "I done it for love."

That's it, is it not? There in the dark shadows of that backyard stable we unwrap the very first Christmas gift, and there on the wrinkled wrapping paper the handwriting of God: "I done it for love." Oh, sure, His grammar would be better—but could you say it any clearer? "I done it for love."

Pause and wonder on this gift of love. What impact has it made on your life?

DWIGHT K. NELSON

A Christmas Miracle

She will bring forth a Son, and you shall call His name Jesus,
for He will save His people from their sins. Matt. 1:21, NKJV.

TUBERCULOSIS WAS killing 23-year-old Eleanor Munro. Physicians had tried everything and had given up hope. Her husband had TB when he returned from overseas after World War II, but before it was detected and checked, they had married, and having no immunity against the disease, she caught it.

It lodged in an almost impossible place to treat—the lower lobe of her lung. The only treatment was for the TB cavity to be forced shut so nature could have a chance to heal it by letting the sides grow together. If it had been in the upper lobe, ribs could have been removed to collapse the lobe, but her body needed the lower ribs for support. They considered removing the lung, but Eleanor was too sick to withstand surgery.

When Dr. MacDougall told Eleanor that there was nothing more they could do, she extracted a promise that if she were alive on Christmas Eve, she be allowed to go home. He promised, but only because he was sure she would be dead by then. But she wasn't. So with warnings to not hold her child and to wear a surgical mask, she was taken home by ambulance.

She came back to the hospital the following night, and her health continued to slip until she could no longer feed herself. But she refused to die. Toward the end of February she was down to 80 pounds when new complications set in. She became nauseated and began to vomit even without food in her stomach. After examining her, a specialist asked if she could be pregnant. Impossible! How could her dying body have conceived? How could it support another life? But the test was positive. Aborting the child wasn't an option; she was so weak the procedure would have killed her.

Then an amazing thing happened: she began to get better. By late March her temperature was coming down. A chest X-ray showed that the growth of the TB cavity had stopped; her diaphragm was pushing up against the lower lobe of her diseased lung to make room for the growing child. The child was saving the mother! What science couldn't do, God did through the miracle of a child!

The greatest miracle of all is ours through another Baby, God's Son. Thank You, Jesus.   KAY KUZMA

Based on the article "Christmas Miracle" by Dr. Joseph A. MacDougall, as told to Douglas How, reprinted in *Women of Spirit,* December 1999.

DECEMBER 26

Witnessing the Impossible

Jesus looked at them and said, "With man this is impossible, but not with God; all things are possible with God." Mark 10:27, NIV.

TINY DEBBIE HAD been sick too long for a simple case of measles. After almost two weeks her worried parents found that their daughter wouldn't arouse when called. She simply lay in bed, eyes staring, unresponsive to mother's murmurs of concern and love. It was time to call the doctor.

I hurried to their home as soon as I could, and made the diagnosis of measles encephalitis. The virus of common measles had invaded the brain of this innocent 6-year-old. The outlook was grim. Settling my little patient in a bed at the hospital, we soon had an intravenous line flowing with vital fluids. Dehydration would soon be corrected. A stomach tube would help provide nutrition.

It was within our power to sustain life, but what about living? Would this innocent little girl ever talk again? Would she shout and play and swim and pray ever again?

Each day, with hope, I made my morning rounds, and each day, following my examination, I quietly closed the door to Debbie's room. A week passed. Then a third, and a fourth. The slender thread of hope was stretched and about to part. It was time, indeed past time, for Divine intervention, an impossible miracle. Centuries ago we had been instructed by the apostle James how to proceed. "The prayer of faith will save the sick" (James 5:15). It was time to call the pastors. Why had I waited so long?

It was evening, going into the sixth week, when we quietly assembled in our patient's room. We were about to plead for a miracle; for healing, perhaps the ultimate act of faith. Prayers were spoken all round. The oil of olives was placed on the forehead of the unknowing patient. We filed out with whispers of mutual comfort.

King Nebuchadnezzar, approaching the den of lions before sunup, could not have rejoiced more than I when I, also at sunup, stole quietly to Debbie's bedside. And wonder of wonders, a timid voice greeted me with "Hi, doctor. The nurses said I'm in the hospital. I want my mommy."

From there on it was a straight and swift road to recovery. James said it most succinctly, "The Lord will raise (her) up."

Is there some impossible thing in your life you'd like changed? A healing? Ask God to make the impossible possible! RAYMOND O. WEST

370

What's Your Purpose for Living?

The Lord will fulfill his purpose for me. Ps. 138:8, NIV.

MY HUSBAND, JAN, had another stroke May 23, 2003. Once again his coumadin (blood thinning) level had slipped so that his irregular heart beat was unable to push the thick blood through his misshapen heart fast enough and a blood clot formed. This time it hit his medulla, the balance center of the brain, resulting in double vision and inability to stand or walk. The term "bouncing off the wall" took on new meaning to those of us watching him trying to get from one place to another. But that didn't discourage Jan, nor did the fall he took rolling down the steep hill into the rocks next to the neighbor's driveway. Regardless of his bruised and bleeding body, the passion to walk drove him to endure two hours of aggressive physical therapy each day. And once again God's healing power coupled with man's determination was a winning combination.

All of us are driven by something. What's driving you? What's your purpose in life? Is it making as much money as possible? Is it getting that next promotion? Or buying that 4x4? Or taking an exotic vacation? Careful! King Solomon said about self-centered goals, "All is vanity."

But even if the driving force in your life is an important short-term goal such as walking again, I propose that its achievement will leave you void of the joy that God promises to you unless you live to fulfill His purpose for your life.

"Without God," Rick Warren writes in his book *The Purpose Driven Life,* "life has no purpose, and without purpose, life has no meaning. Without meaning, life has no significance or hope." Maybe you're like Isaiah, complaining, "I have labored to no purpose; I have spent my strength in vain and for nothing" (Isa. 49:4, NIV). Or like Job, who said, "My life drags by—day after hopeless day. I give up; I am tired of living, Leave me alone. My life makes no sense." (See Job 7:6-16.) Warren concludes, "The greatest tragedy is not death, but life without purpose."

It's healthy to live life with a purpose. Dr. Bernie Siegel found that cancer patients with a purpose to live to 100 years were far more likely to survive than those who didn't care!

Here's the challenge: Live life with a purpose of not just living longer and healthier, but to fulfill God's plan for your existence. I predict the joy of the Lord will grab you!

Lord, why did You create me—with my unique set of genes, personality traits, talents, and interests? What is Your purpose for my life?   KAY KUZMA

Driving Through the Blizzards of Life

Your word, O Lord, is eternal; it stands firm in the heavens. . . . I will never forget your precepts, for by them you have preserved my life. . . . Your word is a lamp to my feet and a light for my path. Ps. 119:89-105, NIV.

I WAS RETURNING from Christmas vacation at home in California to where I was attending college in upstate New York. After spending the night at the home of my brother, Lewis, in Indiana, I was on the last day of the long trip back to school when in mid-afternoon the weather rapidly deteriorated.

Halfway across Ohio it started snowing, and before long the wind began blowing and drifting the snow across the road. Other cars started leaving the freeway to find places to stay for the stormy night, but I was a poor graduate student and had no money for a motel. In the back seat of my Volkswagen "bug" was a very heavy sleeping bag to keep me warm if I got stuck in the snow, so I kept driving.

At times I had to stop and get out of the car to see where the edge of the road was. No one else was on the road except a few large trucks, and they seemed to see through the snow better than I. That's when I discovered a solution to my problem. When a truck passed, I got close behind it so that his taillights were visible to me through the blinding snow.

On we drove through the night, with my eyes glued to those two precious red taillights. Then, just east of Buffalo, New York, the falling snow thinned out, and I could find my way again.

Life has moved on since that blizzard, but other types of storms have sometimes left me wondering which way to go. It's then that I think about the blizzard and the lights that were my trustworthy guide.

How much this is like life. Jesus and His Word are the lights that we can always trust even though we can't see things clearly. They will take us through any problems that life throws at us: health, financial, relational, school, or career. The question is, do we trust enough to keep close to Jesus' light, or do we foolishly lag behind and find ourselves groping alone in the storm?

Every day we must renew our commitment to fix our eyes on Him and allow nothing to distract us from faithfully following Him. Only Christ can lead us safely through the "blizzards."

Have you made following Jesus the first priority of your life?

LEONARD BRAND

How Do You Live Your Dash?

*The days of our lives are seventy years; and if by reason of strength
they are eighty years, yet their boast is only labor and sorrow;
for it is soon cut off, and we fly away. Ps. 90:10, NKJV.*

EVERY SO OFTEN it is good to lean against an old tree or lie down in the
deep grass, gaze up into the sky, and reflect on the way we are living our
lives. We have only one time around on this earth. Are we just treading the
water of self-survival; or are we making a difference in the lives of others?

I find old graveyards fascinating. The stones with the epitaphs—the few
words that sum up the person's life; the word picture that helps to fill in the
blank between the date of birth and that of death. I've often thought how
much the line between the dates represents. One day I came across this
poem by an unknown writer that once again made me reevaluate my life:

> I read of a man who stood to speak at the funeral of a friend.
> He referred to the dates on her tombstone from the beginning to
>   the end.
> He noted that first came her date of birth. He spoke the next with
>   tears,
> But he said what mattered most of all was the dash between those
>   years.
> For that dash represents all the time she spent alive on earth.
> Only those who loved her know what that line is worth.
> It matters not how much we own; the cars, the house, the cash,
> Important is how we live and love; how we spend our dash.
> Think about this long and hard. Are there things you'd like to
>   change?
> You never know what time is left that can be rearranged.
> If we could just slow down enough to know what's true and real,
> And always try to understand the way other people feel.
> And be less quick to anger, and show appreciation more,
> And love the people in our lives like we've never loved before.
> If we treat each other with respect, and more often wear a smile . . .
> Remembering that this special dash might only last a little while.
> When your eulogy is read, your life's actions to rehash,
> Would you be proud of the things they say about how you spent
>   your dash?

How are you living your "dash"?   KAY KUZMA

Grant's Gift of Life to Others

It is God which worketh in you both to will and to do of his good pleasure. . . . Holding forth the word of life; that I may rejoice in the day of Christ, that I have not run in vain, neither laboured in vain. Phil. 2:13-16.

IT WAS NEW YEAR'S EVE. As we began that agonizing trip to the hospital, I began making a mental list of things that would need to be done—call for cost estimates from a couple of mortuaries, make a list of friends and family we should call, keep calm; and then I pleaded again with the Lord to intervene.

A week before, our son, Grant, just 25 years old, was in a motorcycle accident that left him with massive head injuries. Now, despite valiant efforts by the medical team, he was slipping.

My mind raced. How could I go on living without him? He was my pride and joy. Could I be strong enough to face what lay ahead? I knew Grant would hate being an invalid. He was always into physical activities. Was the Lord being merciful by allowing this? Why weren't our prayers being answered? How would his sister be able to face life without the big brother she adored? *Please, Lord, take this cup from us.* On and on my thoughts circled.

Then we were facing the doctor, who told us that Grant was alive only because of life supports. Did we want them shut off? And had we thought about organ donation?

"Yes," our daughter, Jill, piped up, "Grant and I discussed being organ donors some time ago, and we both decided that's what we wanted."

I was shocked. I had never dreamed my children had even thought of such a thing. The decision was quickly made. He would give all his usable organs.

So ended the worst week of our lives and a new chapter began, life without Grant. There was one pinprick of light that entered our darkened souls. What was the result of the organs donated? We had been told that in about three weeks we would receive a letter informing us about the individuals who received the organs. Our lives now revolved around the mail delivery.

Finally it came. We carefully opened the letter and read about the people who were now able to go about their normal lives: A highway patrolman, a construction worker, a medical secretary. regular people, returned home to their families. Some of our sorrow was washed away when we realized that Grant's life was not lost in vain—six people had been given a new chance.

Because of Jesus' death, we all can live. Thank You, Jesus. KAREN LEWIS

Beginning Again

Let each of you look out not only for his own interests,
but also for the interests of others. Phil. 2:4, NKJV.

HE WAS A FAILURE. He messed up his first big assignment. People had admired him; they envied his position; they wondered how someone so young could have risen so high. Then he fell. He had been given the privilege of working with two of the giants in his field, and he blew it. He couldn't take the pressure, and he ran home to mother.

Can you imagine how John Mark felt, walking down the streets of Jerusalem, hearing the whispering, knowing he was a disappointment to his mother and the church members who had seen so much potential in him? Now it was over. He was a has-been. All washed up.

Have you been there? Have you felt like a failure this year? Maybe you started to diet and gained weight. Or got a membership at the fitness center and haven't been there in months. Or vowed you'd read your Bible through, and you're stuck in Leviticus. Have you made decisions you wish you hadn't, and the consequences haunt you? Meet John Mark and take courage.

John Mark was just a kid when Paul and Barnabas, needing an assistant on their missionary journeys, invited him to join them. What a privilege for one so young. But after a few months John Mark got homesick, and Paul quickly sent him on the next boat back to Jerusalem.

Now older, more mature, John Mark once again wanted to go with Paul and Barnabas to visit the churches they had established on their first missionary journey. Paul flatly refused. There are some people like that. They never forget a mistake. They find it hard to grant a second chance. Paul was determined he wasn't going to be burdened down with a crybaby.

But the beautiful part of the story is that Barnabas was just as determined to give John Mark another try. Aren't you glad there are Barnabases in this world, who will stand up for the underdog? Who will say, "You can do it!" Who see potential, regardless of past performance.

At some time everyone needs a second chance. We all long to put our mistakes behind us and begin again. John Mark got that opportunity. And God wants to give you the same opportunity if you'll just take it. As you step into this New Year, why don't you be a Barnabas to someone else? This world needs a whole lot more of his kind!

Thank You, Lord, for new opportunities and new beginnings to feel abundantly alive.   KAY KUZMA

Biographical Sketches

David E. Abbey, Ph.D., is a retired professor of biostatistics at Loma Linda University's School of Public Health. He and his wife, Judy, now live in Millville, California, and are involved in a health mission project in San Jose del Cabo, Mexico. **Sept. 14.**

Tabitha Abel-Cooper, Dr.PH, R.N., C.H.E.S., is a mother, a resource nurse at Loma Linda University Medical Center and Children's Hospital, and a freelance writer. **Feb. 9, Mar. 15, Nov. 16.**

Therese L. Allen, paralyzed since 1974 from an automobile accident, writes from her home in Los Angeles. She passionately enjoys listening to music and watching her favorite teams play hockey at the Forum. **Feb. 20, Apr. 8, Aug. 14, Dec. 8.**

Tim Allston is owner and president of Allston Communications, Inc. He lives in Huntsville, Alabama, with his wife, Elaine. For more information on egoholic recovery, visit www.ego-holicdrecovery.com. **July 13.**

Carole Brousson Anderson, Ph.D., works as a counseling psychologist at Simon Fraser University and as a private therapist. She and her pastor-husband live with their two children in British Columbia, Canada. **Jan. 11.**

George A. Baehm III is a retired former CEO and president of the Baehm Paper Company, Inc. in New York City. He and his wife, Tena, have been active in ASI, Children's Care International, and Maranatha Volunteers International. **June 13.**

Forrest Bailey is an architect who writes from Highland, California, where he lives with his wife, Glenda. His muses wander far, including special interests in the arts, music, culture, cities, and public policy issues. **Jan. 16.**

Leonard L. Bailey, M.D., is professor of surgery at Loma Linda University Medical Center. Known for his pioneering efforts in infant heart transplants, he has performed heart surgery in Greece, Brazil, Korea, China, Saudi Arabia, and Nepal. He and his wife, Nancy, have two sons. **Jan. 1.**

Bernell E. Baldwin, Ph.D., specializes in neurophysiology and taught at Loma Linda University before he came to Wildwood Lifestyle Center and Hospital in Georgia. He coanchors a health news program on 3ABN. **July 1.**

Marjorie V. Baldwin, M.D., taught at Loma Linda University, was editor of the *Journal of Health and Healing,* and a physician at Wildwood Lifestyle Center and Hospital. **Feb. 10, Sept. 20.**

Donna Bechthold, R.N., is vice president of patient care services at Tillamook County General Hospital (Oregon). She teaches for a school of nursing and has authored the book *The Colors of Prayer.* She writes about Ron Bottomly, an ICU registered nurse. **July 18.**

Larry Becker, former editor of *Vibrant Life,* is the executive vice president of university relations at La Sierra University in Riverside, California. He and his wife live in Grand Terrace where Larry enjoys shooting hoops with his son. His devotional reading is taken from an editorial in *Vibrant Life.* **Nov. 25**

Alfred C. Berger, a retired pastor, is a fourth-generation Seventh-day Adventist, and lives in Fagerstrand, Norway. His devotional reading is based on an *Adventist Review* article, "Midnight Meditations" (August 27, 1998). **Nov. 27**

Chris Blake is a professor of English at Union College in Lincoln, Nebraska. His devotional is from an *Adventist Review* article (October 21, 1999). **Aug. 15.**

Alex P. Bokovoy, M.D., F.A.C.S., is a physician who enjoys sharing lifestyle-change information both at home and abroad. **Jan. 13.**

Shawn Boonstra is associate director of It Is Written. He and his wife, Jeannie, have two children. He has written the books *To Your Health* and *The Return.* **May 23, June 26.**

Gordon E. Botting, Dr.P.H., C.N.S., C.H.E.S., C.F.C., is the director of health, community services, and stewardship for the Northern California Conference of Seventh-day Adventists. He and his wife, Margaret, have two grown children. **Apr. 7.**

Charlotte Bowman is an executive assistant at Adventist Health in Roseville, California. She and her husband, Chuck, were missionaries in Bangladesh, Guam, and Russia. They are currently involved in health ministries in the Sacramento community. **Feb. 26.**

Leonard Brand, Ph.D., is professor of biology and paleontology at Loma Linda University, where he teaches and does research. He has chaired the Department of Biology and the Department of Natural Sciences. **Sept. 5, Dec. 28.**

Beverly Chilson Brandstater, R.N., M.F.T., a marriage and family therapist, specializes in depression and anxiety at the Behavior Medical Center at Loma Linda University. **June 1.**

Jim Brackett, M.P.H., is a pastor and health educator. He is currently the director of Church Ministries and the Ministerial departments of the Nevada-Utah Conference of Seventh-day Adventists. **Jan. 2, Feb. 7, Feb. 27, Mar. 18, Mar. 22, Aug. 26, Nov. 19, Dec. 10.**

Rose Nell Brandt received her degree from Pacific Union College in 1947. She and her physician-husband have four adult children. She has been active in church, school, and the Loma Linda University Medical Auxiliary. **July 2, Nov. 17.**

Burton A. Briggs, M.D., is a professor of anesthesiology at Loma Linda University and medical director of operating room services. He lives in Cherry Valley, California, and has two grown daughters. **Apr. 22, Sept. 26, Oct. 1, Nov.7.**

Jennifer Bromley graduated in 2004 from Trinity Western College in British Columbia and plans on becoming a teacher. After marriage she will settle in Portland, Oregon. **Mar. 5.**

Thomas L. Brooks fought a valiant fight against the disease that eventually took his life. His devotional is based on an article he wrote for the *Adventist Review* in December 2000. **May 31.**

Alex Bryan lives in Atlanta, Georgia. **July 6.**

Ruth E. Burke, Ph.D., is an associate professor of French and German at California State University in San Bernadino. She teaches Sabbath school and is a board member of the International Association of Adventist Women. **Oct. 15.**

Diane Burris has two married children and five grandchildren. She loves talking to people and sharing her Christian perspective. She enjoys travel, especially visiting Ireland. **Oct. 19.**

Catherine J. Carpenter is a freelance writer and commercial artist living in Clovis, California, and works in Sierra National Forest near Bass Lake. She is a wife and mother, businessperson, teacher, and an active member of her church. **Aug. 25.**

Michael Cauley is president of Florida Conference of Seventh-day Adventists. His devotional reading is based on an article he wrote for the *Columbia Union Visitor.* **Jan. 4.**

Elden M. Chalmers, Ph.D., now deceased, was an ordained minister, evangelist, licensed psychologist, and professor at Columbia Union College, Pacific Union College, and the Seventh-day Adventist Theological Seminary at Andrews University in Michigan. His devotionals are from his book *Healing the Broken Brain.* **Mar. 9, May 16, Aug. 11.**

Tabasuri Chapman is director of nutritional services at Pacific Health Education Center. Tabasuri has a master's in nutrition, a burden for health evangelism, and a commitment to winning souls for Christ's kingdom. **Jan. 29, Apr. 13.**

Wanda Chipeur, B.S.N., has retired from a career of 38 years in the nursing field. She worked as a supervisor in acute care and as the director of a nursing home. She and her husband, Ed, enjoy their children and grandchildren. **Dec. 9.**

Cheryle A. Chisholm, M.A., was chosen cerebral palsy poster child in 1950 for the Washington, D.C., area. She graduated from Southern Adventist University and studied in Mexico. Since graduating from Middle Tennessee State University with an M.A. in English, she has taught English and Spanish. **Sept. 6.**

Evelyn R. Chisholm, R.N., worked as a critical-care nurse. She and her husband, Darrell, made their home in Cleveland, Tennessee, until her death in 2004. **Mar. 16.**

Jeannine Chobotar is a physical therapist with a specialty in rehabilitation of patients with injuries and disabilities. She and her husband, Todd, make their home in Orlando, Florida, where they are active in health promotion. **Apr. 16.**

Todd Chobotar is director of publishing and creative productions at Florida Hospital in Orlando. The focus of his ministry is assisting 14,000 employees to understand, experience, and share God's gift of whole person health. **May 17, Aug. 9.**

Ed Christian, Ph.D., teaches English and Biblical literature at the Kutztown University of Pennsylvania. His latest book is *Joyful Noise: A Sensible Look at Christian Music*. His devotionals were based on his article in the *Adventist Review* in July 2002. **July 16, Oct. 4.**

Kevin Clay, M.D., is a family practitioner and medical director who lives in Arlington, Washington. Kevin and his wife, Sandy, have two teenage sons, Eric and Jeremy. **May 1, Nov. 2.**

Sandra Clay is an active homemaker, wife, and mother. She is involved with the children's ministries program of the Everett Forest Park Seventh-day Adventist Church, and is editor of the church newsletter. **Jan 26, May 1, Aug. 4.**

Kay Collins is a registered nurse serving God as an evangelistic health educator and Bible instructor in Michigan. She and her husband, evangelist Dan Collins, spent more than 30 years in evangelism. Her greatest joy is sharing Jesus. **Mar. 23, May 8, Nov. 20.**

May-Ellen Colon, Ph.D. is assistant director of the Sabbath school and personal ministries department of the General Conference of Seventh-day Adventists in Silver Spring, Maryland. She and her husband, Gaspar, were missionaries in Africa and the former Soviet Union. **Sept. 28.**

Kathy Corwin is the family life coordinator of the Oregon Conference of Seventh-day Adventists and gives seminars with her husband, Harvey. She volunteers at the Portland Adventist Hospital Cardiac Rehabilitation's Heart Connections program. **June 23.**

Jim Cox is a pastor who also serves as a chaplain for the Dalton, Georgia, police department. He is the Georgia state representative for the International Conference of Police Chaplains and a member of the Whitfield County Juvenile Court. **Mar. 25, Aug. 27.**

Sidney L. Crandall specializes in residential/commercial design and remodel consulting. After completing architectural training at Andrews University, Sidney began his own firm, Freedom Mountain Designs, in Cleveland, Tennessee. **Feb. 15.**

Tim Crosby, Ph.D., is the pastor of Willow Brook Seventh-day Adventist Church in Boonsboro, Maryland. He is a gifted writer and musician. **Sept. 8.**

Des Cummings, Jr., Ph.D., serves as executive vice president at Florida Hospital, the second busiest hospital in America. His lifework of sharing God's gift of whole person health has spanned three distinct phases as a pastor, university professor and health-care administrator. **May 22, June 15.**

Lenna Lee Chase Davidson, M.P.H., R.N., is a retired nursing administrator and assistant professor of nursing at Southern Adventist University. She has three grown children and eight grandchildren. **Apr. 2.**

Michele Deppe is a dietetic technician in Ohio who loves writing, riding horses, gardening, and cooking. She and her husband, Tod, are the proud parents of a Shih Tzu puppy named Chloe. **Apr. 19, Nov. 3.**

Cheryl Woolsey DesJarlais teaches at Salish Kootenai College in Montana. She is an accomplished writer and editor. Some of her books include *Creative Devotions, My Best Friend, Jesus,* and *Moments for Moms.* **Apr. 25, Oct. 31.**

Hans Diehl, Dr.H.S., M.P.H., is founder and president of Lifestyle Medicine Institute in Loma Linda, California. He conducts CHIP (coronary health improvement project) seminars throughout the world. He and his wife, Lily, have two grown children. **Feb. 22, Aug. 16, Oct. 20.**

David Dildine, an entrepreneur in San Diego, repairs rental houses and restores historic homes. His wife, Dana, helped write his devotional reading. **Aug. 20.**

Hildemar Dos Santos, M.D., Dr.P.H., is a physician from Brazil. He has served as a missionary at the San Roque Adventist Clinic, directed the Chino Community Activities Center for the Portuguese, and taught the prevention of substance abuse in jail facilities. **Mar. 31, June 11, July 30.**

Jodi Eulene Dodson is a mother, grandmother, composer, musician, and a retired graphic designer, writer, and speaker. **Feb. 16.**

Rich DuBose is director of Adventist PlusLine for the North America Division of Seventh-day Adventists and Church Support Services for the Pacific Union Conference. He enjoys being with his wife, Linda, writing music, playing his guitar, hiking, and painting. **Oct. 25.**

Roger L. Dudley, Ph.D., is professor of Christian ministry and director of the Institute of Church Ministry at the Seventh-day Adventist Theological Seminary at Andrews University in Michigan. He enjoys writing and presenting marriage seminars with his wife, Margaret. **Feb. 14.**

Dick Duerksen, M.Div., serves as director of mission development at Florida Hospital. He has been a college administrator, high school teacher, principal, campus minister, youth leader, captivating speaker, and author. He and his wife, Brenda, have three grown children. **Mar. 2, June 25, July 20, Sept. 30, Oct. 6, Oct. 12, Nov. 23, Dec. 18.**

P. William Dysinger, M.D., M.P.H., was the senior health advisor for ADRA International and professor of international health at Loma Linda University. Bill and his wife, Yvonne, are retired near Williamsport, Tennessee, where he is president of Development Services International. **July 27.**

Yvonne Dysinger, R.N., M.P.H., has enjoyed traveling extensively with her husband, Bill. Now retired, she enjoys the quiet of their Tennessee farm and keeping in touch with their four children and grandchildren. **Aug. 21.**

Jeanne Ekvall, D.H.S., and her dentist-husband spent 13 years at Taiwan Adventist Hospital, where she was involved in community health programs and being the mother of three children. Currently, she is a preventive care specialist in Brewster, Washington, where she counsels and teaches nutrition, exercise, and lifestyle. **Dec. 11.**

Donna Engbertson, M.A., is a mother, proud grandmother, writer, teacher, and children's mental health advocate. She holds degrees in elementary education and counseling psychology. **May 15.**

Linda Hyder Ferry, M.D., M.P.H., received her medical training at Loma Linda University and the University of Texas at Galveston. She has been highly honored for the outstanding impact she has made in the field of smoking cessation. **Oct. 30.**

Mark Finley and his wife, Earnestine, have been involved in Christian ministry for more than 35 years. He is speaker emeritus of It Is Written Television and director of global evangelism for the Seventh-day Adventist church. **May 26.**

Karen and **Ron Flowers** are codirectors of the Department of Family Ministries for the General Conference of Seventh-day Adventists in Silver Spring, Maryland. They have two grown sons. **May 9.**

Ruthie Flynn loves people, flowers, and living in northern California. **Nov. 30.**

John Gallagher is associate director for the Department of Public Affairs and United Nations liaison director of the Seventh-day Adventist church. **Oct. 29**

Adam David Getchell is working in real estate development. He and his wife, Wendy, live in Charlotte, North Carolina. **Oct. 21.**

Judith Getchell gives Bible studies and teaches adults how to read through the Garland County Laubach Literacy Council in Hot Springs, Arkansas. **Aug. 6.**

Dan Giang's devotional reading is based on his article in the *Adventist Review* (Mar. 21, 2002). At the time of this writing, he was teaching neurology at the University of Rochester in New York. **July 11.**

Eric Gullickson is from Texas and attended Ouachita Hills Academy. He wrote this devotional reading when he was a sophomore. It is said that he has great potential as a future pastor! **Mar. 1.**

Karl Haffner is senior pastor of the Walla Walla College church, in College Place, Washington. **Mar. 27.**

Steven L. Haley, M.Div., is a former police officer who, after studying righteousness by faith, became a pastor. He is ministry director for the northeastern region of the Georgia-Cumberland Conference of Seventh-day Adventists. He and his wife, Malinda (a registered nurse), have three children. **May 20.**

Jean Marie Hametz, R.N., has a background in clinical nursing, management, and health education. While she is convalescing at home because of her chronic illness, she enjoys drawing pictures to accompany Scripture verses. **May 29.**

Tim Hansel is the well-known author of a number of books that include *Holy Sweat, You Gotta Keep Dancin',* and *When I Relax I Feel Guilty.* **Jan. 22.**

Herman Harp and his wife, Sonnie, are involved in a full-time music ministry. You can find information on how to contact them at their Web site: hermanandsonnieharp.com **May 12.**

Feryl E. Harris is a Bible instructor who serves the Mountain View Conference in West Virginia as the director of Sabbath School, Children's Ministries, Women's Ministries, and Trust Services departments. **Dec. 4.**

Freddie Harris and her husband, Cliff, direct the Drug Alternative Program (DAP), a men's drug recovery home, and outpatient drug support groups from their headquarters in Grand Terrace, California. **Dec. 23.**

Toini Harrison, Ph.D., is a professional counselor and educator in human development who taught at La Sierra University and Southern Adventist University. Now retired, she lives in Loma Linda, California. **Nov. 11.**

Marcella Harrom worked as a secretary to Jan W. Kuzma at the Loma Linda University School of Health. She and her husband, Louie, are retired in Redding, California, and are involved in Community Services and lifestyle and cooking seminars. **Oct. 23, Nov. 1.**

LaVerne Henderson is the associate editor of the *Columbia Union Visitor*. Her devotional reading originally appeared in the July 15, 2001, issue and is reprinted with permission. **May 13.**

Gaye Henry is a mother of three who lives in Dayton, Ohio. She works as a private scrub nurse for a plastic surgeon, and enjoys collecting Beanie Babies. **Nov. 3.**

Jim Hinrichs, C.P.A., grew up in Nebraska and Colorado. He worked for Adventist Health System for more than 20 years, and is currently at Shawnee Mission Medical Center in Kansas. **Sept. 16.**

Clarence E. Hodges was vice president of the North American Division of the General Conference of Seventh-day Adventists when he wrote this devotional reading. Presently he is an assistant to the president at Oakwood College in Huntsville, Alabama. **Sept. 23.**

Gladys Hollingsead, B.S.N., P.H.N., R.N., chief executive officer of Pacific Health Education Center in Bakersfield, California, enjoys singing and traveling with her husband, Marshall. **Feb. 18, June 19.**

M. C. Hollingsead, M.D., is medical director of Pacific Health Education Center, **Apr. 18.**

Gary Hopkins, M.D., Ph.P.H., is director of the Institute for Prevention of Addictions at Loma Linda University in southern California. **May 25.**

Cathy Ireland is a writer, speaker, and president of CHATS, an organization presenting hope-filled solutions to life's problems. She lives in Oshawa, Ontario, Canada, where she works with women's ministries and divorce recovery. **Sept. 1, Dec. 21.**

Buddy Ivey returned to Cloudrant, Louisiana, after graduating from Amazing Facts School of Evangelism, where God led him, through many miracles, to establish a Bible study center. **June 7.**

Silvia Jacobsen, C.D.A., a graduate of Amazing Facts School of Evangelism, works for the Northern California Conference of Seventh-day Adventists as a lay evangelism trainer. **Feb. 24.**

Verena Jaggi was working at the Malamulo Hospital in Malawi, Africa, when her devotional reading was published in the *Adventist Review* (July 9, 1998). **July 17.**

Dawn Jakovac is a high school French and English teacher on leave to learn from her three children. To escape the drudgery of housework, she likes to write newsletters or skits for children's church. **Nov. 4.**

Holly Sue Joers is a homemaker, musician, massage therapist, and writer. She and her husband, Skip, are raising their son, Elijah, to be the healthiest little boy in town! **Mar. 14.**

Kim Allan Johnson is the associate treasurer of the Northern New England Conference of Seventh-day Adventists. He has served as a pastor in Massachusetts and Maine, and has written "Spiritual Body Building," a small group lesson series, as well as many articles. **Jan. 8.**

William G. Johnsson, editor of *Adventist Review,* based his devotional reading on an editorial (July 24, 2003). He and his wife, Noelene, live in Maryland, where she directs children's ministries for the North American Division of Seventh-day Adventists. **July 23.**

André V. Jubert, M.D., F.A.C.S., has been a surgical oncologist in Grand Rapids, Michigan, for 30 years. He's married to Bernice, and has written the book *A Doctor's Advice to Keep You Out of His Office.* **Dec. 16.**

Leslie Kay is a wife, mother, and freelance writer who lives in the teaming metropolis of

Kingman, Arizona. Her devotional reading is based on an article that appeared in the *Adventist Review* in Oct. 2001. **Aug. 18.**

Joyce L. Keeler, who processes applications at the retirement office of the North American Division of Seventh-day Adventists, lives in Burtonsville, Maryland. Her devotional reading was based on the *Adventist Review* article "My Battle With Chronic Fatigue" (Aug. 26, 1999). **Dec. 20.**

Carol Kimura teaches English as a second language in Hawaii's public schools and is a ranger at the Seventh-day Adventist Camp Waianae. **Apr. 20.**

Angela Kuzma is an elementary school teacher at Kahili Mountian School in Kauai, Hawaii, as well as a personal fitness trainer and aerobics instructor. Her passion is her husband, Kevin, and daughter, Keana. **Aug. 17.**

Jan W. Kuzma, Ph.D., before his retirement, was chair of the Department of Biostatistics and director of research at the School of Public Health, Loma Linda University. These devotionals readings are based on his book (coauthored with Cecil Murphey) *Live 10 Healthy Years Longer.* **Jan. 19, Feb. 4, Mar. 8, Apr. 5, May 28, June 18, July 21, Aug. 1, Aug. 3, Aug. 7, Sept. 17, Oct. 2, Nov. 15, Dec. 12.**

Kathy Kuzma, R.N., is a homemaker and mother of five grown children. She sews, cooks, reads, and enjoys time with George, her physician husband. **Aug. 28.**

Kay Kuzma, Ed.D., is speaker, author, and founder of Family Matters. She is chair of the 3ABN book division. She and her husband, Jan, have three grown children and six grandchildren. **Jan. 9, Jan. 12, Jan. 14, Jan. 25, Jan. 27, Jan. 30, Feb. 2, Feb. 5, Feb. 8, Feb. 11, Feb. 13, Feb. 23, Apr. 1, Apr. 3, Apr. 6, Apr. 10, Apr. 16, Apr. 27, May 4, May 7, May 19, May 30, June 9, June 14, June 17, June 24, June 27, June 28, July 9, July 21, July 29, Aug. 7, Sept. 11, Sept. 15, Sept. 24, Oct. 7, Oct. 10, Oct. 26, Oct. 28, Oct. 29, Nov. 2, Nov. 8, Nov. 22, Nov. 26, Nov. 29, Dec. 3, Dec. 8, Dec. 9, Dec. 13, Dec. 19, Dec. 22, Dec. 25, Dec. 27, Dec. 29, Dec. 31.**

Kevin Kuzma spent a year in Majuro (Marshall Islands) where he taught third grade. His passion is surfing. He now teaches computer science—and surfing—at Kahili Mountain School in Kauai. **June 8, Aug. 23.**

Elfred Lee taught art at Oakwood College in Alabama and Montemorelos University in Mexico. He is a well-known portrait and mural artist who now lives with his wife, Martha, in Chula Vista, California. **Oct. 13.**

Martha A. Lee, R.N., is a lactation consultant at Paradise Valley Hospital. **Mar. 4, May 10.**

Dr. Ruth Lennox, M.D., a family physician, has several family members who have suffered from depression. She spent nine years in West Africa with her physician-husband and her three children before immigrating to Canada from England. **Mar. 21.**

Molly Lesick, C.R.S., is a health counselor in Chula Vista, California. **July 14.**

Karen Lewis, of Scottsdale, Arizona, is married and has one daughter. After a career in the health-care retirement field, she is administrative secretary for Thunderbird Adventist Academy and directs a women's gospel singing group. **Dec. 30.**

Kenneth H. Livesay is a retired pastor and chaplain. He was personal ministries director and Adventist Laymen's Services and Industries (ASI) director of the Southeastern California Conference. He has also served as executive secretary-treasurer of ASI. **July 15.**

Kathleen H. Liwidjaja-Kuntaraf was the associate director of the General Conference Health Ministries Department. **Jan. 24, Feb. 17, Mar. 19, Apr. 26, Apr. 28, May 24, July 7.**

Edna Maye Loveless, Ph.D., is a professor of English at La Sierra University. She has juggled professional writing, graduate studies, and parenting two lively daughters during more than 40 years of marriage to her husband, Bill. **Jan. 15, Apr. 14, Sept. 3.**

Cezar R. Luchian is a graduate student at the Seventh-day Adventist Theological Seminary in Michigan. Originally from Romania, he plans to return once his studies are completed. **Nov. 6, Dec. 2.**

Aileen Ludington, M.D., is a board-certified physician whose major interest is lifestyle change. She and her physician-husband have worked in Thailand, and now live in Paradise, California. **Jan. 23, Mar. 29, Apr. 29, July 3, Sept. 21, Dec. 7.**

Ben Maxson became director of the Stewardship Department of the General Conference of Seventh-day Adventists after many years as a pastor. Recently he returned to his first love, and is once again a pastor in Paradise, California. **Mar. 6.**

Alberta Mazat, Ph.D., M.S.W., M.F.C.C., R.N., has chaired the Department of Marriage, Family, and Child Counseling at Loma Linda University. She is a well-known speaker and author on the topics of marriage and sexuality. She currently lives in Fletcher, North Carolina. **Apr. 12, Aug. 2.**

Ken McFarland was special assignments editor for Coffey Communication in Walla Walla, Washington, when the article on which his devotional reading is based was published in the *Adventist Review* (July 22, 1999). **July 8.**

Gerard D. McLane, Dr. P.H., C.H.E.S., is a specialist in the therapeutic and motivational approaches to health risk management, disease prevention, and lifestyle interventions. He is president of Reading Institute for Better Living, Inc., in Pennsylvania. **Feb. 25, Mar. 20, May 3, Nov. 14.**

Len McMillan, Ph.D., is a certified family life educator, psychologist, and ordained pastor. After working at Pacific Health Education Center in Bakersfield, he and Karen retired to Florida, where he loves Corvettes and laughs frequently. **Jan. 10.**

Ernie Medina, Jr., Dr.P.H., is a preventive-care specialist at Beaver Medical Group in Redlands, California, and clinical associate professor at Loma Linda University Schools of Public Health and Medicine. **Apr. 11.**

Lonnie Melashenko is the speaker-director for the Voice of Prophecy. His devotional reading is based on his article in the *Adventist Review* (July 3, 2000). **Oct. 16.**

Tom Mostert is president of the Pacific Union Conference of Seventh-day Adventists. His devotional reading is based on his President's Perspective editorial, published by the *Pacific Union Recorder* (September 2003). **June 4.**

Jerry Muncy, D.D.S., has a private dental practice in Safford, Arizona. He is active in his local church and involved with prison ministries. Jerry enjoys flying and volunteering for mission projects. He and his wife, Patti, have three grown children and are enjoying their grandchildren. **Feb. 6, Sept. 18.**

Patti Muncy has been flight instructor and a dental assistant and office manager of her husband's practice. She has her own interior decorating business and is a writer for recovery materials for youth. **Apr. 23, Oct. 3.**

Cecil Murphey is a freelance author who has written more than 100 books. Some of his best sellers include *Gifted Hands* and *Think BIG,* coauthored with Dr. Ben Carson. **Apr. 24, June 18, Aug. 3, Aug. 10, Sept. 17, Oct. 2, Oct. 27, Nov. 15, Dec. 12, Dec. 14.**

Dwight K. Nelson, Ph.D., is senior pastor of Pioneer Memorial church at Andrews University in Berrien Springs, Michigan. He is the speaker for the television broadcast

Evidence. His Christmas devotional reading is based on his article in the *Adventist Review* (December, 2000). **Mar. 17. Dec. 24.**

Nancy Nelson and her husband, Terry, have four children. Evangelism is their family's passion. **Oct. 24.**

Terry Nelson is a pastor-evangelist in the Michigan Conference. He has a dream to train lay leaders to be successful soul winners in their own communities. **Jan 20.**

Velda Nelson is a retired teacher and has four daughters and eight grandchildren. She serves as librarian, Sabbath school teacher, and deaconess at her church, and enjoys quilting, crossword puzzles, needlework, and community service. **Mar. 3, May 18, June 30.**

Nancy Neuharth and her husband, Ruben, are parents of four grown children—three sons and one daughter. Since 1973, Nancy has worked with Ruben for the ABC Prayer Crusade. **June 5.**

Ruben Neuharth attended the ABC Prayer Crusade after a prestigious career with chamber of commerce management. It changed his life. He quit his job so that he could share this message with others. He's conducted more than 200 seminars. **Aug. 19.**

David C. Nieman, D.H.Sc., is a professor in the Department of Health and Exercise Science and the director of the human performance laboratory at Appalachian State University in Boone, North Carolina. His devotionals are based on his book *The Adventist Healthstyle.* **May 2, June 10.**

Yew-Por Ng, Nov. 9.

Svein Nilsen, M.D., has been a family practice physician in San Bernardino for 33 years. He and his wife, Mildred, are now retired. **June 11.**

Pat Nordman writes from DeLand, Florida, where she works for Stetson University. A freelance writer, she has many articles, booklets, and two books to her credit. She and her husband, Charles, have four children. **Mar. 7, Mar. 12, Apr. 9, Apr. 21, May 14, June 6, Aug. 29, Sept. 13, Dec. 1.**

Willie and **Elaine Oliver** are copresenters for the From This Day Forth marriage seminars. Willie is director of family ministries and youth for the North American Division of Seventh-day Adventists. **Aug. 12.**

Victor M. Parachin is an ordained minister and freelance writer who has written several books. His devotional readings are based on his *Adventist Review* article in November 1999. **July 10, Nov. 10.**

Gary Parker, M.Div., and his wife, Donna, spent 22 years in ministry and evangelism. Gary holds master's degrees in theology and social agency counseling, and has his own counseling agency in Iowa. **Aug. 13, Dec. 15.**

Donna Patch lives with her husband, Kenny, in sunny Surprise, Arizona, where she enjoys desert photography, writing, and the exuberant antics of her mini schnauzer, Toby. **Mar. 10.**

Stewart T. Pepper writes from West Virginia, where he is a pastor. He and his wife, Kathy, have three children. **Nov. 12.**

Timothy Pierce has taught developmentally delayed students with behavior problems. He currently teaches third- and fourth-grade children. He and his wife, Tara, have three children and live in Banning, California. **Sept. 9.**

Ray and **Leni Puen** are prayer coordinators at Glendale Filipino Seventh-Day Adventist Church. Leni is staff educator at the White Memorial Medical Center in California; Ray is executive director of EquipNow and Adventist Soul Winners in Action Network (ASIAN). **Sept. 27.**

Risë Rafferty, cofounder of Light Bearer's Ministry, is married to James Rafferty. They have two children. Risë enjoys sharing health messages in articles and through 3ABN television. Her August 8 devotional was taken from *Light Bearer's Ministries Health Nugget* (Sept. 2001). **Jan. 3, Jan. 21, Feb. 21, Apr. 15, May 27, June 21, Aug 8, Nov. 5.**

E. John Reinhold is the executive director of the Christian Care Ministry, an organization of sharing Christians who meet medical needs. He and his wife, Dona, live in Florida, and enjoy family and traveling. **May 21, Sept. 19.**

Larry Richardson, Ph.D., is president of Richardson Health Services. He taught communications and drama at Pacific Union College and La Sierra University. Both he and his wife, Becky, have earned their black belts in karate, and they have two grown children, Damon and Lauren. **Feb. 19, July 19, Aug. 22.**

Joyce Rigsby writes from Loma Linda, California. Her devotional reading is based on her *Adventist Review* article (Oct. 26, 2000). **Oct. 8.**

Nancy Rockey, Ph.D., R.N., and her husband, Ron, are in team ministry. Both Rockeys hold master's degrees in family therapy and doctorates in counseling psychology. They have written a book *Belonging,* and make their home in Phoenix, Arizona. They enjoy their two grown daughters and their grandchildren. **Mar. 13, Oct. 11, Dec. 17.**

Ron Rockey, M.Div., Ph.D., former-pastor-turned-recovery-counselor-and-seminar-leader, is cofounder with his wife, Nancy, of the LifeStyle Renewal Institute, which is dedicated to bringing healing to those suffering from emotional pain. **Oct. 11.**

Ella M. Rydzewski is a retired editor of the *Adventist Review.* **June 3, Sept 12.**

Monte Sahlin is vice president of creative ministries for the Columbia Union Conference and author of a number of books on church growth and the Adventist family. **Jan 6.**

Elmar P. Sakala, M.D., M.P.H., is the former director of medical student education in an OB/GYN department. Elmar has delivered thousands of babies and enjoys making the birthing experience memorable for new parents. He and his wife, Darilee, have two grown children. **Jan. 5, Feb. 2, Feb. 13, May 7.**

Laura Le Salisbury lives in Oregon with her husband, Steve, and enjoys exercising, beach combing, and playing the piano. The Salisburys have four children. **Jan 17.**

Albert Sanchez, Ph.D., is former professor of nutrition at Loma Linda University and Montemorelos University and director of research at Pacific Health Education Center in Bakersfield. He is now retired and lives in California. **July 28, Oct. 5.**

Jon Sandberg attended Ouachita Hills Academy when he wrote this tribute to his dad. His parents, Karland and Jodi Sandberg, have three boys. (Jon is the oldest.) **June 12.**

Richard A. Schaeffer, former director of public relations at Loma Linda University Medical Center, based his devotional reading on material from his book *Legacy, the Heritage of Loma Linda University Medical Center.* **Jan. 18.**

John A. Scharffenberg, M.D., M.P.H., an adjunct professor of nutrition at Loma Linda University, has been assistant director of the Health Department of the General Conference of Seventh-day Adventists, and is now retired in California. **Mar. 11, June 16, July 24, Aug. 30, Dec. 5.**

Blondel E. Senior, Ph.D., is the founder and executive director of Advent Home, a licensed residential treatment program for 12- to 16-year-old boys with learning disabilities (ADHD), located in Calhoun, Tennessee. **Feb.3, Oct. 17.**

Danny Shelton is founder and president of Three Angels Broadcasting Network (3ABN), a satellite television and radio network. **June 2.**

Glenn and **Jerre St. Clair** have dedicated their lives to mission service. After serving for many years at the Masanga Leprosy Hospital in Sierra Leone and in Nepal as hospital administrator and ADRA director, respectively, they are retired in Berrien Springs, Michigan. **Sept. 22.**

Kari St. Clair, P.T., is a physical therapist and the mother of three. She and her husband, Jeff, live in LaFollette, Tennessee. **Apr. 17.**

Lincoln Steed is editor of *Liberty* magazine, a publication of the Seventh-day Adventist Church. **June 22.**

Hal Steenson, a pastor, is the general manager of 3ABN. He lives with his wife, Mollie, in Illinois. **Sept 2.**

Rita Kay Stevens is a medical technologist in Amarillo, Texas. Married to a church administrator, she enjoys traveling, entertaining, walking, reading, and encouraging others. She and her husband have two adult sons. **Mar. 28, July 22.**

Nicole Sydenham has been an administrative assistant at the French School Division and enjoys working in women's ministries and traveling. She and her husband, Ron, have four children. **July 31.**

Bonnie Szumski, R.N., is married to Ed, who is an electronic instructor at San Bernardino Valley College. They have two children, Becky and Eddie. **July 12, Aug. 24, Sept. 29.**

Arlene Taylor, Ph.D., is director of infection control and the risk manager at St. Helena Hospital in California. She is also president of Realizations, Inc.; a brain-function consultant; and creator of The Brain and Innate Giftedness program. **Feb. 28.**

Rob Thomas is happily married and the father of two great teenage sons. He is the chair of physical education at Atlantic Union College, and is an elder at his local church. He enjoys researching his family "roots" and exercising with friends. **July 25.**

Samuel Thomas, Jr., is the author of the "Satisfying Sabbath" e-mail devotional series on which the devotional readings in this book are based. He is the director of Transformation Broadcast Ministries and pastor of the Orchard Park Seventh-day Adventist Church in Chattanooga, Tennessee. **July 4, Oct. 3.**

Agatha M. Thrash, M.D., is cofounder (with her physician-husband, Calvin) of Uchee Pines Institute in Seale, Alabama, and has authored books on natural healing. She practiced pathology for 18 years, then went into general practice. **June 29, Oct. 14.**

Thais Thrasher, M.D., has specialties in both pathology and psychiatry. She taught at the Loma Linda University School of Medicine for 25 years and was on the faculty of psychiatry at the Loma Linda Medical Center. **July 5, July 26.**

Carolyn Towles, R.N., is the director of nurses and inpatient services for Jellico Community Hospital. She graduated from Southern Missionary College (now Southern Adventist University) in 1973, where she met her husband, Doug. They have two grown children. **Nov. 28.**

Eddie C. Towles, D.M.D., is a dentist in LaFollette, Tennessee. He and his wife, Bonnie, and four children live in Jellico. He enjoys outdoor interests with his family. **Mar. 24, May 11, Aug. 5, Oct. 9, Nov. 13.**

Homer Trecartin, a former pastor and teacher, and director of development at Georgia-Cumberland Academy, is now academic dean at Weimar College. He and his wife, Barbara, have three children, and enjoy outdoor activities and traveling. **June 20.**

Bill Tucker is speaker-director of the Quiet Hour in Redlands, California. His devotional is based on material in *Echoes,* a Quiet Hour publication. **Sept. 8.**

Gretchen Turner, P.T., graduated from Andrews University and is a physical therapist in Carlisle, Indiana. **Jan. 31.**

Smuts van Rooyen, Ph.D., is the senior pastor of the Vallejo Drive Seventh-day Adventist Church in Glendale, California. He has a doctorate in counseling psychology and a master of theology. His wife, Arlene, is the light of his life. **Aug. 31.**

Morris Venden, pastor, teacher, author, and evangelist, has been sharing the message of God's love all his life. He and his wife are retired and live in Washington State. **Jan. 28, Nov. 18.**

Céleste perrino Walker, a professional writer-editor, lives in Rutland, Vermont, with her husband, Rob, and children, Joshua and Rachel. She enjoys music, old books, water-color painting, quilting, auctions, and sports. **Sept. 4, Nov. 24.**

Brenda Walsh is director of Kids Time and Kids Time Praise for Three Angels Broadcast Network (3ABN). Her devotional is based on her book *Battered to Blessed.* **May 6.**

Caroline Watkins, C.F.L.E., is a human resource consultant in the Atlanta, Georgia, area. **Sept. 25.**

Arthur Weaver, M.D., retired emeritus professor of surgery at Wayne State University, and his family are actively involved in health education through their nonprofit corporation, Better Living seminars, and short-term mission projects. **Sept. 7.**

Raymond O. West, M.D., who taught in the School of Public Health, Loma Linda University, is the author of the Healthwise column. Though, "semi-retired," he does urgent care in Puget Sound, Washington; travels; and does mission work with his wife, Julie. **Dec. 26.**

David Westbrook, a pastor, is now the director of Back to Enoch Ministry. He and his wife, Laura, and daughter, Allison, live in Malo, Washington. **Dec. 6.**

David White, D.Min., has been a pastor, a hospital chaplain, and vice president for community health programs at Memorial Hospital in Manchester, Kentucky. David and his wife live in Landrum, South Carolina, where he is coordinating the Adventist Health Network and is project coordinator for the North American Division Adventist Development and Relief Agency (ADRA) affiliates. **Sept. 10.**

Ellen G. White, spiritual leader, inspirational author, and cofounder of the Seventh-day Adventist Church, was born November 26, 1827, and died July 16, 1915, at the age of 87. Through her lectures and thousands of written pages, she inspired many to live a more healthful lifestyle. **Jan 7, May 5, Oct. 22.**

Heidi Wiggers, mother of two boys and wife of Marcel, is practicing internal medicine in association with Portland Adventist Medical Center. **Feb. 12.**

Del Wiggins, former teacher, moved to a horse ranch in Walla Walla, Washington, with his wife, Cheryl. After a valiant fight, he finally lost the battle to cancer. **Oct. 14, Nov. 28.**

Donna Willey, along with Rod, her husband, is involved in Bible studies and church planting. **Feb. 1.**

DeWitt S. Williams, Ed.D., M.P.H., is director of the Department of Health and Temperance of the North American Division. He previously served as president of the Central African Union. He and his wife, Margaret, have two grown daughters. **Mar. 26, Apr. 30.**

Gregory R. Wise, M.D., an internist and geriatrician, practiced at Bella Vista Hospital in Puerto Rico and at Loma Linda University before becoming vice president of medical integration at Kettering Medical Center in Dayton, Ohio. He now teaches at Wright State University and is editor of *Primary Care Reports*. **Mar. 30, Oct. 18.**

Melinda Worden has worked at the Review and Herald Publishing Association since 1995. She has her Bachelor of Arts degree in English. She and her husband, Brian, live in Hagerstown, Maryland. **Apr. 4.**

Bonnie Yaw, M.F.C.C., R.N., works at Shriner's Hospital for Children in Sacramento, California. **Nov. 21.**

Topical Index

Aug. 13, 20, 27
Effect of Imaging, Aug. 11
Health,
Education, May 1
Habits, May 19, 29; July 28
Laws of, June 8
Message, Feb. 10
Physical, May 19
Reform, Jan. 7, 27; Mar. 14, 29
Statistics, Feb. 11
Hearing, June 24
Heart Disease, Mar. 16, Apr. 28, June 23
Helping Others, Apr. 8, 20; July 7; Aug.
14; Sept. 6, 10, 12, 20, 29;
Oct. 3, 22; Nov. 28, Dec. 9
Helpers High, Mar. 26
Isaiah's Fast, Apr. 20
Holy Spirit Perspective, July 9
Honesty, Dec. 23
Hope, Jan. 4, 9; Feb. 3, 5, 8; July 29; Oct.
1, 12
Hospital, July 20
Hospitality, Apr. 19
Hurry (sin of) Jan. 22

I

Imaging, July 11
Immune System, Jan. 27; Feb. 22; May 7,
24; July 21; Oct 2; Nov. 9
Immunization, Feb. 9
Intimacy, June 17; Aug. 12
IOUs, June 14

J

Juicing, Apr. 20

K

Kidney Transplant, Aug. 9
Kindness, May 22

L

Laodicea, Jan. 31
Laughter, Jan. 10; Aug. 4
Laws of Health, Nov. 2
Learning Disability, Sept. 9
Lifestyle, Jan. 5, 17, 26, 27, 31; Feb. 7, 10;
Mar. 14, 29, 31; May 1, 19,
29; June 8, 13, 22; July 3, 14;
Aug. 6, 16; Sept. 1, 7, 25; Oct.

20; Nov. 1, 2, 9, 25, 27; Dec.
5, 7, 13, 20, 29, 31
Diseases, Mar. 14
Gift of, Dec. 11
Hawaiian, Nov. 2
Healthy, Jan. 19; May 29; June
13; July 21
Information, July 14
Love, Feb. 14; Mar. 27; May 9, 26; June
6, 8, 13, 14, 17, 20; July 7;
Aug. 22; Sept. 23, 29, 30
Boomerang Effect, July 7
God's Love, Nov. 30

M

Mad Cow Disease, June 21
Marathon, Jan. 26, July 24
Marriage, June 14
Adultery, Apr. 3
Gender Differences, June 1
Intimacy, Aug. 12
Love/Time, Feb. 14
Emotional Anemia, Aug 2
Meat, Jan. 21, Feb. 11, Apr. 29; June 21,
Aug. 30
Mediation, Mar. 12
Melatonin, Apr. 6
Milk, June 21; Oct. 7, 14
Mad Cow Disease, June 21
Miracle, Jan. 20; Feb. 12; Mar. 6, 31; July
18, 31; Oct. 3, 24; Dec. 6, 15,
25, 26
Moderation, Jan. 8, 23; July 24; Aug. 3;
Oct. 27
Monkeys, Jan. 14
MSG, May 27
Music (Healing Effects of), Feb. 13, 16;
Apr. 8; May 8; June 5; July 31

N

Natural Disasters
Blizzard, Dec. 28
Tornado, Mar. 1
Natural remedies, Apr. 4; May 30; June
22; Oct. 14, Dec. 2
Nature, Apr. 2; May 18; Oct. 14, 31;
Nov. 30
Negative Feelings
Aloneness (Abandonment), Apr. 23
Anxiety and worry, July 5